ADVANCES IN CANCER RESEARCH

VOLUME 12

Contributors to This Volume

G. I. Deichman

H. Hanafusa

Karl Erik Hellström

Ingegerd Hellström

Irving I. Kessler

Abraham M. Lilienfeld

G. Pasternak

ADVANCES IN CANCER RESEARCH

Edited by

GEORGE KLEIN

Department of Tumor Biology
Karolinska Institutet
Stockholm, Sweden

SIDNEY WEINHOUSE

Fels Research Institute
Temple University Medical School
Philadelphia, Pennsylvania

Consulting Editor

ALEXANDER HADDOW

Chester Beatty Research Institute
Institute of Cancer Research
Royal Cancer Hospital
London, England

Volume 12

 ACADEMIC PRESS   New York and London   1969

ACADEMIC PRESS, INC.
111 Fifth Avenue, New York, New York 10003

United Kingdom Edition published by
ACADEMIC PRESS, INC. (LONDON) LTD.
Berkeley Square House, London W1X 6BA

LIBRARY OF CONGRESS CATALOG CARD NUMBER: 52-13360

PRINTED IN THE UNITED STATES OF AMERICA

CONTRIBUTORS TO VOLUME 12

Numbers in parentheses refer to the pages on which the authors' contributions begin.

G. I. DEICHMAN, *Institute of Experimental and Clinical Oncology, Academy of Medical Sciences, Moscow, U.S.S.R.* (101)

H. HANAFUSA, *Department of Viral Oncology, The Public Health Research Institute of The City of New York, Inc., New York, New York* (137)

KARL ERIK HELLSTRÖM, *Department of Pathology, University of Washington Medical School, Seattle, Washington* (167)

INGEGERD HELLSTRÖM, *Department of Microbiology, University of Washington Medical School, Seattle, Washington* (167)

IRVING I. KESSLER, *Department of Chronic Diseases, Johns Hopkins University School of Hygiene and Public Health, Baltimore, Maryland* (225)

ABRAHAM M. LILIENFELD, *Department of Chronic Diseases, Johns Hopkins University School of Hygiene and Public Health, Baltimore, Maryland* (225)

G. PASTERNAK, *Institute of Cancer Research, Experimental Station, German Academy of Sciences, Berlin, German Democratic Republic* (1)

97188

PREFACE

It has not been a practice of the editors of this serial publication to include a Preface, feeling that the contributions of the authors should speak for themselves. However, a change in the editorship of this work should not go unheralded; therefore, I am taking this opportunity to welcome George Klein, my new coeditor, and to express my deep appreciation to my previous coeditor, Alexander Haddow.

Alex Haddow is one of a small group of outstanding British experimentalists who have made a series of notable fundamental contributions to our knowledge of carcinogenesis and chemotherapy. Several potent agents developed in their laboratories have found a place in the treatment of human cancer. Under Haddow's guidance, the Chester Beatty Institute has become one of the world-renowned centers of research in cancer. It is a source of satisfaction to me and George Klein that Alex Haddow will continue as a consulting editor.

Alex Haddow and Jesse Greenstein founded the *Advances in Cancer Research* in 1953, and continued coediting the publication through Volume 5, which appeared in 1958. After Jesse Greenstein's untimely death in 1958, it was my privilege to collaborate with Alex Haddow in the editing of Volumes 6 through 11. Despite the rigorous responsibilities of directing an active research program and the Chester Beatty Research Institute, Alex Haddow continued as coeditor until last year, when pressures of his many commitments finally compelled him to resign.

No more worthy successor could have been found than George Klein, who, with this issue, assumes the coeditorship. It is particularly fitting, and is of course no accident, that much of the content of this first issue is devoted to cancer immunology. This is an area of research in which George Klein has attained unique eminence, and it is largely owing to his pioneering work that this field has been thrust into the forefront of the cancer problem.

The years of my association with Alex Haddow as coeditor have been exciting ones indeed for cancer research. With the crescendo of new discoveries in biology there is every reason to hope and to anticipate that in the not-too-distant future this publication will record the unlocking of the secret of the neoplastic cell.

Philadelphia, Pennsylvania　　　　　　　　　　　　　　SIDNEY WEINHOUSE
June, 1969

CONTENTS

Antigens Induced by the Mouse Leukemia Viruses

G. Pasternak

Immunological Aspects of Carcinogenesis by Deoxyribonucleic Acid Tumor Viruses

G. I. Deichman

Replication of Oncogenic Viruses in Virus-Induced Tumor Cells—Their Persistence and Interaction with Other Viruses

H. Hanafusa

Cellular Immunity against Tumor Antigens

KARL ERIK HELLSTRÖM AND INGEGERD HELLSTRÖM

Perspectives in the Epidemiology of Leukemia

IRVING I. KESSLER AND ABRAHAM M. LILIENFELD

CONTENTS OF PREVIOUS VOLUMES

xi

ERRATA

VOLUME 11

Page 49, line 5 should read: The parent cells respond to the antigens of the genetic type of the other parent present within the F_1 hybrid.

Page 49, line 16 should read: Here, the only antigenic type to which the injected A strain cells could mount an immune response was the C57BL/1 of the injected F_1 cells.

ANTIGENS INDUCED BY THE MOUSE LEUKEMIA VIRUSES

G. Pasternak

Institute of Cancer Research, Experimental Section, German Academy of Sciences,
Berlin, German Democratic Republic

I. Introduction

Since the time of the first successful cell-free transfer of a mouse leukemia reported by Ludwik Gross (1951), many laboratories have confirmed his fundamental experiment and have added important new information to this special field in cancer research. Leukemia-inducing agents have been found in a variety of normal and malignant mouse tissues, thus indicating their widespread distribution among mouse colonies of different origin. The viral nature of the agents involved is now beyond all doubt. There are facts such as the serial cell-free transmissions of the disease, neutralization of the leukemogenic activity by specific immune sera, and finally electron-microscopic identification. Using electron-microscopic techniques the localization in tissues and cells of infected and leukemic animals as well as the morphological structure of the leukemia viruses have been thoroughly investigated (for reviews, see Yumoto et al., 1966; Haguenau, 1966). Moreover, methods have been developed for the isolation and purification of virus-containing materials and for the cultivation and propagation of the agents in vitro. On the basis of these results the molecular structure of leukemia viruses is now in process of being elucidated (Mora et al., 1966; Duesberg and Robinson, 1966; Galibert et al., 1966).

In addition to the structural and biochemical characterization of the virus particles, numerous experiments, concerned with epidemiological, morphological, cytogenetic, and pathogenetic problems of the disease have been made or are under way. To study more thoroughly the growth behavior of leukemia cells and particularly the host's reactions against these cells, transplantable leukemia lines have been developed.

From transplantation experiments the first evidence was obtained that a pretreatment of mice induces a state of relative resistance against the outgrowth of syngeneic inocula of leukemia cells. The data indicated a specific antigenicity of leukemia cells in animals otherwise genetically compatible with the primary leukemic host (Klein *et al.*, 1962; Sachs, 1962; Pasternak *et al.*, 1962; Pasternak and Graffi, 1963).

At that time tumor-specific transplantation resistance was known to occur also in several other, experimental, mouse tumor systems (for reviews, see Old and Boyse, 1964, 1965; Sjögren, 1965; Pasternak, 1967c). Sarcomas induced by carcinogenic hydrocarbons had been found strongly antigenic in syngeneic as well as in autochthonous hosts. Transplantation resistance was detected after ligation and regression of subcutaneous or intradermal tumor grafts, surgical removal of temporary growing tumors, and injection of X-ray-killed or subthreshold doses of viable tumor cells. Generally, individual tumors, even when induced by the same carcinogen, did not cross-react. The variation in antigenicity among etiologically identical tumors has now been demonstrated for a number of chemically and physically induced neoplasms. The immunological nature of tumor-specific transplantation resistance was shown by the passive transfer to normal recipients. Lymphoid cells of resistant animals inhibited tumor growth when the cells were admixed *in vitro* before inoculation. Humoral antibodies, however, did not appear to play a predominant role in the defense reactions of the host.

In contrast to chemically and physically induced tumors, the antigens of polyoma virus-induced tumors were found to be identical. After infection of adult mice with polyoma virus, transplantation resistance developed against polyoma tumors of different histological origin. Although the transplantation resistance was produced by the polyoma virus, evidence was obtained that the tumor antigens were of nonviral nature. Thus, virus-free, polyoma tumor homografts were also capable of producing transplantation resistance against polyoma tumors. The lack of antiviral antibodies in these animals suggested the presence of new cellular tumor antigens not related to viral antigens (Sjögren, 1961, 1964b).

It is not surprising that the immunological findings obtained with tumors induced by the deoxyribonucleic acid (DNA)-containing polyoma virus led to similar experiments with another category of virus-induced neoplasms, i.e., with leukemias induced by an agent containing ribonucleic acid (RNA) as genetic material.

A. Review of the Immunology of Mouse Leukemias

Transplantation resistance against leukemia cells was shown to occur after pretreatment of mice with X-ray-killed syngeneic leukemia cells, subminimal doses of cells, allogeneic leukemic tissue, or virus preparations. Immunity was mediated by both lymphoid cells and humoral antibodies as demonstrated by the *in vivo* passive transfer. *In vitro*, antibodies were detectable by the indirect fluorescent-antibody technique with living cells and by the cytotoxic test in the presence of complement. Transplantation tests, as well as *in vitro* experiments, indicated a surface localization of specific antigens of leukemia cells and a common antigenicity of leukemias within the leukemia group investigated. Thus, RNA-containing oncogenic agents also seem to be capable of inducing tumor-specific antigens foreign to the syngeneic, immunologically competent host.

Corresponding data have been reported for mouse leukemias induced by viruses designated as Gross, Graffi, Friend, Moloney, Rauscher, Prigozhina, Mazurenko, Rich, and Breyere viruses. These authors independently isolated leukemia-inducing agents from different sources and, thus, their names came into use in order to recognize the laboratory origin of a given type of leukemia. Three years after the experiments of Gross, a leukemia virus was isolated from transplantable mouse sarcomas and carcinomas including the Ehrlich carcinoma, by Graffi *et al.* (1954). The agent induced predominantly myeloid types of leukemia. Virus-induced myeloid leukemias were also described by Prigozhina (1962) and Jenkins and Upton (1963). Furthermore, in 1956, Friend isolated from the Ehrlich carcinoma an agent which induces reticulum cell leukemias (Friend, 1956, 1957). Agents inducing lymphatic leukemias were detected by Schoolman *et al.* (1957) in Swiss mice, by Moloney (1959, 1960) in mouse sarcoma 37, by Lieberman and Kaplan (1959) in radiation-induced C57BL leukemia, by Breyere (Moloney, 1962; Breyere *et al.*, 1966) in a C3H plasmocytoma, by Tennant (1962) in Balb/c mice, by Rich *et al.* (1963) in Swiss mice inoculated with extracts of Friend virus-infected mice, and by Buffett *et al.* (1963) in Swiss mice. Mazurenko (1960) isolated an agent which induces various hematological forms of leukemia. The virus of Rauscher (1962), isolated from Balb/c, produces erythroblastic leukemia. There are still a number of other laboratories reporting the successful isolation of leukemia virus.

It has often been a point of discussions as to whether these viral leukemias are caused by a single virus or several closely related leukemia viruses. Usually speculations originated from the fact that the structurally identical agents isolated by these authors produce diverse morphological and pathogenetic forms of leukemia, probably depending on the different sources of virus material. With regard to malignant transformation of a certain hematopoietic cell, however, specificity appears to be determined not only by the virus but also by the host. Under certain host conditions, most of the leukemia viruses known at present are capable of inducing more than a single hematological type of leukemia. Therefore, virus differentiation on histological basis, i.e., the classification of an unknown leukemia virus according to the hematological type of the disease induced by this agent, proved to be impossible. Comparison of the viruses based on their sensitivity to treatment with chemical or physical agents likewise indicated common properties. Differences were first detected immunologically by cross-neutralizations of the leukemogenic activity using heterologous immune sera from rabbits. However, contradictory results were frequently reported, probably due not only to the use of different experimental arrangements but also to the relative inaccuracy of this bioassay. Cross-neutralizations with mouse immune sera are also not conclusive at present.

The problem of the relationship between leukemia viruses is now being reinvestigated by immunological methods resulting from studies on the phenomenon of transplantation resistance. It was shown that mice resistant to Graffi leukemia cells when inoculated with Gross leukemia cells succumbed to the progressively growing grafts. Furthermore, pretreatment of animals with preparations of Gross leukemia cells did not afford protection against the outgrowth of Graffi leukemia cells (Pasternak and Graffi, 1963; Pasternak, 1967b). The conclusion was drawn that Graffi and Gross leukemia cells contain different tumor-specific transplantation antigens. The lack of cross-resistance was also demonstrated between Gross leukemias, on the one hand, and leukemias of the Friend, Moloney, and Rauscher type, on the other. In contrast, the latter group displayed a certain degree of cross-reactivity. No doubt, variations among the transplantation antigens reflect differences among the viruses that induce the antigens—all the more since hematologically different leukemias induced by the same agent share common antigens, whereas hematologically identical leukemias induced by different viruses do not. The situation concerning the differences of certain characteristic features among leukemia viruses obviously resembles that of polyoma virus where mutants of different kinds are well known and, thus, can be used as genetic markers. From this point of view the differentation of leukemia viruses may be considered also most important.

At present a number of leukemia-specific antigens detected by different methods are known to develop after virus infection. Not only are there antigens in leukemia cells detected by transplantation studies or by cytotoxic and fluorescent antibody techniques, but there are also antigens that are not restricted to leukemia cells such as soluble antigens demonstrable by adsorption to indicator cells (Stück et al., 1964a), by immunoprecipitation (Geering et al., 1966), and complement fixation (Hartley et al., 1965). Most of the techniques mentioned can also be used for the identification and quantitation of virus infection.

Tumor-specific transplantation antigens of leukemia cells can only be shown by the rejection response of immunized animals. As to the nature of these antigens and their relationship to antigens detected by immunofluorescence or cytotoxicity, there are only preliminary results available leading to speculation. Leukemia viruses mature by budding from the cell surface. During this process the membrane may well contain viral antigens responsible for transplantation resistance as well as the positive immuno-fluorescence reaction and the cytotoxic test. This hypothesis seems to be strengthened by the fact that antiviral antibodies are regularly present in the sera of resistant mice. Moreover, formalin-inactivated preparations of leukemia viruses induce formation of antibodies reacting with leukemia cells *in vitro* (Pasternak, 1965). In any case the latter findings suggest the presence of viral antigens at the surface of leukemia cells. However, there also could be other antigenic specificities at the surface of leukemia cells. As indicated by recent experiments the cells, in addition to viral antigens, may also contain new cellular antigens developing under the influence of virus infection (Pasternak, 1967d). Both antigenic specificities are probably coded by the virus genome so that they can be designated as "virus-induced" antigens. As already mentioned, evidence for the existence of new cellular antigens was first obtained for tumors induced by the DNA-containing polyoma virus (Sjögren *et al.*, 1961; Habel, 1961) and simian virus 40 (Defendi, 1963; Koch and Sabin, 1963; Habel and Eddy, 1963). In the following reports, new cellular antigens of the tumor-specific trans-plantation type, characteristic of each tumor group, were likewise shown for adenovirus 12 (Trentin and Bryan, 1966; Sjögren *et al.*, 1967) and for Rous virus-induced mammalian tumors (Sjögren and Jonsson, 1963; Koldovský and Bubeník, 1964). Distinction of the two antigens induced by the RNA-containing Rous virus was made possible with mouse sarcomas which did not release infectious virus.

Since both primary and transplantable leukemias of viral origin are likely to contain viruses, a distinction between viral and new cellular antigens cannot be achieved with these cell types. This would be possible, however, after isolating cells that carry only one of the antigenic speci-ficities. Sarcoma cells "naturally" harboring the Graffi virus seem to contain only viral antigens at the surface (Pasternak, 1967d). With regard to the antigens measured by different tests, Klein *et al.* (1966b) have found for a number of Moloney lymphomas a rough parallelism between immuno-sensitivity of cells *in vivo* and *in vitro*, i.e., the sensitivity of lymphomas to the rejection response of immunized animals corresponded well with their susceptibility to cytotoxic immune sera. Furthermore, fluorescence and absorption tests indicated that immunosensitivity is related to the con-centration of surface antigen. In contrast, infectious virus released from the lymphomas *in vivo* appeared to be independent of the concentration of surface antigen.

Another type of antigen separable from infective virus and not restricted to leukemia cells was described by Stück *et al.* (1964a). It was termed "soluble" because it could not be sedimented together with the virions by high-speed centrifugation. The antigen was first detected in the plasma of mice bearing transplanted Rauscher leukemias by its ability to adsorb to viable indicator cells, such as cells of a radiation-induced leukemia. The cells then became sensitive to the cytotoxic action of Rauscher-specific immune sera. Soluble antigens cross-reacting with this Rauscher type of antigen were further demonstrated in the plasma of mice infected with Friend virus and of mice with primary or transplanted Moloney leukemias. Since the antigens of Friend, Moloney, and Rauscher leukemia cells detected previously by the cytotoxic technique were found to be identical, this antigenic system was designated the "FMR system" (Old *et al.*, 1964). As pointed out by the authors the cross-reactivities between the soluble FMR antigens provided further evidence that mouse leukemias induced by these three viruses are immunologically related (Stück *et al.*, 1964a). When adsorbed to indicator cells the soluble antigens, which are regarded as a product or a subunit of the virion, completely remove the cytotoxic activity of Rauscher immune sera. It was postulated from these data that soluble antigens and antigens of the leukemia cells detected by the cytotoxic test represent identical antigenic specificities and that the sensitivity of leukemia cells to cytotoxic antibody can be adequately explained by the incorporation of viral antigen into the cell membrane.

Using the indirect fluorescent antibody technique, Aoki *et al.* (1966b) found a soluble antigen, immunologically distinct from the FMR type of soluble antigens, in the plasma of Gross virus-infected mice after adsorbing it to leukemia EL 4 indicator cells. All mice of strains with a high incidence of spontaneous leukemia seem to possess this Gross-specific soluble antigen in their sera before leukemia develops. Thus the test for soluble Gross (G) antigen permits the identification of Gross virus infection.

The antigenic differences observed between the soluble antigens of the FMR type, on the one hand, and the Gross type, on the other, correspond well to those of the tumor-specific transplantation antigens. An antigen common to Gross, Friend, Moloney, and Rauscher viruses was shown with rat immune sera in the immunodiffusion test by Geering *et al.* (1966). Rat immune serum produced by repeated inoculations of adult W/Fu rats with syngeneic grafts of Gross virus-induced rat leukemias, which failed to grow, precipitated ether-treated virus preparations but not preparations of intact virus. Virus materials for this test were isolated from the plasma of leukemic mice. As shown by reactions of identity this antigen appeared to be the same as that from tissues infected with the Gross virus. It was concluded that the cross-reacting antigen is an internal virus component that is present also, in the free state, in virus-infected cells. The authors did not find any correlations between the cytotoxic and precipitating activities of the rat immune sera. There were cytotoxic sera without precipitating activities and vice versa. In general, cytotoxic antibodies were specifically directed against cells infected with the Gross virus.

A common group-specific viral antigen is also measured by the complement fixation (CF) test with sera of rats carrying a transplanted Rauscher leukemia. The CF antigen is present in the fluid of mouse embryo cultures infected with several leukemia viruses, in extracts of virus-induced mouse and rat leukemias, in spontaneous leukemias, and in certain radiation-induced mouse leukemias (Hartley et al., 1965; Rowe et al., 1966). Relationships between precipitating and complement-fixing antigens are still unknown. Possibly they represent identical specificities. Based on the CF reaction, a rapid and sensitive test for leukemia viruses was developed. In general, detection and quantitation of antigens and antibodies can well be applied to the identification and titration of virus since a more direct virus assay does not exist at present.

Unfortunately, in tissue culture, leukemia viruses do not produce cytopathic effects or transformations. Hence such tests cannot be used to quantify virus. On the other hand, titration by induction of the disease is often very time-consuming. Another more rapid assay for virus was developed from the finding that even highly diluted preparations of leukemia viruses, after a prolonged period, induce formation of antibodies reacting with leukemia cells. The latency period of antibody formation was found to be inversely related to the virus dose injected into adults. Generally, high antibody levels persisted so that virus which multiplies in the host cells might be directly or indirectly responsible for antibody production against leukemia cells. This mouse antibody production (MAP) test has been used to titrate the Moloney and Graffi leukemia viruses which, after inoculation into newborns, induce leukemia only several months later (Klein and Klein, 1964b; Pasternak and Pasternak, 1967). In adult mice infected with high doses, antibodies were already demonstrable 7 days after infection. Friend and Rauscher viruses which induce leukemia after latency periods between 2 and 4 weeks can be titrated by infection and more rapidly by the spleen colony assay. From 6 to 9 days after intravenous inoculation of virus, macroscopically visible colonies can be detected in the spleen. Titers are based on the number of foci developing after infection (Axelrad and Steeves, 1964; Pluznik and Sachs, 1964). This test cannot be applied to leukemias having long latency periods.

Virus infection is, furthermore, demonstrable by the fluorescent antibody staining of viral antigens using heterologous antiviral sera. Viral antigen appears as diffuse granular staining in the cytoplasm of infected cells. In tissue culture the test can be adapted to quantify leukemia virus by an end-point dilution method (Pinkel et al., 1966).

Measurement of virus, virus-induced antigens, and antibodies directed against these specificities is most important to the investigation of certain virus–host and virus–cell interactions. Thus, distribution of virus after infection, first appearance of virus-induced antigens, and the host response can be quantitatively followed up. On the cellular level the techniques are suitable to test various cell types of murine and nonmurine origin with regard to differences in their sensitivity to virus infection as well as in the expression of virus-induced antigens. Information on these topics, however, is still incomplete.

Concerning the preconditions of viral leukemogenesis the role of immunological tolerance was studied in several laboratories. It was found that AKR mice, naturally infected as embryos with the Gross virus, failed to develop immunity to Gross virus-induced lymphomas. None of the methods used for immunization was capable of inducing tumor-specific transplantation resistance nor antibodies reacting with leukemia cells (Axelrad, 1963, 1965; Bubeník et al., 1964). Specific Gross virus-induced surface antigens, however, were shown in the AKR leukemia cells by the cytotoxic test with absorbed homologous immune sera (Bubeník et al., 1964) and with specific immune serum against Gross passage A lymphomas of other mouse strains (Wahren, 1965; Old et al., 1965). Moreover, the latter finding suggested a close relationship between the antigens detected in spontaneously developing AKR lymphomas and Gross passage A virus-induced leukemia. Originally passage A virus was derived from a cell-free, transmitted AKR leukemia. Axelrad (1963) was able to inhibit the immune response of C3H adult mice against syngeneic Gross lymphoma cells by injection of Gross virus extract into newborn C3H. Similar findings were reported by Klein and Klein (1966) for the Moloney and by Chieco-Bianchi et al. (1967) for the Graffi system. Mice infected as newborns with Moloney virus did not respond immunologically after reinfection at adult age. There was a parallel lack of virus-neutralizing antibodies and antibodies reacting with leukemia cells. The conclusion was drawn that the animals had been rendered tolerant to the virus and/or virus-induced antigens.

The presence of virus-induced antigens in the "tolerant" animals before leukemias develop was shown by Old et al. (1965) and Wahren (1966a,b) for the Gross system and by Pasternak and Pasternak (1967) for the Graffi system. Because of the relatively low content of the antigens in the preleukemic stage, lymph node and/or spleen cells of infected animals were used to absorb leukemia-specific antibodies. Absorption capacity was taken as a measure for content of antigen. Thus, Gross-specific antigens were also detected in the spleen and in certain other normal tissues of strains with a high incidence of leukemia. These mice did not form antibody. Antibodies with specificity for the Gross antigen were, however, frequently demonstrable in older C57BL/6 mice and their hybrids and were occasionally present in mice of other strains (Aoki et al., 1966a). It was suggested that the capacity to produce Gross-specific antibodies plays an important role in the resistance of mice to the induction of leukemia by naturally transmitted Gross virus. In the Graffi system, spleen cells of animals infected as newborns contain relatively large amounts of virus-induced antigens 14 days after infection, when the animals still appear healthy. Although Graffi virus was shown by the MAP test the virus-induced antigens were not detectable in spleen cells of animals infected as adults.

The isolation of leukemia viruses from sarcoma and carcinoma cells "naturally" harboring these agents and, particularly, electron microscopy of various cell types "artificially" infected with leukemia viruses indicated that multiplication and virus release is not only restricted to cells of the hematopoietic system. In this context it is of great interest to know what cell types are capable of expressing virus-induced surface antigens. Stück et al. (1964b) exposed a variety of ascites leukemias and sarcomas to the Rauscher virus by transplanting tumors lacking the FMR antigen to Rauscher viremic mice. After outgrowth the cells were then tested for their sensitivity to cytotoxic Rauscher serum. Whereas the sarcoma cells and an AKR leukemia showed little or no sensitivity the other leukemias tested, in most cases chemically induced leukemias were sensitive to the cytotoxic action of the serum. This phenomenon, acquirement of virus-induced antigens by infection with an unrelated leukemia virus was termed "antigenic conversion."

During formation and transplantation of tumors, antigenic conversion can certainly occur naturally by infection of the cells with viruses just present in the host. Thus, by the capacity of absorbing cytotoxic antibody, Old et al. (1965) found the Gross antigen in certain transplanted leukemias and chemically induced sarcomas obviously not causatively related to the Gross agent. Breyere and Williams (1964) presented evidence that the presumably normal skin of leukemic mice also contains a virus-induced antigen. Skin grafts from these donors were partially rejected by both unimmunized hosts and hosts immunized with leukemia cells. The pattern of rejection resembled that of skin homografts possessing weak histocompatibility antigens. In our studies (Pasternak and Pasternak, 1967; Micheel and Pasternak, 1968b), spontaneous AKR Gross leukemias were infected with the Graffi leukemia virus and then tested for the production of Graffi virus and the presence of antigens detectable by the phenomenon of transplantation resistance, by the immunofluorescence and cytotoxic tests, and by absorption. Whereas all of the 10 leukemias tested continuously produced Graffi virus, only one appeared to be converted, i.e., the cells were rejected in Graffi immune mice, they were strongly positive in the fluorescence test with Graffi immune sera, and they absorbed Graffi-specific antibodies from immune sera. The other infected Gross leukemias were only slightly positive in the fluorescence and absorption tests. Unfortunately, the presence of Gross virus-induced antigens was not tested. Whether the differences in the antigenicity are qualitative rather than quantitative has to be proven. It seems, however, that full expression of new virus-induced antigens does not necessarily result from infection of a viral leukemia with a leukemia virus capable of inducing distinct antigens.

Leukemia cells can also contain antigens induced by artificial infection with an unrelated tumor virus. This was first shown by Sjögren and Hellström (1965). After infection of a Moloney leukemia with polyoma virus the cells acquired the polyoma-specific transplantation antigen in addition to the Moloney specific antigen.

Antigenic conversion of leukemia cells by natural infection with an unrelated virus was taken into consideration for certain leukemias by Stück et al. (1964c). The antigen was present in several leukemias of the DBA/2 strain and in mammary tumors and lactating mammary tissues of mice infected with the mammary tumor virus (MTV). In view of this distribution it was designated "mammary leukemia" (ML) antigen. Nowinski et al. (1967) then demonstrated that the antigen represents a subunit of MTV.

A different antigenic system, apparently not related to leukemia viruses known at present, is the thymus leukemia (TL) system described by Old et al. (1963b) and Boyse et al. (1963). In mice of certain strains (TL+ strains) the antigen was found in normal thymus cells. However, this antigen is also frequently present in leukemias that develop in mice belonging to TL− strains. Whereas mice of TL− strains are capable of forming TL antibody, mice of TL+ strains are not. The origin of the TL antigen in TL− mice has been explained as release of the TL structural gene from a control mechanism that normally suppresses its formation in TL− mice.

In the following, data on the antigenic specificities induced by the mouse leukemia viruses will be summarized and discussed in detail. Special reference is given to our own studies on Graffi virus-induced antigens.

II. Tumor-Specific Transplantation Antigens

A. Induction of Resistance

From transplantation experiments evidence was first obtained that virus-induced leukemia of mice contains specific antigens not present in tissues of normal uninfected animals. It was found by Klein *et al.* (1962) that syngeneic cell inocula of Gross lymphomas were rejected in highly inbred skin-compatible C3H mice if the animals had been pretreated with allogeneic grafts of other Gross lymphomas or with subthreshold doses of syngeneic lymphoma cells. The leukemias induced by passage A line of the Gross agent were of recent origin so that the antigenicity observed could not be explained by secondary antigenic changes of the cells. This is often demonstrable in tumors with long transplantation history. Furthermore, the lymphomas showed partial or complete cross-resistance indicating that they share common antigens.

After regression of large cell doses of allogeneic lymphomas, a high proportion of the animals was found to be resistant to challenge doses ranging between 10^3 and 10^6 syngeneic cells. In contrast, most of the untreated controls developed progressively growing tumors. The same result was obtained after immunization of the animals by giving increasing doses of syngeneic lymphoma cells. In pretreated animals, not fully resistant to challenge injection with viable cells, tumor-appearance was often delayed. Transplantation resistance was not produced by injection of heavily irradiated cells from syngeneic lymphomas. There was no indication of cross-resistance between a Gross lymphoma and a polyoma virus-induced tumor.

At the same time, Sachs (1962) published data on the transplantability of an X-ray-induced and a Moloney virus-induced leukemia in syngeneic C57BL/6 mice inoculated with the Moloney leukemia virus (MLV). Virus preparations isolated from cultures of Swiss MLV-induced leukemia cells on C57BL/6 spleen feeder layers produced transplantation resistance against viable cells of a C57BL/6 Moloney leukemia. This phenomenon appeared to be very similar to that of polyoma virus-infected animals. Therefore, leukemia cells were also supposed to have acquired a new antigen. On the other hand, growth of the X-ray-induced leukemia was not inhibited in MLV-pretreated animals, thus, showing the absence of the corresponding antigen. Since inoculations with polyoma virus did not influence the growth behavior of Moloney leukemia cells, it was concluded that tumors induced by the two viruses contain different antigens.

It was also shown in our experiments (Pasternak *et al.*, 1962) that specific transplantation resistance can be produced against cell inocula of a virus-induced leukemia. After pretreatment of C57BL mice with X-ray-killed tissue suspensions from a myeloid Graffi leukemia, the outgrowth of viable cells from the same leukemia was inhibited.

Resistance was demonstrable with challenge doses between 5×10^4 and 10^5 cells. Higher cell doses led to tumor growth in both experimental and control animals. In further studies, using a number of different Graffi leukemias, our first result was confirmed (Pasternak and Graffi, 1963).

Resistance was produced by small doses of viable cells, X-ray-killed leukemic tissue, and allogeneic grafts. The effect was marked in all three strains of mice tested. Induction of resistance by allogeneic leukemia grafts indicated common antigens in all Graffi leukemias. After injection of 5 × 10^4 and 10^5 cells, the percentage of resistant animals was between 64 and 79 in pretreated animals as compared with 12 and 34 in the controls.

From studies on the mechanism of homograft rejection, it is known that cell destruction occurring in the course of this process is due to cellular and/or humoral immune reactions against foreign histocompatibility antigens located at the surface of target cells. Reactions against histocompatibility antigens, however, can be ruled out within skin-compatible inbred mice. Thus, inhibition of the outgrowth of syngeneic leukemia cells in pretreated animals reflects reactions against leukemia-specific antigens. These antigens appear to be situated at the cell surface. On the other hand, they are certainly present at membranes of the endoplasmic reticulum, too. With regard to the nature of the antigens involved in the graft rejection, essentially two possibilities were taken into consideration (Slettenmark and Klein, 1962; Sachs, 1962). (1) The antigen could be a virus-induced, new cellular antigen not related to antigens of the virion, and (2) the antigen in question may represent a virion antigen. The concept that a viral antigen could be responsible for cell destruction comes from the fact that leukemia viruses mature by budding from the cell membrane. During this process the membrane may well contain viral antigens. However, it is also conceivable that both viral antigens and new cellular antigens are present in leukemia cells. Problems of differentiation between these antigenic specificities will be discussed later on. Since both antigens are probably coded by the virus genome, the designation "virus-induced" antigens will be used for these antigens to overcome difficulties in terminology. In other words, tumor-specific transplantation antigens of leukemia cells belong to the category of virus-induced antigens.

After the initial experiments concerned with specific transplantation antigens of certain virus-induced leukemias in mice the data were further completed. Using transplantation methods, antigens were detected in leukemias induced by the viruses of Moloney (Klein and Klein, 1964a; Glynn et al., 1964), Prigozhina (Prigozhina and Stavrovskaja, 1964), Rich (Rich et al., 1965), Mazurenko (Stepina et al., 1966), Breyere (Breyere et al., 1966), Rauscher (Bianco et al., 1966), and Friend (Kobayashi and Takeda, 1967). Resistance-inducing capacity was found in all preparations containing leukemia virus, such as viable or X-ray-killed leukemia cells and homogenates and cell-free filtrates from leukemic tissues as well as from virus preparations. There is only one exception concerning the activity of material used for immunization against leukemia cells, namely that

X-ray-killed Gross lymphoma cells did not build up transplantation resistance. Summarized data on methods used for the induction of transplantation resistance against syngeneic cell inocula of several virus-induced leukemia are listed in Table I. It should be mentioned, however, that preparations from virus-containing nonleukemic tissues are equally active in producing resistance.

Among leukemias induced by the same virus, extensive cross-reactions were observed. This is independent of the histology as shown with Graffi leukemia. The virus that predominantly produces myeloid type of leukemia may also produce several other types. Lymphatic and myeloid Graffi leukemia, however, possess the same transplantation antigens. In general, host resistance against leukemia cells has been quantitatively determined by partial or complete growth inhibition of a certain cell dose inoculated subcutaneously. Another quantitative method for measuring host resistance was used by Axelrad (1963) for the Gross leukemia system in C3H mice. The method was based on the observations of Bruce and van der Gaag (1963) that viable AKR lymphoma cells injected intravenously into syngeneic recipients form discrete macroscopic colonies in the spleen. The number of colonies visible between 8 and 12 days after injection was proportional to the cell dose injected.

In Axelrad's experiments (1963, 1965) the number of colonies was considerably reduced in animals pretreated with virus extracts or viable Gross lymphoma cells. Inhibition of lymphoma cell proliferation in spleen, thus, represents a rapid and accurate assay for transplantation resistance. However, the test cannot be applied to all types of leukemia. Graffi leukemia cells injected intravenously may produce generalized leukemia as well as isolated metastases at distinct sites of the body. Each leukemia has its own characteristic transplantation behavior. Spleen colonies have not been observed.

The results obtained by Axelrad (1963, 1965) confirmed those of Klein *et al.* (1962) in that Gross leukemia cells contain specific cross-reacting transplantation antigens. Moreover, the author postulated that if resistance is due to an antigen foreign to the host, it should be possible to induce immunological tolerance to the antigen by pretreatment of newborn immunologically incompetent animals. As shown by a decrease of normal host resistance against transplantation of lymphoma cells, Gross virus extract inoculated into newborns actually produced tolerance, i.e., infected animals challenged later in life developed larger numbers of spleen colonies than untreated controls inoculated with the same cell dose. Suppression of colony formation in normal, untreated C3H mice is probably due to a weak immune response of the recipients against lymphoma cells. The level of host resistance was also reduced by total body γ-radiation with 350 rads.

TABLE I

SUMMARIZED DATA ON METHODS USED FOR THE INDUCTION OF TRANSPLANTATION RESISTANCE AGAINST SYNGENEIC CELL INOCULA OF SEVERAL VIRUS-INDUCED LEUKEMIAS IN MICE

Method, inoculation of adult mice with	Transplantation resistance against leukemia induced by the virus of								
	Gross	Graffi	Friend	Moloney	Rauscher	Prigozhina	Mazurenko	Rich	Breyere
Viable syngeneic leukemia cells in subthreshold doses	+	+		+					+
X-ray-killed syngeneic grafts	−	++		++	+				
Allogeneic leukemia grafts	++	++	+	++					
Virus-containing homogenate or cell-free filtrate (virus preparations)	++				±	+	+	+	

Irradiated animals given Gross virus extract and challenged 38 days later with lymphoma cells developed significantly larger numbers of spleen colonies.

Absence of tumor-specific transplantation resistance was found in the case of lymphomas which had spontaneously arisen from AKR mice (Bubeník et al., 1964; Axelrad, 1965; Pasternak and Hölzer, 1965). Pretreatment of syngeneic as well as semisyngeneic recipients with irradiated leukemic tissue, increasing doses of viable cells, or other preparations from leukemic tissue even failed to produce partial inhibition of lymphoma cell proliferation. Since the AKR strain and its F_1 hybrids are naturally infected with Gross virus, immunological tolerance to Gross virus-induced antigens was supposed to be the cause of nonresponsiveness following pretreatment. The greater colony-forming efficiency of C3H Gross lymphoma cells in "naturally tolerant" (AKR × C3H)F_1 hybrids as compared with "normally reacting" C3H mice was indicative of this hypothesis (Axelrad, 1965). It was also impossible to obtain an increase in the number of spleen colonies by pretreating newborn hybrids with Gross virus extract. Apparently, the animals were already tolerant at the time of injection.

Tolerance is dependent on the temporary or permanent presence of the antigenic stimulus, such as virus and/or virus-induced antigens, in the AKR leukemia system. Particularly, detection of those antigens in certain cells during the preleukemic phase and in lymphoma cells would speak in favor of the tolerance hypothesis. In vitro studies have shown that both lymph node and lymphoma cells of AKR origin are carrying specific antigens (see Section X). They are identical with those induced by Gross passage A virus originally isolated from the AKR strain.

It has not been tested, however, whether AKR lymphoma cells or extracts are capable of producing transplantation resistance against passage A virus-induced lymphoma of C3H mice. Only in this way could the existence of cross-reacting leukemia-specific transplantation antigens be proved.

The concept of tolerance to virus-induced transplantation antigens of leukemia was based on the observation that Gross lymphoma cells grow better in animals "naturally" or "artificially" infected with Gross virus as newborns. In contrast to normal noninfected C3H mice, immune reactions were probably absent. Such animals are also expected to be incapable of reacting immunologically after reinfection if tolerance is really responsible for the effect. In addition to naturally infected AKR mice the influence of reinfection with Gross virus extract was tested in C3H mice (Axelrad, 1965); this experiment was also done with Graffi leukemia by Chieco-Bianchi et al. (1967). Inoculation of virus-containing preparations, while effective in control animals with regard to induction of transplantation resistance, was not followed by resistance in mice already infected with virus as newborns. More detailed data on immunological tolerance to virus-induced leukemia have been obtained with serological methods (see Section X).

B. Significance of Virus-Induced Transplantation Antigens

The significance of virus-induced transplantation antigens is still the subject of speculation. It is not known whether the formation of antigens represents a primary or a secondary event in the process of neoplastic transformation by viruses; a primary one in the sense that the presence of antigens on the cell surface is essential to the acquirement and maintenance of malignancy. Thus, the antigenic change of the surface would allow the cell to escape the mechanisms of growth control exerted by the adjacent tissue. Furthermore, development of immunological tolerance to the virus-induced antigens would favor the outgrowth of the malignant cells. On the other hand, it cannot be also concluded from this hypothesis that all cells having the antigen are malignant cells.

Production of virus-induced antigens as a secondary event would mean that there is no correlation between presence of antigen and neoplastic character of the cell. In this case, both properties might be independent of each other. Although the existence of virus-induced primary or transplanted leukemia, lacking specific transplantation antigens, would be indicative of this possibility, its absence could certainly not speak against the secondary significance of the antigens.

In virus-induced leukemia the situation is complicated by the fact that the transplantation antigens could consist of at least two antigenic specificities, i.e., viral and new cellular antigens. This raises the need for their separate measurement which would be possible if cells carried only one of the antigenic specificities. It is conceivable that, if present in high enough concentration at the surface, only one of the antigens is necessary for the destruction of the target cell. *In vivo* techniques alone, however, are not sufficient to solve the problem.

At present, using the phenomenon of specific transplantation resistance, information can be obtained whether (*1*) all leukemias induced by virus are carrying tumor-specific transplantation antigens, (*2*) there are quantitative antigenic differences among leukemias induced by the same virus, (*3*) antigenicity is retained after serial transplantation, and (*4*) nonleukemic cells infected with a leukemia virus possess virus-induced transplantation antigens.

All Moloney lymphomas tested by Klein *et al.* (1966b; G. Klein and

Klein, 1964) were sensitive to the specific rejection response of pretreated mice. However, there was a considerable variation with regard to immunosensitivity among different lymphomas—several tumors did not grow even when the challenge dose was high (10^5–10^6 cells), and others were not regularly rejected after low doses (10^3–10^4 cells). One lymphoma appeared to be completely resistant to the rejection response; its specific surface antigens could only be detected by *in vitro* methods. This result shows the limitations of *in vivo* techniques. After prolonged transplantation, immunosensitivity of another lymphoma changed from high to low sensitivity, following, however, passage of Moloney lymphomas in pretreated animals.

The same pattern of reactivity was observed with Graffi leukemias of mice. Most of them revealed a certain degree of immunosensitivity *in vivo*. Among 7 Graffi leukemias induced in AKR mice, only 1 appeared to be resistant to the rejection response of immunized animals (Pasternak *et al.*, 1967). In this case the presence of surface antigens was shown by the immunofluorescence technique. Information on the immunosensitivity *in vivo* is also given by the number of "takes" after transplantation of primary leukemias to syngeneic recipients. Although in the first passage high doses of cells were injected, 2 of 15 different Graffi leukemias tested did not grow at all. In 7 other cases, tumors appeared in the minority of animals. Altogether the percentage of tumor takes was 49 (44 of 90 animals). Spontaneous Gross leukemias of the AKR strain, however, were usually accepted by syngeneic recipients. The growth rate was 91% (29 of 32 animals), thus indicating different host conditions, namely tolerance to the virus-induced transplantation antigens (Pasternak, 1967a).

Occasionally, primary grafts were also unsuccessful with leukemias induced by the viruses of Moloney (G. Klein and Klein, 1964), Rauscher (Old *et al.*, 1964), and Breyere (Breyere *et al.*, 1966). Regressions of subcutaneous grafts from early transplant generations of Moloney and Rauscher leukemias have also been reported by Bianco *et al.* (1966).

Regarding the first three points the experimental data obtained can be summarized as follows. Tumor-specific transplantation antigens are demonstrable in the majority of leukemias induced by viruses. Although immunoresistant tumors do exist they contain virus-induced surface antigens as shown by *in vitro* studies. Immunosensitivity *in vivo* varies among different leukemias induced by the same virus. Occasionally immunosensitivity changes after prolonged transplantation. There is no loss of tumor-specific transplantation antigens after passage of leukemia cells through immunized animals. The presence of tumor-specific transplantation antigens in nonleukemic cells will be described separately (see Sections VI and IX). It should be mentioned, however, that such antigens are detectable in cells naturally or artificially infected with a leukemia virus.

C. CROSS-RESISTANCE AMONG LEUKEMIAS INDUCED BY DIFFERENT VIRUSES

Most important to the comparison of leukemia viruses is the question of cross-resistance among leukemias induced by different viruses. In the preceding the phrase "different viruses" was used in the sense that the leukemia viruses were of different laboratory origin. Differences in the specificity of virus-induced transplantation antigens, however, would indicate the existence of genotypically distinct leukemia viruses, i.e., in these viruses at least that part of the virus genome is different which is coding for transplantation antigens. Data on cross-resistance available at present are rather incomplete (Table II). In our experiments we failed to produce transplantation resistance against Graffi leukemia by pretreating the animals with a number of allogeneic Gross lymphomas (Pasternak and Hölzer, 1965). Furthermore, low doses of Gross lymphoma cells grew equally well in controls and in animals highly resistant to Graffi leukemia cells, thus suggesting the absence of cross-resistance. Unfortunately the reverse experiment has not yet been made.

Cross-resistance was also absent between Moloney and Gross lymphomas (Klein and Klein, 1964a). Animals specifically pretreated with allogeneic Moloney lymphomas were not resistant to the two Gross lymphomas tested. Another cross-combination was tested by Bianco et al. (1966). Pretreatment of mice with Rauscher virus-induced leukemia generally produced cross-resistance against Moloney lymphomas. In some experiments, however, cross-resistance could not be detected. It is not known whether this opposite result is due to qualitative or quantitative antigenic differences. There is another fact that cannot be explained to date, particularly in view of the extensive cross-reactions observed between Moloney and Rauscher leukemias *in vitro*. In previous studies the same investigators (Glynn et al., 1964) failed in the attempt to produce transplantation resistance against two different Rauscher leukemias by pretreatment of mice with allogeneic Moloney grafts. More experiments are needed, however, to solve the question of cross-resistance between the two types of leukemia.

Rich et al. (1965) reported that prior inoculations of Rich but not Moloney virus protected against inocula of Rich leukemia cells. Furthermore, injection with Rich virus did not produce transplantation resistance against Moloney lymphoma cells. Although the data suggest certain differences between the two tumors tested, they do not allow any conclusion with respect to antigenic differences. As mentioned by the authors, results strongly depend on quantitative factors such as virus titer, cell number, and interval between virus inoculation and cell transplantation. In addition the concentration of surface antigens of leukemia cells might play an

G. PASTERNAK

TABLE II

Summarized Data on the Cross-Resistance among Leukemias Induced by Different Viruses

Immunized against leukemia induced by the virus of	Challenged with leukemia induced by the virus of							
	Gross	Graffi	Friend	Moloney	Rauscher	Prigozhina	Mazurenko	Rich
Gross						(−)[a]	(−)	(−)
Graffi	−						(−)	
Friend						(−)	(−)	
Moloney					(−)	+	(−)	
Rauscher				+		(−)		
Prigozhina								
Mazurenko								
Rich		−		(−)		+		

[a] Symbols in parenthesis—not conclusively established.

important role. While cross-protection between Rich and Moloney leukemia was absent, *in vitro* studies using cytotoxic immune sera indicated common antigens. Absence of cross-reactions *in vivo* were also observed for the Gross–Prigozhina combination (Prigozhina and Stavrovskaja, 1964). Animals pretreated with extracts from a leukemic AKR mouse were not resistant to challenge inoculation with Prigozhina leukemia. On the other hand, injection of Moloney as well as Mazurenko virus produced transplantation resistance against Prigozhina leukemia. Apparently these types of leukemia share common antigens. Cross-reactions among leukemias of different origin were also tested by Stepina *et al.* (1966). Groups of adult mice were injected with extracts from different leukemias including those induced by the viruses of Mazurenko, Friend, Moloney, Rauscher, Graffi, Prigozhina, and Stepina. Three weeks after the second injection the animals were challenged with Mazurenko leukemia cells. A high degree of resistance was evident only in the group inoculated with extracts of Mazurenko leukemia. Inoculation of extracts from the other types of leukemia did not significantly influence the outgrowth of Mazurenko cells. This result suggests the absence of common antigens. On the other hand, injection with Moloney virus induced weak resistance to Prigozhina leukemia. There was no resistance against this leukemia after pretreatment of animals with extracts from Friend, Rauscher, and Mazurenko tumors. That cross-reactions are also absent between Mazurenko and Prigozhina leukemia is in contrast to the data obtained by Prigozhina and Stavrovskaja (1964).

In summary, all findings of cross-experiments *in vivo* have to be evaluated most critically. Conclusions were frequently based on few experimental data. In consideration of the number of different factors that determine immunogenicity and immunosensitivity of a cell, it is not surprising that contradictory results were obtained.

Standardization of test conditions is certainly difficult; it is needed, however, for the immunological comparison of leukemias of different origin. Although demonstration of cross-protection is suggestive of the presence of common antigens, negative results do not allow conclusion with regard to absence of antigenic relationships. Tumors immunoresistant *in vivo*, for example, do contain virus-induced surface antigens as shown by *in vitro* experiments. Therefore, investigations on the presence or absence of cross-reacting antigens require both *in vivo* and *in viro* experiments. Altogether the present data of *in vivo* cross-studies are incomplete.

III. Passive Transfer of Transplantation Resistance

Methods for the detection of histocompatibility antigens in tumor cells (for review, see Hellström and Möller, 1965) correspond well with those for the detection of tumor antigens. The only difference is the genetic background of the experimental systems. Whereas transplantation resistance induced in foreign recipients is due to immune reactions against isoantigens of tumor cells, the same phenomenon in a syngeneic tumor–host combination indicates specific tumor antigens. Thus, resistance against virus-induced leukemia demonstrated in a skin-compatible mouse system suggests the presence of tumor-specific transplantation antigens. Since transplantation resistance is mediated by humoral and/or cellular defense mechanisms, it was of interest to know whether the same factors are acting in the tumor-specific rejection response against leukemia. *In vivo*, this is detectable by the passive transfer of resistance to normal untreated animals. Lymphoid cells or serum from resistant animals are mixed with tumor cells *in vitro* and then injected into syngeneic recipients (neutralization test). Effectiveness of cells or serum is measured by the inhibition of tumor cell growth. This allows quantitative studies on the degree of immunity (Hellström and Möller, 1965) as well as on the immunosensitivity of target cells. A modification of the neutralization technique is the test for adoptive immunity. For the latter, tumor cells and immune cells are separately injected by different routes. Again inhibition of outgrowth of tumor cells is indicative of the activity of immune cells. Passive transfer of resistance verifies the immunological nature of transplantation resistance.

Although the terms "neutralization" and "adoptive immunity" are preferably applied to experiments with immune cells, there is no reason why they should not be used for experiments with immune serum, too. The effect of humoral antibodies, however, may be either inhibition or enhancement of tumor growth, depending on the experimental system. Several hypotheses have been advanced to explain this opposite effect of antibodies (Hellström and Möller, 1965; Kaliss, 1965). Generally, within H-2 combinations, growth of leukemia cells is inhibited by immune serum while growth of sarcoma cells is enhanced. The growth-inhibiting action on leukemia cells is due to their sensitivity to cytotoxic antibodies. Although enhancement is in the first place restricted to histoincompatible tumors, it has occasionally been found in syngeneic tumor–host combinations (Bubeník and Koldovský, 1964, 1965; Möller, 1965). However, because of the extreme sensitivity of leukemia cells, inhibition of tumor growth is expected to dominate in the leukemia-specific system.

Neutralization of Gross lymphoma cells by lymphoid cells from resistant animals was first shown by Slettenmark and Klein (1962). In these experiments the admixture of lymph node cells *in vitro* inhibited or delayed the outgrowth of a small number of lymphoma cells. Controls were animals injected with the same number of lymphoma cells mixed with lymph node cells from untreated mice. Effective neutralization was demonstrable when the proportion of immune cells to lymphoma cells was higher than 100:1. Cytotoxicity of immune sera was tested by *in vitro* studies alone. Passive transfer of resistance against a syngeneic Gross leukemia of C57BL/6 origin was successful with immune sera from rats (Old et al., 1967). There was a considerable degree of protection against intravenously or intraperitoneally injected leukemia cells if the interval between injection of cells and intraperitoneal administration of serum was short, i.e., between 4 hours and 3 days. Initiation of treatment 5 days after cell inoculation, however, did not influence the growth of leukemia. Complete protection by immune serum was achieved when the number of leukemia cells inoculated was decreased and treatment started at an early time. The relatively strong activity of rat immune serum follows from the fact that 0.1 ml. injected intraperitoneally 4 hours after intravenous inoculation of 10^4 leukemia cells produced complete protection. Animals injected with a leukemia lacking the Gross antigen were not protected.

Reactions against antigens other than leukemia-specific antigens are certainly not responsible for the effect against C57BL/6 Gross leukemia cells since the sera were derived from rats immunized with histocompatible Gross virus-induced rat leukemias. This means that mouse and rat leukemias induced by Gross virus share common antigens. According to Old et al. (1967), effectiveness of passive immunization depends on factors such as (1) titer of antiserum and class of immunoglobulin, (2) extent of disease, (3) disposition of antigen, (4) degree of immunogenicity of leukemia cells, (5) availability of complement, and (6) occurrence of immunoresistant cells.

Passive transfer of resistance against transplantation of spontaneous Gross lymphomas of AKR origin was shown by Bubeník et al. (1964) and by Pasternak (1967b). As a matter of fact, the experiments were performed to demonstrate virus-induced antigens in cells of spontaneous AKR lymphomas. For that purpose histoincompatible recipients were injected with viable AKR lymphoma cells since syngeneic AKR mice were known to be nonreactive against Gross antigens. The immune sera thus obtained were absorbed with normal AKR tissue and then tested for their activity against lymphoma cells. In the experiments of Bubeník et al. (1964) the immune sera were absorbed in vitro and, showing no further effect on normal AKR lymphoid cells, caused prolonged survival of animals when injected in combination with lymphoma cells (neutralization test). Before inoculation the mixture had been incubated for 30 minutes at 37°C. The technique of in vivo absorption was used by Pasternak (1967b). Immune sera from XVII mice were injected in one single dose of 0.3 ml. intraperitoneally into AKR mice; 1 hour later doses of 5×10^2 or 10^3 syngeneic Gross leukemia cells were injected subcutaneously. The outgrowth of cells was considerably delayed in the group inoculated with 5×10^2 cells. Normal serum from XVII mice and a XVII immune serum against AKR Graffi leukemia were ineffective. Particularly in consideration of the inefficacy of the XVII anti-AKR Graffi immune serum, it appears that the reactions obtained with allogeneic anti-AKR Gross serum are specifically directed against the Gross antigen of lymphoma cells. However, normal hematopoietic cells of several highly leukemic strains, including the AKR strain, may also contain the Gross antigen (Old *et al.*, 1965). It is, thus, conceivable that, during absorption of immune sera *in vivo* or *in vitro*, antibodies with Gross specificity are completely or at least partially eliminated. In general, the concentration of Gross antigen in cells of preleukemic animals is, indeed, very low (Wahren, 1966a,b) so that the remaining activity of absorbed sera can be explained on the basis of insufficient elimination of Gross-specific antibodies. In contrast, H-2 antibodies were no longer present after *in vitro* absorption since the sera did not affect normal AKR lymphoid cells.

Passive transfer of transplantation resistance was also successful in the Moloney and Graffi leukemia systems. Using mouse immune serum, Klein and Klein (1964a) were able to transfer resistance against Moloney lymphomas. Tumor outgrowth was inhibited if immune serum was repeatedly given intraperitoneally to mice inoculated with serum and lymphoma cells which had been mixed *in vitro* before inoculation. Serum from animals resistant to Gross leukemia had no effect on Moloney cells. Furthermore, immune serum prevented active immunization. Animals showing no tumor growth after passive immunity were not resistant against reinoculation of lymphoma cells.

The outgrowth of Graffi leukemia cells was considerably delayed in animals if injected with admixed lymph node cells from Graffi resistant animals (Pasternak, 1967b). A proportion of lymph node cells to leukemia cells higher than 50:1 was found to be effective. A similar dose effect has also been found for the passive transfer of resistance by immune sera. Two intravenous injections of 0.25 ml. immune serum on two successive days inhibited the growth of 10^3 Graffi leukemia cells inoculated subcutaneously. This effect was not demonstrable after injection of 10^4 cells.

In summary, transplantation resistance against virus-induced leukemia of mice can be passively transferred to untreated recipients by both serum and lymphoid cells from resistant animals (see Table III for summarized data).

IV. Virus-Induced Surface Antigens of Leukemia Cells Detected by Immunofluorescence

A. Indirect Immunofluorescence Test with Viable Cells

Sera of mice resistant against transplantation of virus-induced leukemia contain antibodies reacting with leukemia cells *in vivo* and *in vitro*. Re-

TABLE III

SUMMARIZED DATA ON THE PASSIVE TRANSFER OF TRANSPLANTATION
RESISTANCE AGAINST VIRUS-INDUCED LEUKEMIA

Leukemia	Neutralization		Adoptive immunity	
	Immune cells	Serum	Immune cells	Serum
Gross	+	+[a]		+[b]
Graffi	+			+
Moloney		+		

[a] Neutralization of AKR Gross lymphomas.

[b] Demonstrated in mice by rat immune serum against histocompatible rat leukemia and by absorbed mouse immune sera derived from histoincompatible donors (see text).

actions between humoral antibodies and leukemia cells *in vitro* are detectable by the indirect fluorescent antibody technique with viable cells and by the cytotoxic test in the presence of complement. Both techniques are applicable to the detection of antigens located at the cell surface. Results of immunofluorescence tests on leukemia cells are presented in the following. Hitherto this technique, originally introduced for the demonstration of mouse isoantigens by Möller (1961), has been applied to leukemias induced by the viruses of Moloney, Graffi, Gross, Mazurenko, and Friend. In principle, it is based on the fact that antibodies specifically bound to virus-induced surface antigens are demonstrable by heterologous antibodies against mouse γ-globulin if the latter are marked with a fluorescent label. According to Klein and Klein (1964a) and Pasternak (1965), viable leukemia cells are mixed with immune serum and then incubated for 20 to 30 minutes at 37°C. After washing the suspension 3 times with buffered saline solution (BSS), one drop of fluorescein isothiocyanate-labeled rabbit anti-mouse γ-globulin is added to the cell sediment. The mixture is again incubated for 20 to 30 minutes and subsequently washed 3 times to eliminate free labeled serum. Finally a small amount of BSS is given to the sediment, the cells are suspended, and examined in the fluorescence microscope. About 150 cells of each preparation are counted to determine the percentage of stained and unstained cells. Diffuse fluorescence of the whole cell indicates death of the cell. The dead cells are not taken into consideration. All cells showing punctiform or semicircular fluorescent patterns at the membrane may be considered positive. Frequently the entire membrane is stained and the cells show an annular fluorescent pattern.

Using this technique, specific antibodies as well as virus-induced surface antigens can be at least semiquantitatively measured. For comparison of antibody activity of different sera, either a fluorescence index (FI) is calculated or the titer is estimated by diluting the serum to an end point.

For calculation of the index, the percentage of negative cells in the sample containing immune serum is subtracted from the percentage of negative cells in the control sera, and the quantity thus obtained is divided by the latter value; $FI = (a - b)/a$. Indices higher than 0.2 or 0.3 may be regarded as positive. The cause of nonspecific background staining by control serum will be described later on.

Antigen is measurable by comparing the intensity of surface fluorescence at different serum dilutions as well as by the absorption capacity of the cells. Absorption is evident if the FI is significantly decreased as compared with unabsorbed serum. More precise information about concentration of surface antigens is obtained if the number of cells necessary to decrease the index to a certain value is known. Since measurement of antigen or antibody by immunofluorescence is based on visual evaluation of the tests, all quantitative statements have to be considered with caution. Provision has to be made for avoidance of subjective interpretations during cell count. For example, only coded samples should be used. Measurement of fluorescence intensity by photometry is not practicable on account of the considerable variability of components participating in the reaction.

B. SURFACE ANTIGENS DETECTED BY IMMUNOFLUORESCENCE

Specific antibodies against Moloney lymphoma cells were detectable by the immunofluorescence test 5 days after two inoculations of 10^5 lymphoma cells (Klein and Klein, 1964a). Immune sera cross-reacted with all other lymphomas induced by the same agent. The reactions appeared to be most sensitive and highly specific for Moloney lymphoma cells. Cross-reactions were not observed with lymphomas induced by the Gross agent, long-transplanted lymphomas of no known viral origin, and normal lymphoid cells. Specificity was further proved by the absence of positive reactions between Moloney lymphoma cells and Gross-specific immune sera as well as antipolyoma virus serum. Complete absorption of Moloney immune sera was obtained only with Moloney lymphoma cells. In an attempt to detect differences in the concentration of surface antigens measurable by immunofluorescence, different target cells were tested against serial dilutions of the same serum. Two of the lymphomas compared showed stronger differences in their capacity to bind antibodies. In general, the serum dilutions required for the staining of 50% of cells in excess of control background varied by one or two steps for the different lymphomas (Klein et al., 1966b).

The immunofluorescence test was likewise applied to Graffi leukemia of mice (Pasternak, 1965; Pasternak and Hölzer, 1965). A number of different Graffi immune sera were found to react specifically with Graffi leukemia cells. The sera tested did not react with normal bone marrow or spleen and lymph node cells. Reactions were also negative with cells of spontaneous AKR Gross leukemia. By the use of only syngeneic cells throughout the experiments, reactions of immune sera with H-2 isoantigens were eliminated. After absorption of sera with cells of various Graffi leukemias the FI decreased. In most experiments, antibodies were completely absorbed after incubation of 0.1-ml. samples with 60 to 80 million cells. The relative decrease of the FI after absorption with normal spleen and lymph node cells is probably due to the weak dilution of immune sera during the absorption procedure. As to be expected, Gross leukemia cells did not absorb Graffi-specific antibodies.

Studies on cross-reactions between leukemias induced by the Moloney and Graffi viruses are not yet completed. It is indicated, however, that both types of leukemia show a certain degree of antigenic relationship (E. Klein and G. Pasternak, unpublished results). Summarized data of immuno-fluorescence tests are presented in Table IV.

In the experiments with Moloney and Graffi leukemia cells, interpretation of nonspecific background staining after incubation of cells with control serum has been often a point of discussion. It is impossible, for example, to differentiate between specific and "nonspecific" staining of the cell membrane by the fluorescent pattern. Leukemia cells stained by normal mouse serum show the same picture of fluorescence as when stained by immune serum, although the intensity of the staining is usually lower in the controls. In general, the background level depends on the rabbit fluorescence serum. A strong serum is capable of staining 100% of normal mouse cells as well as leukemia cells when the cells had been incubated with normal mouse serum only. This serum would not distinguish between immune and normal mouse serum. The staining of both normal and tumor cells decreases with the dilution of the rabbit serum, provided that the cells had been incubated with normal mouse serum. After further dilution of the rabbit serum to the point where leukemia cells incubated with normal serum do not show any fluorescence, the rabbit serum still gives a positive reaction with leukemia cell that had been incubated with mouse immune serum. At this point of dilution a "nonspecific" staining apparently does not exist. To have a distinct, well-visible, specific reaction, however, a certain background is desirable. According to Klein (personal communication) there is, as a rule, no significant difference between the background obtained with BSS and with control serum. This fact indicates that the nonspecific staining is not an immunological reaction. In our experiments with Graffi leukemia cells the background staining of fluorescent sera was adjusted to give 20–30% positives. However, the background staining of a given fluorescence serum varies according to the cell type used as target (Pasternak and Pasternak, 1967).

TABLE IV

Summarized Data of Immunofluorescence Tests

Immune sera against leu-kemia of	Cells used for the immunofluorescence test										
	Moloney	Graffi	Gross	Mazurenko	Friend	Rauscher	6C3HED[a]	EL 4[b]	Normal lymph node	Spleen	Bone marrow
Moloney	+	+?	−				−	−	−	−	−
Graffi	+?	+	−				−		−	−	
Gross	−										
Mazurenko				++	++	++			−		
Friend				++	++	++			−		

[a] Originally induced by estradiol.
[b] Originally induced by dimethylbenzanthracene.

In studies of Dirlugyan and Stepina (1966, 1967) the surface antigens of Mazurenko, Friend, Rauscher, and Graffi leukemia cells were compared by the immunofluorescence test. Immune sera against Mazurenko and Friend leukemia reacted strongly with homologous cells. They did not react with normal cells.

Cross-experiments demonstrated the presence of common antigens in both types of leukemia, i.e., Mazurenko immune sera reacted with Friend leukemia cells and Friend immune sera with Mazurenko leukemia cells. Furthermore, previous absorption of Mazurenko immune serum with Friend leukemia cells completely eliminated antibodies against Mazurenko leukemia. Normal cells did not influence the antibody activity. These *in vitro* findings, showing common antigens in Friend and Mazurenko leukemia of mice, are in contrast to those obtained *in vivo* by the same group of investigators (Stepina *et al.*, 1966). In these experiments, Friend virus was incapable of producing transplantation resistance against Mazurenko cells. The discrepancy of results may be due to (*1*) different sensitivities of the techniques or (*2*) different qualities of antigens detected by transplantation and by immunofluorescence tests. On the other hand, it is also conceivable that cross-reactions between leukemias may occur after uncontrolled infection of one type of leukemia with another unrelated leukemogenic virus.

Dirlugyan and Stepina (1967) were able further to show that Mazurenko immune sera also reacted with Rauscher leukemia cells. Immunofluorescence test was negative, however, when testing Graffi leukemia cells with both Mazurenko and Friend immune serum. Summarizing these studies, common antigens appear to be present in Mazurenko, Friend, and Rauscher leukemia, whereas Graffi leukemia has distinct antigenic specificities.

Finally, the immunofluorescence technique was used for the demonstration of antibody with specificity for the Gross leukemia antigen (Aoki *et al.*, 1966a). It was found that specific antibodies are present in the serum of some untreated mice from strains with a low incidence of spontaneous leukemia. This natural antibody was shown in sera of older C57BL/6 mice and C57BL/6 hybrids. In contrast, mouse strains with a high incidence of leukemia did not contain Gross-specific antibodies. Presence of antibodies as well as development of spontaneous Gross leukemia in certain strains gives evidence of the widespread distribution of the Gross agent among mouse colonies.

In a first attempt to apply the membrane immunofluorescence test to the search for antigens in human tumors, Klein *et al.* (1966a) focused their interest on the Burkitt lymphoma of African patients. As indicated by various criteria, this tumor is suspected to be of viral origin. As a matter of fact, the sera of certain patients reacted with Burkitt lymphoma cells.

Specificity of the reaction, however, was not regarded as conclusively established.

V. Virus-Induced Surface Antigens of Leukemia Cells Detected by Cytotoxic Tests

A. MICROSCOPIC EVALUATION OF CYTOTOXIC EFFECTS

Cytotoxic reactions produced by antibodies in the presence of complement are first characterized by irreversible morphological changes of the cell surface. This is accompanied by an increase of membrane permeability, leading to the cellular release of cytoplasmic macromolecules as well as uptake of water. The cells begin to swell and, finally, disintegration may occur (Ellem, 1958). During this process the target cell is killed. In general, there are no major differences in the mode of action between antibodies of heterologous or homologous origin if their activity is specifically directed against surface antigens. The strength of cytotoxicity is determined by the concentration of both antibodies in the serum and antigenic receptors at the cell surface. An increase in the ratio of antibody to tumor cells as well as an increase in the number of reactive antigen–antibody sites at the surface increases the cytotoxic efficiency of isoantisera (Hellström and Möller, 1965). These latter findings were obtained with isoantibodies in the mouse.

As a rule, normal and malignant cells of the lymphoid system are most sensitive to antibodies. Susceptibility of mouse leukemia cells to cytotoxic isoimmune sera, as compared with sarcoma and carcinoma cells, can be ascribed to the relatively high concentration of surface antigens. In the presence of H-2 antibodies, leukemia cells are thus rapidly killed (Gorer and O'Gorman, 1956; Boyse et al., 1962). The effect can be shown by exposing the treated cells to trypan blue or eosin. Dead cells are stained and are, therefore, distinguishable from unaffected, living cells. From the proportion of stained and unstained cells after antibody–complement action, antigen and antibody can be semiquantitatively measured. It was shown by Slettenmark and Klein (1962) that this cytotoxic test is also applicable to the leukemia-specific system.

Sera from mice resistant to syngeneic Gross leukemia were cytotoxic for Gross lymphoma cells in vitro. Positive reactions were then obtained with leukemias induced by the viruses of Friend (Old et al., 1963a; Wahren, 1963), Mazurenko (Zueva, 1964), Moloney (Klein and Klein, 1964a; Old et al., 1964), Rauscher (Old et al., 1964), Rich (Rich et al., 1965), and Graffi (Pasternak, 1965). Before specification and discussion of experimental findings, some methodological details will be described for the detection and measurement of cytotoxic antibodies against specific surface antigens of leukemia cells. The method used by Slettenmark and Klein (1962) was based on the technique of Gorer and O'Gorman (1956). Lymphoma cells in doses of 5×10^5 cells per 0.05-ml. diluted or undiluted serum were incubated for 1 hour at 37°C. in the presence of 0.05 ml. undiluted guinea pig complement. Controls were lymphoma cells incubated with normal mouse sera or normal lymphoid cells incubated with immune sera. At various intervals the percentage of stained and unstained cells was determined by exposing the cells to eosin. According to the FI of the immunofluorescence technique (see Section IV), a cytotoxicity index (CI) was calculated. The percentage of unstained cells in the samples containing immune serum was subtracted from the percentage of unstained cells in the control, and the difference thus obtained was divided by the percentage of unstained cells in the normal serum controls. A CI $\geq$ 0.2 or even 0.15 was arbitrarily regarded as positive. The number of dead cells does not accurately indicate the activity of immune sera because some cells may undergo complete lysis. In the cytotoxic tests of Klein and Klein (1964a) the activity of immune sera was not evaluated unless the control sera showed more than 60% surviving cells after incubation. There are minor modifications of the test concerning cell number, serum volume, time of incubation, and staining procedure. In all experiments, however, guinea pig complement was used in excess to increase the sensitivity of the cytotoxic reaction.

Occasionally the guinea pig serum must be absorbed with mouse tumor cells before use as complement in order to remove from the serum those components that are toxic to mouse cells (Pasternak, 1965). Cytotoxic activity is also measurable by titration of immune sera. The titer is given by the serum dilution producing roughly 50% viability of cells (Old et al., 1963a). Activity is, furthermore, demonstrable by plotting the percentage of dead cells vs. serum dilution (Boyse et al., 1962). Antigens are measurable by the capacity of cells or tissue homogenates to absorb cytotoxic antibodies. The absorption effect is indicated by the decrease of CI or titer of immune serum.

B. CHROMIUM-51 TECHNIQUE

A modification of the cytotoxic test is based on $Na_2{}^{51}CrO_4$-labeled target cells releasing the isotope after antibody–complement action. This test was developed to obtain a more accurate and objective measurement of cytotoxic antibodies. Originally introduced by Goodman (1961) and applied to H-2 antigens of mice by Wigzell (1965), the chromium-51 technique was, then, also used for the measurement of Moloney antigens by Haughton (1965) and by Klein et al. (1966b). For this purpose a certain number of Moloney lymphoma cells was labeled for 30 minutes with the isotope (20 μcuries/ml. for 5×10^7 cells) at 37°C. After washing the cells in saline solution and suspending them in 5% calf serum, they were ready for the cytotoxic test. Labeled cells were incubated with diluted antiserum for 15 minutes at 37°C., the unfixed antibody was removed by centrifugation, and guinea pig complement was added to the cell pellet. After 45 minutes at 37°C., the cells were again sedimented and the supernatant was removed for estimation of liberated ^{51}Cr with a scintillation counter. Titration is possible by plotting percentage of radioactivity released vs. serum dilution. The technique is also applicable to the measurement of antigens. Previous addition of antigen-containing cells or subcellular fractions to the immune serum inhibits liberation of radioactivity from the target cells. The degree of inhibition is related to the concentration of antigens. Using this technique, high numbers of serum samples can be simultaneously investigated. Moreover, in the inhibition test, antigen-containing cells or preparations need not be removed before addition of labeled target cells.

C. FLUOROCHROMATIC TEST

Another new technique for the measurement of immunocytotoxicity, the fluorochromatic test, was developed by Celada and Rotman (1967). The first data presented included those obtained with Moloney immune sera. Target cells were imbedded in a thin layer of agarose. Small pieces of filter paper containing the immune sera were then deposited on the agar, and the plates were incubated for 60 minutes at 37°C. Complement was added and the plates were again incubated for 30 minutes. After washing, a solution of fluorescein diacetate was given to the plates. Finally the dye was poured off. Living cells accumulate fluorescein intracellularly as a result of enzymic hydroloysis of the fluorogenic substrate. Thus, cytotoxicity caused by immune serum is indicated by a dark area in the agar surrounding the filter paper if examined under blue light, whereas living cells show bright fluorescence. Agarose plates with living cells could be stored for 3 days at 4°C. without loss of viability. This technique allows simultaneous measurement of many serum samples, and minimum amounts of serum are needed. A general application of the fluorochromatic technique to leukemia-specific surface antigens, however, remains to be seen. The majority of cytotoxic tests has been performed in the usual way by evaluating the effect under the microscope.

D. SURFACE ANTIGENS DETECTED BY CYTOTOXIC TESTS

1. *Gross Antigen*

Virus-induced surface antigens of leukemia cells detectable by cytotoxic tests generally revealed the same degree of specificity as compared

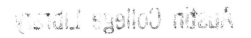

with antigens detected by immunofluorescence. Lymphomas induced by the Gross agent showed extensive cross-reactions *in vitro* when tested with immune sera derived from animals which were resistant to syngeneic, Gross leukemia grafts. For example, of 17 Gross immune sera tested, 16 were active against Gross leukemia GHA (Slettenmark and Klein, 1962). On the other hand, only 4 of 12 sera were active against lymphoma GHB. Generally, most of the immune sera tested reacted with one or more of the Gross lymphomas. Differences in the reactivity are in the first place due to differences in the concentration of antigenic receptors at the cell surface and to the different strengths of the sera. The latter factor usually depends on the immunization schedule. Gross-specific antibodies were not cytotoxic for normal lymph node cells and 6C3HED lymphoma cells, nor did these sera, obtained from C3H mice repeatedly inoculated with normal lymph node cells, 6C3HED, or LNSF*) lymphoma cells, exert any effect on Gross lymphoma cells. Specificity of cytotoxic reaction was further shown by absorption of immune sera with Gross lymphoma cells. The cells completely removed cytotoxicity.

Electron microscopically the damaging effect of immune serum on Gross lymphoma cells was shown by Jakobsson and Wahren (1965). Slightly damaged cells had a swollen outer membrane which was lacking in more heavily damaged cells. Lesions of the cell membrane were also seen in the absence of virus budding. Of course, it cannot be concluded from this fact that antibodies are specifically directed to a new cellular antigen only. Possibly viral antigens might be present in the membrane before the virion is formed.

Using the direct cytotoxic technique and absorption, specific antigens were also demonstrable in spontaneously developing AKR lymphomas (Bubeník *et al.*, 1964; Wahren, 1965, 1966a). Bubeník *et al.* (1964) immunized allogeneic hosts with spontaneous AKR leukemic tissue. After absorption with normal AKR cells the immune sera were still cytotoxic for AKR lymphoma cells *in vitro*. In the experiments of Wahren (1965, 1966a), 6 of the 10 spontaneous AKR lymphomas tested were sensitive to immune sera produced in C3H, C3H hybrids, or C57BR mice against Gross passage A virus-induced lymphomas. The other 4 also contained Gross antigens as was shown by absorption. Although AKR lymphomas were not capable of inducing antibodies in AKR mice which are naturally tolerant to the Gross antigens, they produced tumor-specific cytotoxic antibodies in allogeneic hosts. The immune sera obtained reacted with cells of syngeneic lymphomas induced by Gross passage A virus. Spontaneous AKR lymphomas and passage A virus-induced tumors of other strains are, thus, caused by the same virus. In experiments of Old *et al.* (1965), C57BL/6

---

* Spontaneous leukemia of (A $\times$ A.SW)F$_1$ origin.

immune sera against AKR leukemia were cytotoxic for Gross virus-induced C57BL/6 leukemias. The G antigen which is detected by these sera, was present in spontaneous leukemias of the AKR, AKR.K, C58, and F strains, too.

2. *Friend, Moloney, Rauscher Antigens*

Formation of cytotoxic antibody against Friend leukemia was shown by Old *et al.* (1963a) and Wahren (1963). Immune sera were obtained from mice belonging to both resistant and susceptible strains. In the experiments of Old *et al.* (1963a), immunization was achieved by injection of histoincompatible Friend leukemia tissue. The sera reacted with syngeneic Friend leukemia cells but not with normal spleen cells, spontaneous lymphatic A strain leukemias, or leukemias induced by X-rays. Reaction was also negative with one leukemia induced by passage A Gross virus and with a chemically induced leukemia. However, Friend-specific immune sera were cytotoxic for syngeneic spleen cells prepared from mice that had been infected with Rauscher virus. This cross-reactivity corresponds well with results of immunofluorescence tests. By using the cytotoxic technique, Old *et al.* (1964) were able to show that leukemias induced by Friend, Moloney, and Rauscher viruses share related antigens. Cells of different leukemias were tested for their sensitivity to cytotoxic antibodies and for their absorption capacity. In the direct cytotoxic test, cross-reactions were found with Moloney and Rauscher immune sera. The sera were usually more active against cells of the leukemia used for immunization. Sensitivity of individual leukemias to cytotoxic antibodies ranged from complete sensitivity to resistance. Furthermore, a Rauscher typing serum was found to be cytotoxic to Friend leukemia cells. Antigenic relationship among these leukemias was confirmed by absorptions. Adequate absorption of Friend, Moloney, and Rauscher immune sera with any other leukemia of these types produced complete elimination of cytotoxic antibodies. There was a parallelism between absorption capacity of a leukemia and its sensitivity to cytotoxic antibodies. Because of the antigenic similarity the designation "FMR antigen(s)" was proposed for this cross-reacting system. Gross leukemias did not contain FMR antigenic specificities as was shown by direct cytotoxic tests and by absorptions. Most interesting in this context are the findings of Rich *et al.* (1965). They compared the FMR and Gross antigens, on the one hand, with the antigens of Rich leukemia, on the other. Direct cytotoxic and absorption tests showed cross-reactions with both FMR and Gross antigens, i.e., Rich immune sera did not only react with Rich cells but also with Friend, Moloney, Rauscher, and Gross cells. Thus, the Rich leukemia may be placed antigenically between the two distinct FMR and G groups.

Absence of cross-reactions between Friend and Gross leukemia was also shown by Wahren (1963). Gross-specific immune sera known to be cytotoxic for Gross lymphoma cells did not react with Friend leukemia cells. Likewise, no cytotoxic effect was observed when Gross lymphoma cells were tested with Friend immune sera. In these studies of Wahren (1963), specificity of cytotoxic antibodies to Friend virus-induced antigens was demonstrated by the direct cytotoxic test and by absorption of antibodies with Friend leukemia cells *in vivo* and *in vitro*. The *in vivo* absorption was done by inoculating the immune serum intravenously into tumor-bearing hosts. One hour after injection, blood was taken and the serum was tested for cytotoxic activity. There was a complete absorption of antibodies. On the other hand, cytotoxic activity of immune serum inoculated into normal animals did not decrease significantly. Friend immune sera did not react with normal spleen or lymph node cells and cells of other leukemias not known to be of viral origin.

Cytotoxic reactions of antibodies to the Moloney leukemia have been investigated by Klein and Klein (1964a). Most of the lymphomas tested were sensitive to the cytotoxic action of Moloney hyperimmune sera. Antibodies detectable by cytotoxic tests appeared later in the serum as compared with those detectable by immunofluorescence. Antibodies cross-reacted with other Moloney lymphomas. One lymphoma resistant to cytotoxic antibodies contained surface antigens as demonstrated by the immunofluorescence test. Cytotoxic activity of immune sera could be removed by absorption with Moloney leukemia cells. The cytotoxic test, however, did not reveal the same degree of specificity as the immunofluorescence test. Some Moloney hyperimmune sera gave positive reactions with Gross lymphomas and with lymphomas such as EL 4 and 6C3HED, while others were not affected. Activity against non-Moloney cells could be removed by all sensitive cells but not normal lymph node cells. On the other hand, sensitive non-Moloney cells did not completely absorb activity against Moloney cells. The conclusion was drawn that hyperimmune Moloney sera may contain antibodies against at least two different antigenic specificities one of them only present in sensitive non-Moloney cells.

3. *Measurement of Moloney Antigen*

In the Moloney leukemia system, cytotoxicity of antibodies was also measured by the chromium-51 technique (Haughton, 1965; Klein *et al.*, 1966b). By using a standard immune serum the latter authors compared 10 different lymphomas. As indicated by the liberation of ^{51}Cr from the target cells in the presence of antibodies and complement, lymphomas of different sensitivity to cytotoxic antibodies could be distinguished. The lymphomas ranged from highly sensitive to moderately sensitive and resistant tumors.

By inhibition of cytotoxic antibody, tumor-specific antigen was quantitatively measured. Immune serum was diluted to a concentration that liberated about 25% of total radioactivity from the target cells. This immune serum was incubated with various numbers of cells to be measured for Moloney antigen. After that the labeled target cells were added to measure residual antibodies. The number of cells that caused 50% inhibition of cytotoxicity was used as a measure of the amount of Moloney antigen per cell, i.e., the amount of antigen per cell was expressed as the reciprocal of the cell number causing 50% inhibition.

In other experiments the amount of antigen was measured taking into consideration cell size which differs among the lymphomas tested. This included cell size measurements by means of a Coulter counter and establishment of "antigen units." When calculated from an arbitrary value of 10 of a certain lymphoma, the units of antigen per tumor cell ranged from 2 to 25 for the different lymphomas. By using as a basis the units of antigen per tumor cell, it was possible to calculate units of antigens per unit surface area.

This method confirmed that lymphomas with a high concentration of surface antigen were also highly susceptible to cytotoxic antibodies; tumors with a low concentration were resistant. Particularly cells of lymphomas growing as generalized leukemias were found to have a high concentration of antigens as compared to cells of leukemias growing as ascites. The lowest concentration was found in two generalized primary lymphomas having latency periods of over 500 days.

4. *Mazurenko and Graffi Antigen*

Cytotoxicity specifically directed to Mazurenko leukemia cells was first described by Zueva (1964), and for the Graffi leukemia system, cytotoxic antibodies were shown by Pasternak (1965). In the latter system differences could also be shown with regard to sensitivity of leukemia cells to cytotoxic antibodies. Out of 3 Graffi leukemias used as targets, 1 was most sensitive, another moderately sensitive, and the third one was relatively resistant. Resistant cells, however, were capable of absorbing specific antibodies from immune sera. The sera did not react with normal cells or with Gross leukemia cells.

E. COMPARISON OF IMMUNOFLUORESCENCE AND CYTOTOXIC TESTS

Special attention was drawn to the comparison of immunofluorescence and cytotoxic reactions. It is not known whether they measure the same or different antigens, i.e., viral and new cellular antigens. There are several facts, however, indicating that both techniques are detecting the same antigenic specificities. In our experiments with more than fifty different immune sera, we did not observe any positive cytotoxic reaction in the absence of a positive immunofluorescence reaction. Using sensitive target cells, a strong fluorescence reaction was always paralleled by a strong cytotoxic reaction. Weak sera could only be detected by the fluorescence test. However, this effect of weak sera could also be produced artificially by diluting strong cytotoxic immune sera to that point where antibodies did not exert any cytotoxic effect on the cells but were still demonstrable at the cell surface by immunofluorescence. The only difference between the two techniques, therefore, appears to be their sensitivity to the detection of virus-induced surface antigens, i.e., the difference is quantitative rather than qualitative. This does not rule out that two different antigens are present at the cell surface. Provided that leukemia cells contain viral and new cellular antigens, cytotoxicity might be obtained if one of the two or both antigens are present in high enough concentration. All tests hitherto performed in this way do not allow a differentiation of the tumor-specific virus-induced surface antigens.

F. ANTIGENIC RELATIONSHIP AMONG LEUKEMIAS INDUCED BY DIFFERENT VIRUSES

Considering the antigenic relationship of different types of leukemia as measured by immunocytotoxicity, there are at least two distinct groups, the FMR and G antigenic groups. In other words, there are leukemia viruses coding for distinct tumor-specific surface antigens. Hence, distinct leukemia viruses do exist. On the other hand, Rich virus-induced antigens appear to be cross-reactive with both antigenic groups. However, the few data published up to now are still inconclusive. It is conceivable that leukemia cells can be naturally superinfected with an unrelated leukemia virus and acquire the antigens characteristic of the superinfecting agent (see Section IX).

Three of the leukemias tested by cytotoxicity were found to share common antigens. From these data the viruses of Friend, Moloney, and Rauscher might be considered identical. Identity, however, could only be postulated for that portion of the viral genome coding for the specific surface antigen.

Detection of common antigenicity does not necessarily indicate complete identity of antigens. Although cross-reactions were regularly obtained by cytotoxic tests the cells of Mazurenko and Friend leukemias contained also antigens specific for each type of leukemia (Zueva, 1967). After *in vitro* absorption of Mazurenko immune sera with Friend leukemia cells, there were still antibodies in the sera reacting with Mazurenko cells but not with Friend cells. On the other hand, Mazurenko cells removed from Friend immune sera those antibodies that reacted with Mazurenko cells.

Activity against Friend cells remained in the sera. These data are suggestive for the presence of two types of antigens in Friend and Mazurenko cells—one common to both and one specific to each of the leukemias. Direct cytotoxic and absorption tests indicated that Graffi and Mazurenko leukemias are antigenically different.

It would be most important to know whether cross-reacting leukemias, such as Friend, Moloney, Rauscher, and Rich leukemias, also contain distinct antigenic specificities. As has already been discussed by Zueva (1967), the possibility could not be completely ruled out that her data obtained by absorption experiments reflect quantitative rather than qualitative differences, although the weaker cytotoxic effect of immune sera to cells of the cross-reacting type of leukemia would also speak against this assumption. Quantitative absorptions are needed to get more information on the relationship among virus-induced leukemias. However, supposing that immunologically distinct viral and new cellular antigens may occur in different concentrations at the cell surface the problem can hardly be solved without being able to measure these antigens independently of each other. According to Geering et al. (1966) the G antigenic system appears to be a complex group of distinct antigens. This was shown with sera from rats resistant to syngeneic grafts of Gross virus-induced rat leukemia. The animals had been further treated by up to twelve intraperitoneal inoculations of 8×10^6 to 300×10^6 viable leukemia cells. Immune sera were cytotoxic to both Gross rat leukemias and mouse leukemic and nonleukemic cells containing the G antigen. However, there were several, presumably Gross virus-induced, mouse leukemias negative for G antigen in the mouse test system but positive with rat serum, as demonstrated by absorption of cytotoxic activity. Apparently these cells lack a determinant that can only be detected in the mouse system. Thus, at least two antigenic specificities are present in Gross virus-induced leukemia. The component detectable in the mouse system was designated as G(a), and the component of the rat system G(b). Concerning the nature of these antigens the authors discussed that they may represent viral coat proteins that are incorporated in the cell membrane.

To sum up, the virus-induced surface antigens of leukemia cells can be detected by cytotoxic reactions of immune sera in the presence of complement. Cytotoxic immune sera are obtainable from mice specifically resistant to cell inocula of virus-induced leukemia. Leukemia cells differ in their sensitivity to cytotoxic antibodies. There are cells completely resistant to the antibody–complement action. Antigens of these cells, however, are detectable by their capacity to absorb cytotoxic activity from immune sera. Leukemias induced by different viruses, such as Friend, Moloney, and Rauscher, show extensive cross-reactions. Gross leukemia of mice apparently occupies an exceptional position in that cross-reactions with most of the other leukemias are lacking. Summarized data of direct cytotoxic and absorption tests with mouse immune sera are presented in Table V. Immune sera from rats resistant to syngeneic Gross rat leukemia are cytotoxic to cells of both rat and mouse leukemias having the Gross antigen. Certain data indicate that the cytotoxic test may detect distinct antigenic components at the cell surface of leukemias induced by the same virus.

VI. Virus-Induced Surface Antigens in Nonleukemic Cells of the Hematopoietic System

By means of transplantation tests *in vivo* and immunofluorescence, cytotoxicity, and absorptions *in vitro*, specific surface antigens have been first demonstrated in leukemic cells. To understand the significance of these antigens in viral leukemogenesis, it is most important to know whether they are restricted to leukemia cells only or might be present in nonleukemic cells, also. In the true sense the term "nonleukemic" includes all cells other than leukemia cells. The data presented in the following, however, shall be limited to those nonleukemic cells belonging to the hematopoietic system. After virus infection the cells of spleen, lymph nodes, thymus, or bone marrow are the targets that are potentially susceptible of being transformed to leukemia cells. Although formation of the first leukemia cell is by no means detectable and might appear early after infection, there is certainly a period, the preleukemic stage, where the animal is still free from leukemic cells. Considering our *in vivo* cloning experiments using Gross (G. Pasternak and Pasternak, 1968) and Graffi (Pasternak and Pasternak, unpublished data) leukemia cells, it takes less than 35 days in tolerant baby mice until leukemia is evident after transplantation of a single leukemia cell. Leukemias with long latency periods, such as Gross, Graffi, and Moloney leukemias, hardly arise within this short time. Usually they develop after latencies of several months so that at least early after infection the cells of the hematopoietic system are still nonmalignant. Otherwise leukemia would have developed within a few weeks. Demonstration of virus-induced antigens in these "preleukemic" cells would indicate that antigen induction is not connected with neoplastic transformation.

The situation is more obscure with leukemias having short latencies. For example in the case of Friend and Rauscher leukemias, malignant transformation of cells probably occurs early after virus infection since manifestation of the disease is evident within a few days or weeks. The difference between leukemias having long and short latency periods cannot be explained by different doses of virus or by the hypothesis that the former develop from a few transformed cells only, whereas the latter arise multi-

TABLE V

SUMMARIZED DATA OF DIRECT CYTOTOXIC AND ABSORPTION TESTS WITH MOUSE IMMUNE SERA

Immune sera against leukemia of	Cells used for the cytotoxic test								
	Gross	Friend	Moloney	Rauscher	Mazurenko	Graffi	Rich	6C3HED	Norman spleen or lymph node cells
Gross	+	−	−	−			+	−	−
Friend	−	+++	+++	+++	+		+++		−
Moloney	±	++	++	++			+++		−
Rauscher	−	+	+	+			+		−
Mazurenko					+	−			−
Graffi						+			−
Rich	+	+	+	+			+		−

centrically from large cell numbers. In any case, the preleukemic stage, defined as the period between virus infection and formation of leukemia cells, appears to be very short in the Friend and Rauscher systems. Therefore it is nearly impossible to decide whether target cells infected with these viruses are transformed or are still nonmalignant.

In general, animals infected with Gross, Graffi, or Moloney viruses as adults do not develop leukemia because they are capable of reacting immunologically against virus and virus-induced antigens. Formation of virus-induced antigens in these animals is indicated by the presence of antibodies against surface antigens of leukemia cells. There are obviously cells in the body which behave immunologically like leukemia cells, although they cannot be detected by histological methods or by transplantation. However, it is not known whether the cells are really leukemia cells developing in the course of viral infection and are then eliminated by immunological attack. The alternative is that certain nonmalignant cells like leukemia cells are also capable of expressing virus-induced surface antigens. Then the fate of these cells might not differ from that of leukemia cells. By all means, search for antigens in resistant animals appears to be most interesting.

A. GRAFFI ANTIGEN

Since virus-induced surface antigens of nonleukemic cells cannot be detected by transplantation methods, the *in vitro* techniques, such as immunofluorescence and cytotoxicity, have to be applied to the measurement of antigens. In most cases, however, the more sensitive absorption test has been used. For example, the direct immunofluorescence test failed to demonstrate Graffi virus-induced surface antigens in spleen and lymph node cells of 3-month-old animals infected with virus as newborns. By absorption, however, we were able to show that spleen cells of 14-day-old infected animals already contained high amounts of virus-induced surface antigens. One single absorption of a Graffi immune serum sample with about 60 million living spleen cells totally removed antibody activity against leukemia cells (Pasternak, 1969). Absorption capacity of spleen cells corresponded well with that of leukemia cells. In contrast, thymus, liver, and brain did not contain measurable amounts of antigens although at this time the virus titer in these organs was not much different from the titer in spleen. In other words, despite the fact that virus is present in about the same quantity, spleen does contain virus-induced surface antigens whereas other organs do not. Even 100 days after infection of newborn mice, these organs appeared to be free from virus-induced surface antigens. In previous studies of Fey and Graffi (1958) the spleen was shown to play an important role in the leukemogenesis of myeloid leukemia. Splenectomy of infected animals early in the postnatal period prevented the development of myeloid leukemia. Thus, spleen cells appear to be the targets susceptible to be transformed by Graffi virus. The early appearance of virus-induced surface antigens in spleen cells supports the hypothesis that spleen is important to myeloid leukemogenesis. Absorption experiments with lymph node cells were not successful since the absorbed sera were nonspecifically toxic to leukemia cells.

As measured by absorption, virus-induced surface antigens were lacking in spleen cells of animals infected as adults, whereas virus was found in spleen, thymus, lymph nodes, and bone marrow (Micheel and Pasternak, 1968a). Data of the experiments are listed in Table VI.

Virus-induced antigens were apparently absent in cells of spleen, lymph nodes, and thymus from young adult rats infected with Graffi virus as newborns (Micheel and Pasternak, 1968a). The cells did not remove the antibodies from Graffi, mouse, immune sera reacting with mouse leukemia cells in the immunofluorescence test. On the other hand, Graffi virus was demonstrable in spleen and liver of infected animals. It should be men-

TABLE VI

RESULTS OF ABSORPTION EXPERIMENTS FOR THE DEMONSTRATION OF GRAFFI
VIRUS-INDUCED ANTIGENS IN DIFFERENT CELLS OF INFECTED ANIMALS

Cells used for absorption	No. of tests[a]	Decrease of FI[b] after absorption		Presence of virus
		>50%	<50%	
Leukemia (positive control)	12	12	0	+
Normal[c] (negative control)	13	0	13	−
Spleen	2	2	0	+
Lymph nodes of animals	3	e	e	+
Thymus infected as (100)[d]	1	0	1	+
Liver newborns	2	0	2	+
Brain	2	0	2	+
Spleen of animals infected as newborns	3 (45)[d]	3	0	+
	1 (36)[d]	1	0	+
	3 (14)[d]	3	0	+
Spleen of animals infected as adults	5	0	5	+

[a] Before and after absorption of the Graffi immune serum pool, leukemia cells L 414/2a were used as targets.

[b] Fluorescent index (see Section IV).

[c] Spleen, thymus, liver, or brain cells.

[d] Number of days after inoculation of Graffi virus-containing homogenate.

[e] Absorbed serum is toxic to leukemia cells.

tioned in this context that cells of rat leukemias induced by Graffi virus contain certain virus-induced surface antigens, as was shown by immuno-fluorescence tests with Graffi, mouse, hyperimmune sera (Micheel and Pasternak, unpublished data).

B. Gross Antigen

The distribution of Gross virus-induced antigens of lymphoid cells among low- and high-incidence strains has been thoroughly investigated by Old et al. (1965). Using a number of separately prepared immune sera, of C57BL/6 origin, against a transplanted AKR leukemia, a variety of normal and leukemic tissues of many mouse strains were tested for the presence of G antigen by means of absorption. Specificity of immune sera for G antigen had been shown previously by their direct cytotoxic action on Gross virus-induced C57BL/6 leukemias and by elimination of the activity after absorption with leukemias induced by passage A Gross virus as well as after absorption with spontaneous leukemias of the AKR and C58 strains.

Gross antigen was found in normal spleens of young adult mice with a high incidence of spontaneous leukemia. These included the AKR, AKR.K, C58, PL, and F strains. The antigen was not demonstrable in spleen cells of fourteen low-incidence strains, although certain spontaneous and induced leukemias of these strains were positive for G antigen. Absence of Gross antigen or reduction of its quantity was shown for hybrids from certain crosses between AKR or C58, on the one hand, and C57BL/6 or C3Hf/Bi, on the other. Data are summarized in Table VII. With regard to the tissue distribution of Gross antigen in AKR and C58 mice, it was found that spleen, lymph nodes, bone marrow, and liver from 2-month-old animals contain approximately equal amounts of G antigen. The concentration of antigen appeared to be lower in thymus and some other organs such as kidney and brain as well as erythrocytes were negative. Gross antigen was also demonstrable in cells of spleen and thymus from 34-day-old animals which had been infected as newborns.

Studying the Gross virus-induced antigens, Wahren (1966a,b) was also able to show that lymphoid cells of 2 to 9 months old, AKR mice contain the Gross antigen. Whereas direct cytotoxic tests were unsuccessful the antigens were demonstrable by absorption. By means of quantitative absorption with graded cell doses, evidence was obtained that antigen concentration is considerably lower in lymph node cells of healthy AKR mice which have not yet developed primary lymphoma than in lymphoma cells. Small doses of lymphoid cells had only little or even no absorption effect, whereas larger cell doses caused a clear absorption of Gross-specific

TABLE VII

Occurrence of G Antigen in Normal Spleen from
Young Adult Mice of Various Strains[a]

Gross antigen +	Gross antigen −
C58	C3Hf/Bi
AKR	C57BL/6
PL	C57L
F	C57BR/cd
AKR.K	RF/J
	SJL/J
	Swiss Ha/ICR
	DBA1
	DBA2
	CE
	MA
	R III
	CBA
	A
	BALB/c
(C58 × C3Hf/Bi)F₁	(C58 × C57BL/6)F₁
	(AKR × C57BL/6)F₁

[a] According to Old *et al.* (1965).

antibodies. Lymphoid cells from mouse strains with a low incidence of leukemia did not produce any absorption effect.

As discussed by Wahren (1966b) the absorption properties of AKR lymph node cells are either due to a small number of cells with high antigen content, present in an otherwise normal cell population, or to all lymphoid cells possessing the antigen in a low concentration only. A distinction between these two alternatives on a quantitative basis, however, seems to be impossible at present. Transplantation assays indicated that the fraction of malignant cells did not exceed 0.5% in the "preleukemic" cell populations and was probably not more than 0.05%. Calculations based on the fact that 10^3–10^4 primary AKR lymphoma cells cause tumor growth, whereas absence of tumor growth was observed when 2×10^6 "preleukemic" cells had been inoculated. Therefore, the conclusion was drawn that the cell suspension used for absorption could have contained 0.05–0.5% of strongly antigenic leukemia cells. On the other hand, strongly antigenic cells do not necessarily have to be malignant. In any case, since the direct cytotoxic test permits detection of sensitive cells only if they are present in concentrations higher than 5–10%, the proportion of strongly antigenic cells in preleukemic cell populations must have been lower than 5%.

Gross antigen was also found in infected animals that do not develop leukemia. This was shown with lymph node cells from animals infected with Gross virus at birth and thymectomized 2 months later. Such animals remain free from leukemia although virus is demonstrable in different organs. Thus, the absorption capacity of lymph node cells from thymectomized animals indicates that the Gross antigen is present in non-leukemic cells.

In the Friend leukemia system, sensitivity of spleen cells to cytotoxic antibodies increased during 15 to 20 days after infection. The maximum was reached around the twentieth day. Before the tenth day, sensitivity could not be detected (Wahren, 1963). However, the experiments have not been compared with absorptions so that Friend virus-induced antigens possibly present at an earlier time could not be shown.

In summary, absorption experiments indicate that lymphoid cells from mice in the preleukemic stage contain virus-induced surface antigens. Lymphoid cells remove those antibodies from mouse immune sera reacting with leukemia cells in the immunofluorescence or cytotoxic tests. Antigen-containing cells are supposed to be nonmalignant. The early appearance of antigens a short time after infection and their presence in lymphoid cells of thymectomized animals which do not develop leukemia speak in favor of this hypothesis. Apparently, the presence of virus-induced antigens at the surface does not necessarily render the cells neoplastic.

Antigens were not detectable in spleen cells of animals infected as adults although their presence, at least temporarily, is indicated by the fact that the mice had produced antibodies against them. Obviously, antigen-containing cells are eliminated by the immunologically competent host. The nature of the virus-induced antigens, viral vs. new cellular antigens, cannot be decided on the basis of the results presented.

VII. Virus and Viral Antigens in Infected Cells

A. TITRATION OF INFECTIVITY

In contrast to tumors induced in different animal species by the DNA-containing viruses as well as to Rous virus-induced mammalian tumors, primary and transplanted mouse leukemias of viral origin are continuously producing virus. Viral components are probably synthesized in the cytoplasm of infected cells and the particles forming at membranes of the endoplasmic reticulum are released by a budding process into intracellular vacuoles or into the extracellular space. Synthesis of infectious virus is not restricted to leukemia cells only but may also occur in cells of different histologic origin. This could be shown mainly by electron-microscopic and tissue culture studies.

Methods for the detection of virus and viral antigens are not only important for the quantitative virus determination but also for the elucidation of certain virus–cell and virus–host interactions. Measurement of mouse leukemia viruses proved to be impossible by direct methods since the agents did not reveal agglutinating, cytopathic, or transforming properties *in vitro*. Therefore, quantitation is based on indirect methods such as titration of leukemogenic activity of virus-containing preparations or measurement of certain immunological events induced by the virus. Because titration of leukemogenic activity is not directly related to immunological problems the techniques will be described only briefly. After inoculating groups of susceptible mice with equal volumes of serially diluted virus-containing preparations, the resulting leukemias are recorded, and from this the effective dose can be estimated which produces leukemia in 50% of the mice (ED_{50}). Results obtained at different times can be compared by taking as a basis that result obtained with a standard preparation. For details of virus titration and statistical analysis, reference is given to Bryan (1957) and Dougherty (1964). In the case of leukemias having long latency periods, estimation of ED_{50} takes a long time, usually more than 10 or 12 months. The time required for virus quantitation is considerably reduced when testing leukemia viruses that produce the disease after latencies of a few weeks only. Friend and Rauscher leukemias which belong to the latter type are further characterized by splenomegaly. Enlargement of spleen is detectable and measurable by palpation (Rauscher, 1962; Zeigel and Rauscher, 1964). Spleen weight increases with virus dose and time after infection so that it may serve as a quantitative criterion of virus infection (Rowe and Brodsky, 1959; Fieldsteel *et al.*, 1961). Finally, another quantitative test was elaborated—the spleen colony assay (Pluznik and Sachs, 1964). The method is based upon focal proliferation of spleen cells after intravenous injection of adult mice with Rauscher virus preparations. Colonies can be detected macroscopically at 6 to 8 days after inoculation. There is a linear relationship between virus concentration and number of colonies. At the same time, Axelrad and Steeves (1964) developed independently the spleen focus assay for the Friend leukemia virus. However, with regard to focus formation, Gross passage A, Graffi, and Moloney viruses, are ineffective.

B. NEUTRALIZATION

Leukemia viruses are immunologically detectable by neutralizing antibodies producing inhibition of leukemogenic activity. Antigenicity of a leukemia virus in heterologous species was first shown by Graffi and Fey (1955) and Graffi *et al.* (1957) for the myeloid leukemia virus. Immune sera obtained by injection of rabbits with virus-containing cell-free filtrates completely inhibited leukemogenic activity of such filtrates when the mixture was incubated *in vitro* before inoculation into newborn mice.

Rabbit sera against normal mouse tissues did not reveal any neutralizing activity.

Neutralization by rabbit immune sera was also shown by Friend (1959) for the virus that she had isolated from the Ehrlich carcinoma. Moreover, the agent was antigenically active in mice. Sera derived from animals that had survived the original injection with cell-free filtrates were found to neutralize infectivity. At the same time neutralizing antibodies against Gross passage A virus were induced in rabbits and guinea pigs (Gross, 1961).

Antigenicity in heterologous and/or homologous species was then demonstrated for the Moloney (Moloney, 1962), Rauscher (Fink and Malmgren, 1963; Fink and Rauscher, 1964), and Rich leukemia viruses (Rich, 1966). However, attempts to produce neutralizing antibodies against Gross virus in mice have been unsuccessful (Wahren, 1964). Although the mouse immune sera tested were strongly cytotoxic for Gross lymphoma cells *in vitro*, they did not inhibit leukemogenic activity of a virus-containing homogenate. Obviously the antibodies present in the sera are not directed against antigens which participate in the neutralization reaction. In general, those mouse immune sera reacting in the cytotoxic and immunofluorescence tests with virus-induced surface antigens of leukemia cells also possess virus-neutralizing properties. This has been shown for the Friend, Moloney, and Graffi leukemia systems (Wahren, 1963; Klein and Klein, 1964b; Pasternak, 1965). The sera used in these experiments were from mice which had been pretreated with materials containing active virus. However, neutralizing antibodies can also be obtained from animals immunized with formalinized virus preparations. Quantitation of viruses by neutralization with immune sera is quite possible, but the method is not frequently used because of its relative inaccuracy.

Most difficult with regard to interpretation are results of cross-neutralization experiments designed to compare the antigenic specificities of leukemia viruses. Quantitative differences in neutralization do not necessarily indicate that two viruses are antigenically different, particularly, if data such as virus dose and antibody titer are unknown. Many results of cross-experiments published in the past must be considered most critically since the tests could not be sufficiently controlled by quantitative criteria.

Exact comparison by neutralization is best possible by studying the neutralization kinetics. Using this experimental arrangement, Steeves and Axelrad (1967) thoroughly investigated the antigenic relationships between Friend and Rauscher viruses. Neutralization was measured by the spleen colony method, i.e., inhibition of focus-producing potency of virus preparations was taken as evidence of antibody activity. Thus, Steeves and Axelrad (1967) were able to show that the antigenic sites on the two viruses which participate in the neutralization reaction are identical. The cross-reactions resemble those obtained by the immunofluorescence and cytotoxic tests. Namely Friend, Moloney, and Rauscher leukemia cells have been found to share common virus-induced surface antigens (see Section V). This does not necessarily mean that the antigenic specificities present in the virus and in the membrane of leukemia cells are the same.

Inhibition of focus-producing potency of Rauscher virus by immune sera was also used by Sinkovics *et al.* (1967) for the immunological characterization of virus sublines. It was found that higher dilutions of a mouse immune serum against photodynamically inactivated, stock preparation of the virus inhibited about 90% of the focus-producing potency of both stock and control virus preparations from untreated leukemic mice. The same serum dilutions failed to inhibit Rauscher virus preparations obtained from leukemias that recurred after irradiation treatment and adoptive immunization. Apparently sublines of virus developing from recurrent leukemia display a certain degree of resistance to neutralizing antibodies. Decreased sensitivity to antibodies is supposed to be related to changes in the capsid of infectious particles. However, explanations other than those of antigenic changes have not been ruled out by the authors.

The action of antiviral antibodies can be made visible by electronmicroscopic techniques. Like other viruses, such as erythroblastic, polio, vaccinia, and influenza viruses, the leukemia viruses are agglutinated by immune sera derived from heterologous or homologous species (Mayyasi *et al.*, 1965, 1966). A precondition of the test is that plasma or tissue culture virus must be available in sufficient quantity. The test is applicable to the titration of the agglutinating capacity of immune sera as well as to the immunological comparison of leukemia viruses. By this way a common antigenic component was detected in the Friend, Moloney, and Rauscher viruses.

C. Mouse Antibody Production Test

A relatively precise immunological test for leukemia viruses is the MAP test. Inoculation of virus-containing materials into adult mice induces formation of antibodies reacting with leukemia cells in the cytotoxic or indirect fluorescent antibody tests (Klein and Klein, 1964b; Stück *et al.*, 1964a; Pasternak, 1966). It was found that the latency of antibody appearance is inversely related to the virus dose. In the experiments of Klein and Klein (1964b) and Klein *et al.* (1966b), several materials containing Moloney virus were assayed for antibody formation in adult animals. Antibodies were measured by the indirect immunofluorescence test since the cytotoxic test appeared to be less sensitive. After one single inoculation of adult mice with equal doses of irradiated cells prepared from different lymphomas, antibodies were detected after latency periods varying between

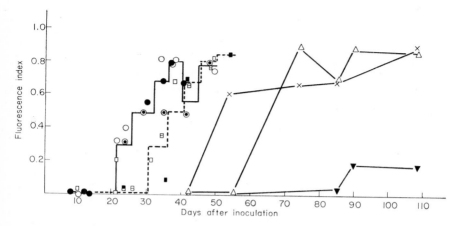

Fig. 1. Antibody response of (C3H × C57BL)F₁ mice after the inoculation of virus-containing homogenate, as detected by immunofluorescence. Symbols: circles, 10^{-1}; rectangles, 10^{-2}; crosses, 10^{-3}; empty triangles, 10^{-4}; filled triangles, 10^{-5}. Shadings within symbols represent different experiments. (From Klein and Klein, 1964b.)

20 and 40 days. The time interval between inoculation and antibody appearance was characteristic of each lymphoma. When varying numbers of lymphoma cells were injected, the length of the latency period and the number of irradiated cells inoculated were inversely related. Then, virus-containing homogenates were inoculated in serial ten-fold dilutions. Doses of 0.1 ml. of 1:10 diluted virus produced antibodies after a latency of 3 weeks. A ten-fold further dilution delayed the response by approximately 10 days. In Fig. 1 the antibody response of (C3H × C57BL)F₁ mice is shown after inoculation of virus-containing homogenates. As measured by the fluorescence index, high antibody levels persisted during the observation period of several months. The regularity and persistence of antibody development, even after inoculation of highly diluted homogenate, is evidence that virus which multiplies in the host cells might be directly or indirectly responsible for antibody formation against leukemia cells. Hydroxylamine, which is known to inactivate virus, prevented antibody formation as well as mouse immune sera admixed *in vitro* with the virus-containing homogenates (MAP neutralization).

Summarizing the experiments with Moloney lymphomas, all tumors tested were found to release virus although the amount of virus varied considerably as indicated by variations in the latency of antibody appearance.

The same technique was used for the detection and measurement of Graffi leukemia virus in leukemic and nonleukemic tissues of mice (Pasternak and Pasternak, 1967). Like the Moloney system, primary and

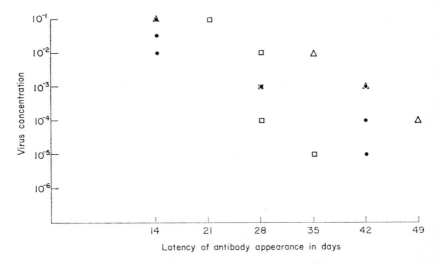

FIG. 2. Relationship between virus concentration and latency of antibody appearance as measured by the mouse antibody production test. Fluorescence indexes $\geqq$ 0.5 were arbitrarily taken as positive. Cell-free filtrates per animal: 0.3 ml. (circles); 0.1 ml. (squares and triangles).

transplanted Graffi leukemias were shown to release virus. Cell-free leukemia filtrates as well as viable and X-irradiated cells were tested for virus. Virus-containing cell-free filtrates were titrated in adult XVII mice. As expressed by the fluorescence index, already 14 days after inoculation, antibodies reacting with L 414/2a Graffi target cells were detected in the sera of animals which had received the more concentrated filtrates (10^{-2} and 10^{-3} dilutions). The highest dilution inducing antibodies was 10^{-5}. Results obtained with three different filtrates prepared from primary leukemias are presented in Fig. 2. In one case the titer was 10^{-4} only. Comparison of immunogenicity between viable and X-irradiated cells of the L 414/2a Graffi leukemia is shown in Fig. 3. Irrespective of the presence or absence of growing tumor grafts, antibodies appeared at all doses of viable leukemia cells inoculated. As little as one hundred viable cells were sufficient to produce antibodies after a latency period of 28 days. When using irradiated cells, a 10^6-fold increase in cell number was required to attain a comparable antibody response. From this the conclusion can be drawn that titration of viable cells is a more sensitive test for virus detection. Obviously proliferation of leukemia cells for a certain period following inoculation is an optimal condition for virus multiplication. In this case high amounts of virus are formed in the donor's target cells which are rapidly multiplying in the host. After inoculation of X-ray killed cells, however,

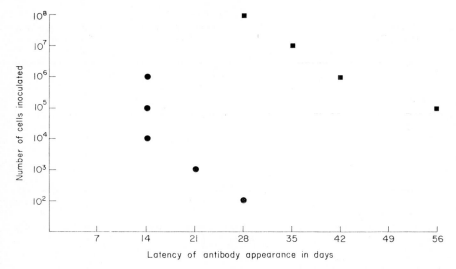

Fig. 3. Relationship between cell dose and latency of antibody appearance as measured by the mouse antibody production test. Comparison of immunogenicity between viable and X-irradiated Graffi leukemia cells. Fluorescence indexes > 0.3 were arbitrarily taken as positive. Symbols: circles—viable Graffi leukemia cells (leukemia L414/2a); squares—X-irradiated Graffi leukemia cells (leukemia L414/2a).

virus has to reach new host target cells. Disregarding the resulting temporal delay in virus multiplication, many particles are certainly inactivated in this way. It should be mentioned that certain rapidly growing leukemias are not suitable to the MAP test with viable cells. The animals are killed before antibodies can develop.

The MAP test was further used to investigate the distribution of the Graffi virus in different organs at certain intervals after newborn mice were infected. For this purpose, groups of animals inoculated with virus-containing cell-free filtrates were killed at 1, 3, 5, 14, and 21 days and homogenates were prepared from their brain, liver, lymph nodes, spleen, and thymus. The homogenates were then used for the MAP test. Summarized data of the experiments are shown in Table VIII. It was found that Graffi virus was already detectable in liver, spleen, and brain 1 day after infection of newborns. Homogenates from lymph nodes and thymus prepared from the same animals did not contain measurable amounts of virus, i.e., they could not elicit antibody formation. Obviously the Graffi virus leaving the site of injection at first settles specifically and multiplies in cells of spleen and liver. Then, secondarily, virus spreads from these organs via the vascular system and infects all other tissues and organs. Spreading occurs very rapidly. Three and 5 days after infection, virus was detected

TABLE VIII

DEMONSTRATION OF GRAFFI VIRUS AS MEASURED BY THE MOUSE ANTIBODY
PRODUCTION TEST IN DIFFERENT ORGANS DERIVED AT CERTAIN INTERVALS
FOLLOWING INFECTION OF NEWBORN XVII MICE

	Latency of antibody appearance[b] in days				
Days[a]	14	21	28	35	42
1	—	LS	—	—	B
3	N	S	BL	T	—
5	—	ST	LN	B	—
14	LNST	—	B	—	—
21	LNST	—	B	—	—

[a] Time interval between infection of newborn mice and preparation of organ homogenates.

[b] Fluorescence indexes $\geqq 0.3$ were arbitrarily taken as positive. B = brain, L = liver, N = lymph nodes, S = spleen, T = thymus.

in all organs tested, although, if the delay of antibody appearance were taken as a measure, some quantitative differences might be observed. The final concentration of virus in the organs was reached 14 days after infection. As measured by the latency of antibody appearance, there was no further increase of virus concentration in the organs tested until leukemias developed.

Animals infected with Graffi virus as adults develop virus-neutralizing antibodies and antibodies against surface antigens of leukemia cells. Despite the fact that virus-induced surface antigens were absent in spleen cells from these animals, virus was detectable in spleen as well as in thymus, lymph nodes, and bone marrow. Liver and brain did not contain measurable amounts of virus (Micheel and Pasternak, 1968a). Obviously the virus is present in the immunologically active organs. At this site, specific surface antigens are induced in certain target cells so that the animal can develop antibodies against them. However, the antigens induced by the virus are not detectable since the cells containing such surface antigens are too low in concentration or they are rapidly eliminated by the defense mechanisms of the host. Absence of virus in liver and brain can be explained by inhibition of hematogenic virus spreading caused by neutralizing serum antibodies.

Graffi virus is capable of producing leukemia in rats (Graffi and Gimmy, 1958; Graffi et al., 1962). It was, therefore, of interest to know whether virus is demonstrable in rat cells and whether it multiplies in cells of other species. Rats, hamsters, and rabbits infected with Graffi virus as newborns were killed between 8 and 13 days after inoculation, and homogenates from their spleens and livers were subjected to the MAP test. Whereas spleen and liver from infected rats were shown to contain virus, the same organs from infected hamsters and rabbits were negative. It is most important in this context that attempts to produce Graffi virus-induced leukemia in hamsters or rabbits have failed as yet. Lack of infectivity for hamster and rabbit cells could be due to the absence of virus receptors at the cell surface or to certain mechanisms causing inhibition of intracellular virus multiplication. The results of the MAP tests are very similar to those obtained by tissue culture studies. Whereas Graffi virus is produced by mouse embryonic and spleen cells for several cell-free tissue culture passages, virus in the medium appeared to be of considerably lower titer 2 weeks after *in vitro* infection of calf kidney or rat embryonic cells. There was a more rapid disappearance of virus from the tissue culture media if human kidney cells were used as targets. The experiments do not allow the conclusion that Graffi virus is capable of multiplying in cells other than mouse cells (Graffi and Schramm, 1963; Schramm and Graffi, 1963).

Finally the MAP test was negative for a rat leukemia induced by Graffi virus. Unfortunately, the leukemia was first tested after its sixth transplantation generation. Despite the absence of virus, certain virus-induced surface antigens were demonstrated on the cells by the indirect immunofluorescence test with Graffi mouse immune sera (Micheel and Pasternak, unpublished results). Experiments on the measurement of Graffi virus in "naturally" or "artificially" infected tumors are shown in Section IX.

In summary, not only development of virus-induced surface antigens but also multiplication of virus in cells of immunologically incompetent hosts seems to be a prerequisite to leukemia induction. This hypothesis is strengthened by the fact that mouse leukemia viruses apparently induce the disease only in those animal species in which virus multiplies at least for a certain period. Graffi virus was found in various organs of mice and rats which are sensitive to leukemia induction if infected as newborns. It was absent in spleen and liver of hamsters and rabbits resistant to leukemia induction. Adult mice which are infected with virus and thus develop immunity contain the virus in immunologically active organs. Most probably, however, the presence of infectious virus in leukemia cells is not required for the maintenance of malignancy. Whereas cells of all primary and transplanted mouse leukemias were shown to contain virus, it may be absent in rat leukemia cells or it is at least decreased in concentration.

D. Complement Fixation Test

Another immunological technique for the detection of mouse leukemia viruses is the CF test. Originally developed by Sarma *et al.* (1964) as an assay for noncytopathic, avian leucosis virus infection of tissue culture, the test was modified by Hartley *et al.* (1965) for mouse leukemia viruses. Leukemia viruses grown on mouse embryo tissue culture (METC) cells produce a CF antigen that reacts with sera of rats carrying transplanted Rauscher virus-induced leukemia. Complement-fixing antigen is detectable after infection of METC cells with Friend, Moloney, and Rauscher virus. It is also present in extracts of mouse and rat tumors induced by these viruses and the Gross virus. The cross-reactions obtained indicate that the CF test measures an antigen that is apparently common for all mouse leukemia viruses.

After infection of METC cells with tissue extracts containing high doses of virus, the antigen is produced within 6 days and increases in titer by 14 days. With lower doses of virus the highest titer appears between 18 and 21 days; this is the time required for the evaluation of the test. Essentially the antigen is prepared from infected METC cells by homogenization or sonication of the repeatedly frozen and thawed cells. In the centrifuge, sedimentation of the antigen occurs at 12,000–15,000 g for 60–90 minutes. Chloroform treatment destroys the activity. After heating at 56°C. for 30 minutes activity is partially reduced, and trypsin or periodate did not affect CF activity. It is supposed from these data that the CF antigen represents the virion. Moreover, rat sera with high CF antibody also contain high titer of neutralizing antibody. By means of the CF test, virus titration and neutralization tests were carried out. For titration purposes, serial ten-fold dilutions of virus preparations were used for the infection of METC cells. The plates were assayed for CF antigen at 3 weeks after infection, and the titer was expressed as the 50% tissue culture infective dose (TCID$_{50}$). Titers in Swiss embryo cells of $10^{4.5}$ to 10^6 were obtained for several Rauscher virus fluid pools, and for cell homogenates or sonicates the titer was $10^{5.5}$–$10^{7.0}$. Complement-fixing antigen did not develop in hamster and chick embryo, in bovine embryonic spleen, nor adult rabbit kidney.

For neutralization, dilutions of inactivated serum were mixed with virus and the mixture was incubated at 37°C. for 1 hour before inoculation into METC cells. Reduction of infective titer was used as a measure for neutralization activity. Seventeen of 19 rat sera with high CF titers inhibited CF antigen production by Rauscher, Friend, and Moloney virus.

Potent antisera, however, did not neutralize Gross virus or an isolate from AKR leukemia (Rowe *et al.*, 1966). This is an indication that the antigens measured by CF and neutralization tests are of different specificity.

In addition to the CF test the rat sera were subjected to the fluorescent antibody test (Rowe *et al.*, 1966). Comparable group specific reactions for leukemia viruses were obtained. The antigen appeared to be located in the cytoplasm of infected cells. Diffuse or finely granular staining was observed.

Rauscher rat immune sera were also applied by Duc Nguyen et al. (1966) to the detection of CF antigen in a kidney cell line derived from a rat with lymphoid leukemia. The antigen was present at various passages. At the same time viral buds and virus particles were found by electron microscopy.

In the course of screening several murine, tissue culture, cell lines for virus infection, Hall et al. (1967) used the CF test in correlation with the electron microscope for the detection of mouse leukemia viruses. Immune sera were from rats bearing a Gross virus-induced thymic lymphoma. It was found that there was a strong correlation between presence of mature C-particles, on the one hand, and presence of CF antigen or ability of the preparations to induce CF antigen in Swiss METC cells, on the other. With one exception, all of the cell lines containing leukemia virus had also undergone "spontaneous" neoplastic transformation in vitro. However, transformation was also found to occur in the absence of detectable mouse leukemia virus.

Another CF test, the quantitative CF test, was used by Gerber et al. (1966) for the comparison of Friend and Rauscher viral antigens. Homologous antisera were from BALB/c mice immunized with formalin-inactivated, virus-infected, BALB/c spleens. Purified plasma preparations of the viruses fixed complement. Reciprocal reactions indicated similarity of the Friend and Rauscher antigens. In all preparations of purified antigens even after two cycles of density-gradient centrifugation, small amounts of host components were demonstrable, i.e., Rauscher virus preparations reacted with guinea pig antiserum to normal mouse plasma.

Although incorporation of host components into the virion is conceivable the latter result of CF tests does not allow this conclusion. It cannot be ruled out without using electron-microscopic studies that host components having the same density as the virions are present in such preparations.

Gerber and Birch (1967) then applied the quantitative CF test to the detection of antibodies in sera of human and nonhuman primates against viral antigens derived from Burkitt's lymphoma cells. Partially purified viral antigens from the P_3 Burkitt lymphoma line, which contains herpeslike virus particles, reacted with 90% of sera from healthy adults and patients with malignant diseases. Thus, the widespread distribution of such antibodies was shown. The reactions were negative with an antigen prepared from a virus-free Burkitt lymphoma line. Although the virus-specificity of the CF reaction with sera of humans is evident, the relationship of this agent to the Burkitt lymphoma or other malignancies is as yet unknown.

As discussed by the authors the frequent demonstration of the particles in neoplasms or cells of the lymphoid system may reflect a preferential site of multiplication.

E. IMMUNOPRECIPITATION

Sera from rats repeatedly inoculated with syngeneic Gross virus-induced rat lymphoma cells were shown to contain also precipitating antibodies against a group-specific antigen of murine leukemia viruses (Geering et al., 1966). In the immunodiffusion test the antibodies precipitated extracts from G+ (Gross antigen-containing) cells as well as ether-treated preparations of Gross, Friend, Moloney, and Rauscher leukemia viruses. There was no precipitation with intact virus or with the mammary tumor virus, nor did mouse immune sera typing for G antigen show any precipitating activity. Reactions of identity in the immunodiffusion test have shown that the antigenic specificity of cell extracts and ether-treated virus preparations is the same. Possibly the antigen represents an internal component of the virus which is also present in the free state in cells infected with Gross virus. Certain immune sera are capable of producing distinct precipitin lines with extracts from a variety of G+ sources.

Rat immune sera also possess strong neutralizing activity against passage A Gross virus. Little or no neutralizing activity, however, was found against Rauscher virus. The rat immune sera tested thus contained (1) cytotoxic antibodies to G+ cells (see Section V), (2) precipitating antibodies to a group specific antigen of leukemia viruses, and (3) Gross virus-neutralizing antibodies. The results obtained by Hartley et al. (1965) with Rauscher rat immune sera in the CF test and those of Geering et al. (1966) with Gross rat immune sera in the precipitation test both demonstrate group-specific antigens of mouse leukemia viruses. Most probably the tests are measuring the same antigenic specificity although immunoprecipitation and CF activity have not been compared in the same experimental system. However, Hartley et al. (1965) and Geering et al. (1966) differ in their concepts with regard to the nature of the antigen. It was taken into consideration by Hartley et al. (1965) that the antigen is the virion. This hypothesis appears to be unlikely if it is meant for the intact virion. In the case of chicken leucosis virus, for example, it is known that the group-specific CF antigen is located within the virion and that it is released by freezing and thawing (Bauer and Schäfer, 1966). Freezing and thawing of cell suspensions containing leukemia virus was also used for the preparation of CF antigen by Hartley et al. (1965). During the procedure at least a partial breakup of virions might have occurred so that the CF reaction could become positive. Actually, there is no argument speaking against the identity of CF and precipitating antigen. Neutralizing activity of rat immune sera was tested by both groups of investigators. Apparently the antigen participating in the neutralization reaction is not the group-specific antigen of leukemia viruses. Gross rat immune sera caused a stronger neutralization effect on Gross than on Rauscher virus, and Rauscher rat immune sera did not neutralize Gross virus. Unfortunately, cytotoxic activity of Rauscher rat immune sera has not been investigated.

Immunodiffusion techniques are also applicable to other experimental systems designed for the antigenic characterization of leukemia viruses. Fink and Cowles (1965) and Fink et al. (1966) prepared immune sera in several animal species against the Rauscher virus. For immunization purposes they used concentrated plasma virus obtained from Rauscher-infected mice. Before testing the sera, Forssman antibody was removed by absorption with sheep red cells. Moreover, the sera were also absorbed with BALB/c plasma and erythrocytes. Immune sera derived from BALB/c mice, guinea pigs, rabbits, rats, and monkeys produced up to four precipitation lines with the homologous plasma virus, and one or two lines with Friend virus. Moloney virus was positive with the Rauscher monkey immune serum alone. This Moloney antigen cross-reacted with one of those present in both Rauscher and Friend virus. Each of the immune sera contained neutralizing antibodies against Rauscher virus. Although it is evident from the findings that Rauscher virus can be detected and identified by using the immunodiffusion technique with several immune sera, definite results on antigenic relationships among leukemia viruses have not been obtained.

Rabbit immune sera against Mazurenko virus-containing extracts from leukemic tissue were produced by Shershulskaya and Ievleva (1964). In the immunodiffusion test the sera reacted with leukemic organ preparations but not with preparations from normal animals. The significance of the antigen concerned is unknown.

Finally, the immunodiffusion technique was used for the detection of precipitating antibody in human sera against an antigen present in Burkitt's lymphoma cells (Old et al., 1966). The antigen was prepared from a culture line of Burkitt's lymphoma that is known to contain herpeslike particles. A high incidence of positive reactions was found among patients with Burkitt's lymphoma as well as with carcinoma of the postnasal space. Sera of patients with acute leukemia did not contain the precipitating antibody. The question whether the precipitating antibody is directed against a component of the herpeslike particles could not be answered by the authors.

F. Viral Interference Test

A new technique for the detection and titration of murine leukemia viruses is the viral interference test (Sarma et al., 1967) which was developed from a similar test for avian leucosis virus. In tissue culture, leukemia viruses were found to induce resistance to superinfection with the focus-forming Moloney sarcoma virus (Hartley and Rowe, 1966). None of the mouse embryo cultures infected with Friend, Moloney, Rauscher, and Gross viruses developed any foci, even after challenge inoculation with 10^3 to 10^4 focus-forming units of the sarcoma virus. Reduction of focus-forming titer in comparison with uninfected control cultures can be used as a measure for virus. Addition of immune serum to leukemia viruses before infection of cultures resulted in a loss of interference.

G. IMMUNOFLUORESCENCE

Infection of cells or tissues with a leukemia virus is, furthermore demonstrable by the immunofluorescence technique. Unlike the immunofluorescence test with viable cells which is applicable to the detection of surface antigens only, the technique with acetone-fixed cells allows examination of intracellularly located antigen. Cryostat cut sections, cover-slip cultures, as well as cell smears are likewise suitable for the tests. In the case of positive reactions, however, it is not possible to decide whether the fluorescence indicates the virion or a viral antigen.

By means of the direct immunofluorescence test with rabbit sera against preparations of cultured leukemia of viral origin, Ichikawa and Notake (1962) detected specific antigens at the surface and within the cytoplasm of leukemia cells. The direct test was also used by Fink and Malmgren (1963). Fluorescein-labeled rabbit sera against plasma virus of Rauscher infected BALB/c mice, which contained sufficient amounts of neutralizing antibody, stained malignant lymphoid tissues of BALB/c mice and Osborne-Mendel rats infected with Rauscher virus. Stainable antigen appeared to be located intranuclearly and less constantly in the cytoplasm. Mature megakaryocytes of rat bone marrow had the fluorescence only in the nucleus. However, viral particles have not yet been observed at this site by electron microscopy. In view of the extensive control experiments of Fink and Malmgren (1963), nuclear fluorescence cannot be explained on the basis of nonspecific reactions.

Contrary to this, nuclear fluorescence of infected cells was completely absent in the experiments of Osato et al. (1965) and Pinkel et al. (1966). Both groups of investigators used the indirect technique. However, the antiviral sera were from rabbits as in the experiments of Fink and Malmgren (1963). After infection of monolayer cover-slip cultures of mouse embryonic tissue with Friend virus, first appearance of fluorescence was observed in a small number of cells at 24 hours (Osato et al., 1965). Fluorescence was limited to the perinuclear area of the cytoplasm. Most of the cytoplasm was stained in about 20 to 30% of the cells at 48 hours. At 6 days about

50% of the cells were stained. By 10 days the fluorescence was bright at the cell periphery. Progression of viral synthesis is dependent on the multiplicity of virus inoculum. Friend virus-infected cells adsorbed chicken erythrocytes. First adsorption was observed at about 1 week after infection.

Pinkel *et al.* (1966) used the immunofluorescence technique for an *in vitro* assay of murine leukemia viruses. Monolayers of mouse fetal cells were infected with Moloney or Rauscher viruses. Fluorescent cells appeared at 11 days after inoculation of Moloney plasma virus concentrate. Higher dilutions delayed development of fluorescence. Rauscher virus-infected cultures showed first fluorescence at 1 day after inoculation. As in the experiments of Osato *et al.* (1965), initial fluorescence was in the perinuclear area and appeared later in the peripheral cytoplasm. There was a linear relationship between percentage of fluorescent cells and dilution of virus inoculum. On the basis of these findings, an end-point dilution test was developed.

Presence of fluorescence in the cytoplasmic area of cells infected with a leukemia virus was also confirmed by Brown *et al.* (1966a). They used convalescent mouse sera in the direct and the indirect complement fluorescent test.

Like other techniques, immunofluorescence was also applied to the examination of human leukemia. Fink *et al.* (1964) produced a rabbit immune serum against concentrated plasma pellets of individuals with leukemia. For immunization, only those pellets were used that contained viruslike particles. After absorption with normal human antigens the labeled rabbit serum was found to react specifically with leukocytes of the peripheral blood and with bone marrow cells of a significant number of individuals with acute lymphocytic leukemia. There was no reaction with cells from normal humans. Anti-Rauscher leukemia immune serum cross-reacted with the human leukemia cells. In later studies the results of first experiments were confirmed (Fink *et al.*, 1965). Cross-reactions between mouse leukemia antibody and human leukemic antigen were also reported by Brown *et al.* (1966b).

Interpretation of the results is most difficult. Despite the fact that the tests apparently included satisfactory controls there is not sufficient evidence that the fluorescence detected in human leukemia cells is due to an antigen which was induced by a leukemia virus.

H. Persistence of Virus and Viral Antigens in Leukemia Cells

Application of different techniques to the detection of leukemia viruses and viral antigens has shown that mouse and rat leukemias induced by the mouse leukemia viruses as well as infected nonleukemic cells contain virus or viral antigens. Presence of only virus-induced antigens in the absence of virus was shown for a transplanted Graffi rat leukemia. However, there are reports also on the establishment of virus-free virus-induced leukemias (Fieldsteel et al., 1966; Kobayashi et al., 1967). Although infectivity of both Friend tumor lines, investigated independently by these groups, was completely lost, Kobayashi et al. (1967) were still able to detect an antigen in the "virus-free" tumors that induced virus-neutralizing antibodies. Furthermore, electron-microscopic studies revealed type A particles which accumulated intracellularly (Kobayashi et al., 1966). Maruyama and Oboshi (1967) then demonstrated by combined biological, electron-microscopic and serological studies that the "virus-free" Friend cells of Kobayaski et al. (1967) belong to those tumors that persistently produce attenuated virus. These particles are not capable of inducing the Friend disease.

Production of high yields of particles with decreased infectivity was first observed by Wright and Lasfargues (1965, 1966) after long-term tissue culture propagation of a chronically Rauscher virus-infected cell line. Attenuation of Rauscher virus after long-term propagation in vitro was also obtained by Sinkovics et al. (1966). In such cultures both C- and A-type particles could be seen, and mice pretreated with this material resisted challenge with virulent Rauscher virus (Barski and Youn, 1965, 1966; Wright and Lasfargues, 1966). Highly concentrated preparations were infectious for BALB/c mice, indicating a very low proportion of infectious virus which is mixed with a high concentration of noninfectious virus (Wright and Lasfargues, 1966). The nature of the decreased infectivity was hitherto unknown.

In contrast to these findings, Fieldsteel et al. (1966) could not produce protection with the tumor against challenge inoculation with virulent Friend virus. Electron microscopy has not been applied to the investigation of this line, nor did the authors test the cells for virus-induced surface antigens. It would be very helpful to know that there are really no viral activities in this cell line.

VIII. Soluble Antigens

Mouse and rat cells infected with a murine leukemia virus generally contain the virus as well as virus-induced antigens which are detectable by a variety of in vivo and in vitro techniques. Specific surface antigens have been demonstrated by the phenomenon of transplantation rejection for leukemic cells and by immunofluorescence with viable cells and cytotoxicity in the presence of complement for leukemic and nonleukemic cells. Absence of cross-reactions at least between the FMR and G as well as Graffi (Gr) and G antigens indicates that type-specific differences do exist among murine leukemia viruses. Viral neutralization experiments with sera from rats carrying transplanted virus-induced rat leukemia are in line with this concept although the antiviral antibodies could be directed against antigenic specificities other than those present at the cell surface. As shown by immunofluorescence, virus or viral antigens appear to be localized within the cytoplasm of infected cells.

Virus-induced antigens, however, are not only detectable at the cellular level alone. The concentrated serum or plasma of leukemic animals was found to react in the immunodiffusion test with sera from leukemia-bearing rats. Identical reactions were obtained with concentrated leukemic extracts from which the virus was removed by centrifugation, and with ether-treated preparations of Friend, Moloney, Rauscher, and Gross viruses. The antigen could be identified as a group-specific viral antigen which is apparently not related to the "type-specific" antigen participating in the neutralization. Taking as a basis the antigenic differences observed between cells of the FMR and G types of leukemia the group-specific antigen is certainly not an integrated part of the cell membrane. Group-specific antigens of leukemia viruses are, furthermore, measured by the CF test. In all probability, precipitating and CF antigens are identical.

A. Friend, Moloney, and Rauscher Soluble Antigen

Another antigen that may also occur outside of virus-infected cells was found by Stück et al. (1964a). After incubation of certain Rauscher antigen-negative indicator cells with the plasma of Rauscher virus-infected mice, the cells became susceptible to the cytotoxic action of Rauscher-specific antibodies. The antigen which is present in the plasma and serum was termed soluble because it was not sedimentable under conditions where all infective activity is in the pellet. Whereas centrifugation at 105,000 g for 2 hours left the antigen in the supernatant, centrifugation for 16 hours caused its sedimentation. Heating to 56°C. for 30 minutes reduced the adsorbing activity; the activity was completely abolished at 65°C.

Indicator cells from a transplanted radiation-induced C57BL/6 leukemia, which had adsorbed the soluble antigen, were sensitive to Rauscher immune serum as well as to Friend and Moloney immune sera. These cells removed the cytotoxic activity of Rauscher immune sera against both antigen-sensitized indicator cells and leukemias induced by Rauscher virus. Thus, it is indicated that the soluble antigen and the virus-induced surface antigen of Rauscher leukemia cells, which is detected by cytotoxicity, are of the same specificity. This is strengthened by the fact that cytotoxic tests with sensitized indicator cells and Gross-specific immune sera were negative. As has already been mentioned, Rauscher and Gross leukemias possess different virus-induced surface antigens. Furthermore, the cells of the radiation-induced leukemia also acquire sensitivity to

Rauscher-specific immune sera after incubation in the plasma of mice with primary Friend or Moloney leukemia. However, the plasma of mice with primary or transplanted Gross leukemias did not render the cells sensitive to cytotoxic Rauscher immune sera.

All cross-reactivities observed among the soluble antigens of virus-induced leukemias correspond well with those among virus-induced surface antigens of leukemia cells, i.e., both types of antigen characterize the Friend, Moloney, and Rauscher leukemias as an immunologically closely related group distinct from the Gross leukemias.

Soluble antigen of the Rauscher type was also capable of sensitizing the EL 4 leukemia of C57BL/6 origin and a Gross virus-induced BALB/c leukemia. Several other leukemias, two ascites sarcomas, and normal spleen cells of certain mouse strains adsorbed the soluble antigen as shown by absorption of cytotoxic antibody, but they were not lysed by cytotoxic Rauscher antibody. Spleen cells of BALB/c, C3H/An, AKR, I, and C57L mice even failed to adsorb antigen. Rauscher soluble antigen did not sensitize cells from 4 cases of human leukemia. Apparently, specific receptors must be present at the cell surface to get adsorption of soluble antigen. However, there was no correlation between presence of the receptors on cells from various strains, on the one hand, and susceptibility or resistance of these strains to the development of Rauscher leukemia, on the other. The fact that certain cells are sensitized to cytotoxic antibody and others adsorb antigen without being sensitized indicates differences with regard to surface concentration and distance of receptor sites. It is not known whether cells lacking receptors of FMR specificity are lacking receptors of G specificity, also, or whether the receptors of both FMR and G specificity are identical. The soluble antigen is assumed to be a product or subunit of the leukemogenic virus (Stück et al., 1964a). Its type-specific reactivity, which corresponds to that of virus-induced surface antigens, distinguishes the soluble antigen, however, from the group-specific viral antigen detectable by CF and immunodiffusion tests.

Most important for the characterization of soluble antigen would be to know whether or not antigen is capable of inducing virus-neutralizing antibodies or of absorbing antibodies from mouse immune sera. Results of such experiments in the Graffi leukemia system are not yet conclusive.

B. GROSS SOLUBLE ANTIGEN

Soluble antigens possessing Gross specificity have been shown by Aoki et al. (1966b). Since the indicator cells used did not acquire sensitivity to cytotoxic antibody the authors applied the more sensitive indirect immuno-fluorescence test to the detection of adsorbed antigen. The possibility was considered that G soluble antigen was present in the plasma of mice with

Gross leukemia but that it was adsorbed onto the cells in insufficient quantities. Evidence was then obtained by positive immunofluorescence reactions that EL 4 leukemia as well as other C57BL leukemias adsorbed soluble G antigen. Gross soluble antigen was demonstrable in all mouse strains with a high incidence of spontaneous leukemia. The pattern of distribution was the same as that of G cellular antigen. The conclusion was drawn that the test for soluble G antigen in the plasma permits the unequivocal identification of mice from strains with high incidence of leukemia, long before they develop leukemia. Soluble antigen could also be separated from suspensions of leukemia cells. Apparently, the antigen appears to be adsorbed *in vivo* onto cells of infected mice. For separation the cells were only slightly homogenized to avoid considerable disruption. Thus, soluble antigen was obtained in a relatively pure state.

C. Graffi Soluble Antigen

Mice infected with Graffi leukemia virus also contain a soluble antigen which appears about 4 weeks after virus inoculation into newborns. Indicator cells were from various methyl nitrosourea (MNU)-induced leukemias of strain XVII/Bln. Adsorption was demonstrated by the indirect immunofluorescence test. Results of the experiments are shown in Table IX.

TABLE IX

Adsorption of Graffi-Specific Soluble Antigen onto Cells
of Methyl Nitrosourea-Induced Leukemias

Designation of leukemia	FI before adsorption[a]	FI after adsorption[a]	Adsorption
LME 3	0.01 ⟶ 0.97		+
	0.03 ⟶ 0.95		
LME 16b	0.00 ⟶ 0.86		
	0.01 ⟶ 0.77		+
	0.00 ⟶ 0.73		
LME 8	0.00 ⟶ 0.00		
	0.02 ⟶ 0.00		−
	0.04 ⟶ 0.07		
	0.00 ⟶ 0.00		
LME 42a	0.00 ⟶ 0.00		
	0.00 ⟶ 0.02		−
	0.05 ⟶ 0.02		
	0.07 ⟶ 0.15		

[a] FI = fluorescence index.

Whereas two of the leukemias adsorbed considerable amounts of soluble antigen, two others were negative. In view of the high sensitivity of the indirect immunofluorescence test, it is indicated that cells of the latter type of leukemia are not capable of adsorbing the Graffi-specific antigen. The conclusion can be drawn that leukemias even when induced by the same chemical carcinogen differ in their adsorption capacity for soluble antigen. Furthermore, there was no correlation between adsorption capacity and histological type of the leukemias tested. Preliminary data indicate, however, that adsorption capacity of an MNU-induced leukemia is related to its ability to express certain virus-induced surface antigens after artificial infection with Graffi virus. Leukemias LME 3 and LME 16b behaved immunologically like Graffi leukemia cells when they had been infected with Graffi virus, whereas leukemias LME 8 and LME 42a, although actually producing Graffi virus, did not reveal the same degree of antigenic change.

IX. Virus-Induced Antigens in "Naturally" and "Artificially" Infected Cells

It has been shown in the preceding that surface antigens induced by leukemia viruses are present in leukemic as well as nonleukemic cells of the hematopoietic system. By use of a sensitive technique, such as the absorption, appearance of virus-induced surface antigens is detectable in cells of spleen or thymus less than a month after infection of newborn mice with Graffi or Gross virus. However, kidney or brain of infected animals does not contain measurable amounts of virus-induced surface antigens. This raises the question whether infected cells other than those of the hematopoietic system are at all capable of expressing leukemia-specific surface antigens. From electron-microscopic studies, it is known that virus is released from epithelial cells or cells of liver, parotis, or genital organs. Thus, at least viral antigens are expected to be present at their surface. Independently of the mode of infection, i.e., inoculation or vertical transmission of virus, such cells may be considered "naturally" infected as a consequence of viral spreading in the organism.

In addition, natural infection is supposed to take place by chance in the case of tumors arising in, or transplanted to, animals harboring a certain virus. In this regard, the history of infection is obscure, and very often the question whether or not the agent is causally related to the tumor cannot be answered. As an example, most of the leukemias that develop in mice after X-irradiation are transmissible by cell-free tumor extracts.

In the course of serial transplantation, tumors of viral and nonviral origin may also pick up unrelated viruses including tumor viruses, i.e., they may become naturally infected. Both the Landschütz sarcoma I and the Ehrlich carcinoma from which the Graffi virus was originally isolated and which still produces the virus belong to that category of naturally infected tumors.

Simulation of such events under controlled laboratory conditions is possible by artifical infection of tumors. This is obtained by passaging the tumor in virus-infected animals or by infecting the tumor cells in tissue culture. The methods allow consideration of quantitative aspects of infection, selection of suitable tumor types, as well as repetition of the experiments. Immunological analysis, particularly of cells artificially infected with an oncogenic virus, gives a chance to get more information on virus–cell interactions and the mechanism of malignant transformation.

Sjögren (1964a) was able to demonstrate that methylcholanthrene-induced sarcomas of mice contain the polyoma-specific transplantation antigen provided that the tumors had been infected with polyoma virus. Sensitivity to virus-induced transplantation resistance was also described by Svet-Moldavsky and Hamburg (1964) and Hamburg and Svet-Moldavsky (1964) for chemically induced tumors infected with herpes simplex, Sendai, SV 40, or polyoma virus. They designated this phenomenon as "artificial heterogenization" of tumors. It is noteworthy in this context that non-oncogenic viruses, such as herpes and Sendai, apparently like tumor viruses induce formation of specific transplantation antigens in infected cells. However, unlike polyoma- and SV 40-infected cells where the transplantation antigen was shown to be a nonvirion antigen, the antigen of herpes and Sendai viruses-infected cells have not yet been identified. Transplantation resistance could be due in this case to antiviral immunity and the presence of viral antigens at the surface of infected cells.

In the meantime, several other virus–cell combinations have been tested for the appearance of new virus-induced antigens including CF antigens of SV 40 or polyoma tumors. A summary of experiments is given by Sjögren (1966).

A. Virus-Induced Surface Antigens in the Skin of Infected Animals

In the virus leukemia system, Breyere and Williams (1964) presented evidence that the presumably normal skin of leukemic BALB/c mice contains an antigen that is not present in the skin of normal graft donors. After immunization against leukemia induced by Breyere virus, recipient mice rejected a high number of syngeneic skin grafts derived from leukemic animals. The average survival time of rejected grafts was 18 days. In general, the rejection response did not differ from reactions against minor histocompatibility antigens. In nonimmune recipients, skin grafts from leukemic mice were only partially rejected. Under grafts in normal mice, tumors often developed, i.e., leukemia cells are present in the donor skin grafts. All skin grafts derived from normal BALB/c mice healed into place and did not show any sign of rejection irrespective of transplantation into immunized or nonimmunized recipients. The authors concluded that in animals infected with a leukemia virus, the cells of normal tissues may acquire virus-associated antigenic properties.

A similar skin graft rejection phenomenon was observed by Svet-Moldavsky et al. (1967). Skin grafts taken from mice with certain transplanted, chemically induced sarcomas were completely rejected in syngeneic recipients. Moreover, the rejection phenomenon was transmissible to normal recipients by skin grafts from mice which had already rejected the skin of tumor-bearing donors. Although the data suggest the participation of virus, there is no indication as yet that the agent is related to the leukemia viruses.

B. Virus-Induced Surface Antigens in Leukemia Cells Artificially Infected with Rauscher Virus

Leukemia cells can also acquire new antigenic specificities which are characteristic of leukemias induced by an unrelated virus. Stück et al. (1964b) artificially infected with the Rauscher virus a variety of transplanted ascites leukemias and sarcomas lacking the FMR antigen. For this purpose the cells were inoculated into mice that had been infected 5–16 days previously with the leukemia virus. At various intervals after inoculation the tumor cells were tested for their sensitivity to a Rauscher typing serum. The following tumors were found to have acquired the Rauscher antigen after passage in infected animals: leukemia EL 4 (chemically induced), urethan-induced leukemia U 15, and BALB/c Gross leukemia No. 2. Another ascites leukemia of AKR origin and the three ascites sarcomas tested showed little or no sensitivity to Rauscher immune serum. Rauscher antigen persisted in infected leukemia cells as was shown by serial cellular passages in normal uninfected animals. Acquisition of the new antigenic specificity induced by an unrelated virus was termed "antigenic conversion."

C. Virus and Virus-Induced Surface Antigens in Malignant Cells Artificially or Naturally Infected with Graffi Virus

In our experiments with the Graffi leukemia virus, various tumors of different etiology have been artificially infected. They included leukemias induced by MNU, spontaneous Gross leukemias of the AKR strain, as well as sarcomas induced by methylcholanthrene and ultraviolet light. For infection the tumors were repeatedly transplanted to Graffi virus-infected animals. In the case of AKR Gross leukemias, five successive intramuscular passages were performed in infected mice. Subsequently, the presumably infected sublines were further passaged in normal uninfected animals. Later on, one single passage of the tumors in infected mice was found to be sufficient for artificial infection of the cells.

All infected and noninfected sublines of the tumors were tested for the following characteristic features: (*1*) persistent production of Graffi virus— after several passages in normal mice, in some cases after more than fifty generations of transplanting, the infected tumors were subjected to the MAP test; (*2*) presence of tumor-specific transplantation antigens of the Graffi leukemia type—for this purpose the cells were transplanted to Graffi resistant animals; (*3*) presence of Graffi virus-induced surface antigens detectable by immunofluorescence; (*4*) absorption capacity for Graffi-specific antibodies detectable by immunofluorescence; and (*5*) passive transfer of Graffi-specific resistance by the neutralization test. This experiment was performed with sarcoma cells only.

1. *Methyl Nitrosourea-Induced Leukemia*

Summarized data on the antigenic specificities of MNU-induced leukemias artificially infected with Graffi leukemia virus are presented in Table X. Evidence of infection was obtained by the MAP test. In contrast to the noninfected leukemias, all infected sublines tested produced Graffi virus. After infection, transplantation antigens of the Graffi leukemia type were demonstrable; infected cells did not grow in the majority of Graffi-resistant animals. Noninfected cells grew equally well in Graffi-resistant and normal mice. In the immunofluorescence test, however, considerable differences were observed among infected leukemias with regard to intensity of staining reaction. Two of the leukemias (LME 8 and LME 42a) were negative or had only a faint surface fluorescence when incubated with Graffi hyperimmune serum and stained with labeled, rabbit, anti-mouse γ-globulin. Obviously the surface concentration of the Graffi virus-induced antigen is very low in these cells. However, it is not known whether the staining intensity of the immunofluorescence test reflects qualitative rather than quantitative differences. Repeated infection experiments had the same result. Moreover, both noninfected leukemia lines did not adsorb measurable amounts of soluble Gr antigen. Absorption capacity for Graffi-specific antibodies was correlated with the staining intensity of the immunofluorescence test. The differences in immunological behavior among Graffi virus-infected MNU-induced leukemias is subject to further studies.

2. *Spontaneous AKR Gross Leukemia*

In another series of experiments (Micheel and Pasternak, 1968b) spontaneous Gross virus-induced leukemias of the AKR strain were infected

TABLE X

Summarized Data on the Antigenic Specificities of Methyl Nitrosourea-Induced Leukemias Artificially Infected with Graffi Leukemia Virus

Designation of leukemia[a]		Production of Graffi virus[b]	Transplantation antigens of the Graffi leukemia type[b]	Graffi virus-induced surface antigens (detected by immunofluorescence)	Absorption capacity for antibodies against Graffi virus-induced surface antigens[b]	Adsorption of soluble Gr antigen[b]
LME 3	I	+	+	+	+	N.t.
	NI	−	−	−	−	+
LME 8	I	+	±	± or −	±	N.t.
	NI	−	−	−	−	−
LME 16b	I	+	+	+	+	N.t.
	NI	−	−	−	−	+
LME 39	I	N.t.	N.t.	+	N.t.	N.t.
	NI	−	N.t.	−	N.t.	N.t.
LME 42a	I	+	+	± or −	−	N.t.
	NI	−	−	−	−	−

[a] I = infected; NI = noninfected.
[b] N.t. = not tested.

by repeated cellular passages in AKR or AKR-F₁ hybrids which had been inoculated with Graffi virus as newborns. Altogether, 10 different Gross leukemias were tested. It is shown in Table XI that all of them produced permanently the Graffi virus. One of the leukemias still released this virus on its fifty-second cellular passage following infection. As compared with primary Graffi leukemias, the virus titer was about 10- to 100-fold lower.

The transplantation antigens which are characteristic of Graffi leukemia, however, were detected in only 1 out of 9 infected leukemias tested. This leukemia differed from the other 9 leukemias only in that it had a very short latency period of 196 days. Doses of 10^4 cells were rejected in Graffi resistant animals, whereas the same doses of cells prepared from the original noninfected line produced progressively growing tumors in resistant as well as in normal mice. In the immunofluorescence test the cells were strongly positive with Graffi immune sera; the reaction was negative with cells of the original line. Cytotoxic tests were unsuccessful owing to the extreme sensitivity of both infected and noninfected cells to guinea pig complement. Graffi virus-infected cells of this leukemia, however, completely absorbed those antibodies from Graffi immune serum that react with the virus-induced surface antigens of Graffi leukemia cells. For this particular case the conclusion can be drawn that infection with Graffi virus rendered Gross leukemia cells immunologically indistinguishable from cells of Graffi leukemia.

With the exception of this leukemia, all other 9 Graffi virus-infected

TABLE XI

SUMMARIZED DATA ON THE ANTIGENIC SPECIFICITIES OF THE AKR GROSS
LEUKEMIAS ARTIFICIALLY INFECTED WITH GRAFFI LEUKEMIA VIRUS

Leukemia	Production of Graffi virus[a]	Transplantation antigens of the Graffi leukemia type[a]	Graffi virus-induced surface antigens detected by immuno-fluorescence[a]	Absorption of antibodies against Graffi virus-induced surface antigens[a]
Spontaneous AKR Gross leukemia	0/10	0/6	0/9	0/2
Graffi virus-infected AKR Gross leukemia	10/10	1/9	7/9[b]	1/7[c]

[a] Number of positive cases of leukemia per total number tested.

[b] Only those leukemias were considered positive in which at least 50% of the tests performed with the cells had indexes > 0.3.

[c] Absorption is considered positive if at least 50% of antibody activity is removed from undiluted immune serum (as measured by fluorescence index).

Gross leukemias showed a different behavior. Growth of the cells was not inhibited in animals resistant to Graffi leukemia. In contrast in some cases the tumors even appeared earlier in immunized than in normal mice. However, there is no indication as yet whether the better growth is related to the phenomenon of immunological enhancement. Slightly enhanced growth can also be observed after inoculation of AKR Gross leukemia cells into syngeneic recipients pretreated with X-ray-killed Gross leukemia homogenate. It is known that this does not immunize the AKR animals because they are naturally tolerant to Gross virus-induced antigens. In certain tumor–host combinations, tissue extracts are apparently capable of inducing a nonspecific stimulation of tumor growth.

Surface antigens characteristic of Graffi leukemia cells were not demonstrable in infected Gross leukemia cells by the cytotoxic technique. Immunofluorescence tests, however, yielded some positive results. Depending on the strength of Graffi immune serum, in 7 out of 9 cases investigated, a certain number of cells revealed a weak, but distinct, surface fluorescence. Further, the absorption capacity of the cells for Graffi virus-induced surface antigens was very low. Except for the 1 Gross leukemia which was immunologically indistinguishable from Graffi leukemias, all other 7 leukemias produced only a very slight reduction in antibody activity. Specificity of the absorption effect as measured by immunofluorescence could not be exactly established.

The difference between infected and noninfected cells, regularly detectable in the immunofluorescence staining with Graffi hyperimmune sera, however, indicates the presence of a certain Graffi virus-induced antigen at the surface of infected Gross leukemia cells. Original, noninfected, Gross leukemias transplanted simultaneously with their infected sublines did not spontaneously acquire Graffi virus or Graffi virus-induced antigens.

In some but not in all of the experiments performed, Graffi virus apparently disappeared from artificially infected Gross leukemias after one single passage of the tumors in Graffi-resistant animals, i.e., homogenates prepared from the outgrowing tumors no longer induced formation of antibodies reacting with Graffi leukemia cells (negative MAP test). It was postulated with regard to the mechanism of virus elimination that only those cells containing Graffi virus and virus-induced surface antigens are attacked and destroyed by the Graffi-specific immune response of the host (G. Pasternak and Pasternak, 1968). In this case, however, the tumor would consist of two different cell populations, one containing Graffi virus and the other not. The Graffi virus-containing population then must represent a minor population since there were no significant differences between the growth behavior of Graffi virus-infected cells in immunized and nonimmunized mice, i.e., selection of virus-free cells in resistant animals was not detectable by growth inhibition of the tumor. A low number of Graffi virus-producing cells in infected Gross leukemias could also explain the relatively low virus titer demonstrated by the MAP test.

Clones of the Graffi virus-infected, Gross ascites leukemia GGr 4967b were established to test whether cells lacking Graffi virus do exist in artificially infected Gross leukemia. All clones grew from single cells which had been isolated from microdroplets with a glass capillary and inoculated intraperitoneally into newborn (C57BL × AKR)F$_1$ or (XVII × AKR)F$_1$ hybrids. After 4 weeks, leukemia ascites developed in about 10% of the animals inoculated with one single cell. Previously five cell clones had been obtained which were then passaged in normal mice and which have now been analyzed in the same way as the original GGr 4967b leukemia. It was found that three of them produced Graffi virus in about the same amount as GGr 4967b, but the other two were negative in the MAP test. Graffi virus-containing as well as virus-free clones, however, did not differ in their growth behavior when injected into Graffi-resistant or normal animals. They even had the same growth rate as the original leukemia GGr 4967b. *In vitro*, using Graffi hyperimmune sera, a number of cells of the virus-infected clones revealed weak membrane staining in the immunofluorescence test; cells of clones lacking Graffi virus did not show any positive reaction. It should be mentioned that Graffi virus-free clones were not resistant to reinfection with Graffi virus.

Progressive growth of Graffi virus-containing clones on resistant animals is an interesting phenomenon. Provided that only those Gross leukemia cells lacking Graffi virus are capable of multiplying in Graffi-resistant animals, the clone derived from a single Graffi virus-infected cell must again consist of virus-free and virus-containing cell populations. If Graffi virus is multiplying at a low rate in Gross leukemia cells this could be explained by segregation. However, more than fifty cellular passages of Graffi virus-infected Gross leukemia in normal mice were not sufficient to get complete natural elimination of Graffi virus. Obviously there is a relatively stable equilibrium between the proportion of virus-free and virus-containing cells. It cannot be ruled out at present that mechanisms other than selection are responsible for immunological elimination of Graffi virus from infected Gross leukemia. Problems of virus-cell interactions in the Graffi–Gross combination of leukemia are being investigated further. Special attention is dedicated to the measurement of Gross antigen in Graffi virus-infected Gross leukemia cells.

3. *Chemically and Physically Induced Sarcomas*

Artificial infection with Graffi virus was also applied to chemically and physically induced sarcomas (L. Pasternak and Pasternak, 1968a). The

TABLE XII
DEMONSTRATION OF TRANSPLANTATION ANTIGENS OF THE GRAFFI LEUKEMIA
TYPE IN SARCOMAS "ARTIFICIALLY" INFECTED WITH GRAFFI VIRUS

Pretreatment	Challenge tumor		Cell dose	Animals with progressively growing tumors per total number inoculated
Graffi virus-containing cell-free filtrate	UV	14306[a]	2×10^5	10/10
—				10/10[d]
Graffi virus-containing cell-free filtrate	UVGr	14306[b]	2×10^5	0/10
—				6/10[d]
Graffi virus-containing cell-free filtrate	MC	11504[c]	2×10^5	8/9
—				8/9[d]
Graffi virus-containing cell-free filtrate	MCGr	11504[b]	2×10^5	0/14
—				9/14[d]

[a] Sarcoma induced by ultraviolet light.
[b] Graffi virus-infected subline.
[c] Sarcoma induced by methylcholanthrene.
[d] Nonimmunized.

experiments included one sarcoma induced by methylcholanthrene (MC 11504) and another induced by ultraviolet light (UV 14306) in XVII mice. Both tumors continued to produce Graffi virus after one cellular passage in Graffi viremic animals. In agreement with results from Graffi virus-infected Gross leukemias, the titer was 10- to 100-fold lower than in primary Graffi leukemias. In Table XII it is shown that the Graffi virus-infected sarcomas, designated as UVGr 14306 and MCGr 11504, did not grow in animals immunized against Graffi leukemia by inoculation of Graffi virus-containing cell-free filtrates. The resistance effect was very striking and did not differ from that observed after challenge inoculation of Graffi leukemia cells. Infected sarcoma cells thus behaved like leukemia cells in immunized animals. Recent experiments have shown that both infected sublines still contain their original tumor-specific transplantation antigens. For ultraviolet-induced sarcomas, antigenicity was previously found to be of the "individual-specific" type just as for chemically induced tumors (Pasternak et al., 1964).

The clear-cut resistance effect stimulated experiments on the passive transfer of immunity. Lymphoid cells derived from lymph nodes of Graffi-resistant mice, indeed, completely inhibited the outgrowth of Graffi virus-infected sarcoma cells if they had been admixed with the lymphoid cells before inoculation. Normal lymphoid cells, however, did not influence the outgrowth of sarcoma cells. In all experiments, 2×10^5 sarcoma cells were mixed with 2×10^7 immune or normal lymphoid cells. Immune serum was less if at all effective against sarcoma cells.

Immunofluorescence tests were rendered more difficult since the trypsinization method had to be used for the preparation of cell suspensions from the solid tumors. During this procedure surface antigens may undergo some changes so that the negative results hitherto obtained are still inconclusive. Homogenates from infected sarcomas removed only little antibody activity from Graffi immune sera.

Results of transplantation experiments, however, are evidence of the presence of certain Graffi virus-induced surface antigens in infected sarcoma cells.

In the course of typing mouse tumors for Gross antigen, Old et al. (1965) examined a number of chemically induced sarcomas. Three of 5 transplanted BALB/c sarcomas, in their twenty-fifth, twenty-seventh, and fifty-second transplant generations, and a long-transplanted C3H ascites sarcoma, originally induced by benzpyrene, contained G antigen. Three other long-transplanted ascites tumors, including Sarcoma I and a methylcholanthrene-induced tumor, were negative. Five different spontaneous mammary tumors were also lacking demonstrable G antigen. Presence or absence of G antigen in the tumors was determined by the absorption capacity of the tissues for cytotoxic Gross antibodies.

Since the G antigen is normally absent in BALB/c mice it is a surprising fact that transplantable tumors of this strain may contain the antigen, i.e., infection with Gross virus must have occurred. It was taken into consideration by the authors that Gross virus exists in a masked or integrated state in some low-incidence strains and that it can be activated by certain stimuli such as chemical carcinogens. On the other hand, Gross virus may have natural infectivity for low-incidence strains when virus-containing strains are maintained in the same quarters.

4. Landschütz Sarcoma I and Ehrlich Carcinoma

Natural infection with a leukemia virus was also investigated immunologically in the case of Landschütz sarcoma I (Sarcoma I) and the Ehrlich carcinoma (Pasternak and Pasternak, 1967). Both tumors harbor the Graffi leukemia virus. The MAP test revealed virus in about the same titer as in artificially infected tumors. In control experiments, a transplanted sarcoma originally induced by implantation of polyvinyl chloride platelets, and a chondroma, which had developed spontaneously about 30 years ago, were found to be inactive in the MAP test.

To test the sensitivity of Graffi virus-containing tumor cells to the virus-induced rejection response, Sarcoma I cells were injected into Graffi-resistant animals. Progressively growing tumors occurred in both immunized and control groups, showing no significant differences in the tumor mean diameter. Antibody activity against Graffi leukemia cells did not decrease in immunized animals despite the development of large tumors. Moreover, after tumors in the control animals became palpable, antibodies reacting with Graffi leukemia cells appeared (positive MAP test with viable cells).

Sarcoma I cells reacted with Graffi immune sera in the immunofluo-rescence test. In 13 of 16 tests, the FIs were higher than 0.3. However, only 7 had indexes higher than 0.5. As expressed by the FI, Ehrlich car-cinoma cells reacted less strongly than Sarcoma I cells. Both tumors absorbed only little antibody activity from Graffi immune sera. Absorption was measured by the immunofluorescence test.

In summary, natural or artificial infection with a leukemia virus may cause an antigenic change of both normal as well as malignant cells. They acquire certain virus-induced antigens characteristic of leukemias which are produced by that particular virus. The change in antigenicity is demon-strable by the sensitivity of the infected cells to the virus-induced rejection response, by the indirect immunofluorescence test, and by absorption. These particular methods proved to be more or less suitable for the detection of antigens, depending on the cell type tested. Immunofluorescence and absorption tests are considered the most sensitive for antigen detection. Certain tumors infected with a leukemia virus may grow equally well in immunized and normal animals. In general, naturally and artificially infected cells are continuously producing leukemia virus.

D. Virus-Induced Surface Antigens of the Leukemia-Specific Type in Tumors Induced by the Murine Sarcoma Virus

Tumors induced by the murine sarcoma virus (MSV) of Moloney (Moloney, 1966) apparently contain antigenic specificities characteristic of virus-induced leukemia (Fefer et al., 1967a). Like the sarcoma virus of Harvey (1964) which induces tumors in mice, rats, and hamsters the Moloney MSV was derived from a passage line of Moloney mouse leukemia virus. Sarcomas were originally obtained in BALB/c mice after inoculation of high doses of the leukemia virus (Moloney, 1966). Cell-free extracts prepared from BALB/c sarcomas produce rhabdomyosarcoma at the site of injection in 100% of infant mice within 3 to 5 days. The agent can be maintained in this strain by cell-free transmissions. Morphologically it is not different from the leukemia viruses (Dalton, 1966). Moreover, the density of the agent as measured by gradient centrifugation also corre-sponds with that of leukemia viruses (Moloney, 1966). However, unlike these viruses the agent is capable of producing *in vitro* morphological transformation of mouse embryo cells (Hartley and Rowe, 1966) and rat embryo cells (Ting, 1966). Transformation of hamster embryo cells was shown for the Harvey MSV by Simons *et al.* (1967).

The agent is apparently defective in the sense that it requires the presence of a mouse leukemia virus for focus production in mouse tissue cultures (Hartley and Rowe, 1966), i.e., leukemia viruses serve as helpers for the defective MSV particles and presumably for virus production. The helper effect was also found with leukemia viruses other than the Moloney type. Studies of Huebner *et al.* (1966) indicate that the focus-forming viruses have the envelope antigens of the helper virus.

Antigenicity of Moloney MSV-induced sarcomas of mice was investigated by Fefer *et al.* (1967a). Pretreatment of histocompatible hosts with preparations of MSV or with X-ray-killed sarcoma cells induced tumor-specific transplantation resistance against sarcoma cells. Even primary tumors were found to regress in a high proportion of animals. Serum from these animals neutralized the oncogenicity of MSV (Fefer *et al.*, 1967b). Animals pretreated with MSV were also resistant to Friend, Moloney, and Rauscher leukemia cells. Tumors of non-FMR origin were not rejected in MSV-immunized mice. Furthermore, cross-experiments demonstrated that Moloney leukemia virus or X-ray-killed Moloney lymphoma cells can immunize against sarcoma cells. The data indicate that leukemia induced by the FMR viruses and Moloney MSV-induced sarcomas share common antigens.

In vitro, the immunofluorescence reaction was positive with FMR leukemia cells and immune sera from animals pretreated with X-irradiated sarcoma cells. Since attempts to prepare suspensions of viable sarcoma cells for the immunofluorescence test were unsuccessful the authors measured the absorption capacity of packed cells for FMR antibody. It was found that sarcoma cells but not EL 4 leukemia cells removed antibody activity from FMR immune sera.

Transplantation and immunofluorescence tests strongly suggest that Moloney MSV-induced sarcoma cells share common antigens with Friend, Moloney, and Rauscher leukemia cells. Both types of tumors, however, are known to release virus particles. Common antigenicity could be explained by the simultaneous presence of Moloney leukemia virus and MSV in the sarcoma cells as well as in the MSV preparations although such preparations are obviously not leukemogenic in mice. Neutralization experiments with mouse immune sera have shown that both agents possess antigens in common. Presence of common antigens was further confirmed by use of rat anti-Gross sera (Fefer *et al.*, 1967c).

E. Antigenic Change of Leukemia Cells Caused by Agents
Other Than Leukemia Viruses

It is now well established that leukemia viruses may cause an antigenic change of normal as well as neoplastic cells including those of leukemias induced by other agents. Leukemia cells, however, can also be modified in antigenicity by infection with agents other than leukemia viruses.

1. Mammary Leukemia (ML) Antigen

Stück et al. (1964c) detected an antigen in certain DBA/2 leukemias that is associated with presence of the mammary tumor virus (MTV). Association was concluded from the fact that mammary tissues and mammary tumors of mouse strains infected with this virus contain the same antigenic specificity. The term "mammary leukemia" (ML) was suggested for the antigen to characterize its tissue distribution. Immune serum with ML specificity was first obtained by immunizing histoincompatible strains with DBA/2 spontaneous leukemias. Cytotoxic isoantibodies were absorbed *in vivo* by injection into DBA/2 recipients. Absorbed sera were cytotoxic for spontaneous DBA/2 leukemias and for a urethan-induced DBA/2 leukemia. These leukemias were capable of removing ML antibodies from immune sera. Antibody absorption was also positive with a DMBA leukemia and with two long-transplanted ascites leukemias which did not show sensitivity to cytotoxic ML antibody in the direct test. Furthermore, absorption data demonstrated that ML is different from Gross and FMR antigens.

Presence of ML antigen in mammary tumors and MTV-infected mammary tissue was also measured by their absorption capacity. Mammary leukemia antibody was removed by mammary tumors of different mouse strains as well as by MTV-infected DBA/2 and C3H/An mammary tissue, but not by agent-free C57BL/6 and BALB/c mammary tissue.

A number of DMBA-induced DBA/2 leukemias failed to induce antibody with ML specificity. They did not even absorb ML antibody from immune sera; ML is also absent from leukemias of MTV-infected strains other than DBA/2 (Old and Boyse, 1965). This latter finding is somewhat surprising since natural infection with MTV might have occurred at least in certain cases. The authors, therefore, take into consideration that the DBA/2 strain could carry a variant leukemogenic virus which arose by recombination with the MTV.

Nowinski et al. (1967) were then able to show that ML represents a subunit of MTV. Rabbit immune serum against MTV preparations from infective milk of RIII mice was found to precipitate in the immunodiffusion a soluble antigen which is present in concentrated extracts of primary and transplanted mammary tumors and of ML-containing DBA/2 leukemias. Mammary tumor and ML leukemia extracts gave reactions of identity. Precipitation with fresh pellets from homogenates was positive only after freeze-thawing of the preparations or after treating them with ether. Treatment with ether released the antigen from intact MTV which was isolated by density-gradient centrifugation of RIII milk. Reaction was negative before ether treatment. This is evidence that the antigen is a virus subunit. It is not sedimented by centrifugation at 96,500 g for 4 hours. The same antigen, which is named MTV-s1, is also detectable by precipitation with mouse immune sera against mammary tumors or against ML-containing leukemias.

2. *Moloney Lymphoma with Polyoma Tumor Antigen*

Antigenic change of leukemia cells induced by artificial infection with polyoma virus was described by Sjögren and Hellström (1965, 1967). Moloney leukemia cells were incubated with polyoma virus *in vitro* and subsequently inoculated into genetically compatible recipients. Cells from developing tumors were repeatedly infected. After 10 serial infections one of the three YAA Moloney sublines infected became highly sensitive to the virus-induced rejection response of polyoma-immunized animals. Two single cell clones from this subline were both found to be sensitive. Thus, the cells had acquired the polyoma tumor-specific transplantation antigen. Virus release from the cells could not be detected. Despite the presence of polyoma antigen the cells had not lost the Moloney-specific antigen. The polyoma tumor antigen in antigenically changed lymphoma cells could also be detected by an *in vitro* assay. Incubation with immune sera and complement reduced the plating efficiency of tumor cells. Cells of this Moloney line were also suitable as targets for the distinction between the effects of antiviral and anticellular polyoma antibodies. Antibodies of the latter type only caused a significant reduction in plating efficiency (Hellström, 1965).

F. Thymus Leukemia Antigens

Another leukemia-specific antigen not related to G, FMR, or ML antigenic specificities was detected by means of C57BL/6 immune sera against spontaneous or radiation-induced leukemias of the A strain or of (C57BL × A)F1 hybrids (Old *et al.*, 1963b; Boyse *et al.*, 1963). The sera were found to be cytotoxic for cells of C57BL/6 radiation-induced leukemias. Normal tissue of C57BL/6 origin did not contain this antigen. On the other hand, the antigen was present in normal thymus cells of A mice. The authors proposed the name "thymus leukemia" (TL) for this antigen.

Since TL is apparently not determined by a virus it will be described only briefly.

On the basis of the presence or absence of TL, mouse strains may be classified as TL+ or TL−. Mice of TL+ strains have the antigen in the thymus; they cannot form TL antibody. Thymus leukemia is a leukemia-specific antigen in TL+ leukemias of TL− strains of mice. Genetic experiments have shown that TL is determined by a single dominant gene with its locus in linkage group IX in close proximity to the D end of the H-2ᵃ group of alleles (Boyse et al., 1964).

Thymus leukemia antigens can be extracted and purified by methods that have also been used for H-2 antigens. However, TL soluble antigen can be separated from H-2 soluble antigen by column chromatography (Davies et al., 1967).

The appearance of TL antigen in leukemias of TL− mice is regarded as a disturbance of the mechanisms normally controlling the expression of TL antigen. With regard to possible viral participation in expressing TL antigen, Boyse et al. (1966) reviewed their findings on TL antigen and stated that it would be necessary to resort to concepts such as viral integration to account for the inheritance in normal mice or to transduction to account for its appearance in leukemias of TL− mice. The possibility is considered that the normally inert gene of TL− strains could be activated by a product of the genome of certain leukemogenic viruses. These mechanisms, however, seem to be rather unlikely.

The outgrowth of TL+ leukemia cells is not inhibited in animals containing cytotoxic TL antibodies. During growth of TL+ leukemia cells in immunized mice, the antigen completely disappears, but it is fully restored after further passages in normal recipients. This phenomenon is termed "antigenic modulation." It is supposed that an adaptational change affecting the whole cell population is the basis of antigenic modulation. This phenomenon is also producible by passive immunization.

The apparently complex TL locus determines further antigenic specificities (Boyse et al., 1966). Except for the first TL component, which is termed TL 1, there are two other TL antigens, TL 2 and TL 3. All TL antibodies are present in C57BL immune serum against a spontaneous leukemia of the A strain. The TL 2 is demonstrable in the normal thymus of three TL 1− strains by the direct cytotoxic test with this immune serum absorbed in vivo in normal A mice. Antigens TL 2 and TL 3 have not yet been detected in leukemias of TL 2− or TL 3− strains. Thus, only TL 1 represents a leukemia-specific antigen in TL− mice.

X. Immunological Tolerance to Virus-Induced Surface Antigens

Immunological tolerance to virus-induced surface antigens is apparently an important precondition for the outgrowth and spreading of cells transformed to malignancy by leukemia viruses, i.e., generalization of leukemia depends on or is promoted by the host's tolerance to leukemia-specific antigens. This is evident at least in the case of viral leukemias having long latency periods such as Gross, Moloney, and Graffi leukemias. Adult mice infected with these viruses form antibodies against virus and virus-induced antigens, whereas generalized leukemia develops following infection of newborns when antibodies are absent. Newborn animals, however, are known to be most sensitive to tolerance induction if an antigen is present in an optimal concentration. Indeed, there are indications in the leukemia system that concentration of viral and virus-induced antigens increases within a short period after virus inoculation. It was found that Graffi virus rapidly spreads and multiplies in the newborns and that as early as 2 weeks after infection, virus-induced surface antigens were detectable in spleen cells (Pasternak and Pasternak, 1967).

Similar observations were made by Old et al. (1965) and Wahren (1966a,b) studying the distribution of Gross virus-induced antigens in preleukemic mice naturally infected with Gross virus. They found the antigens already present in lymphoid cells of 2-month-old animals which are still free from leukemia at this time (Section VI). These data, however, are not sufficient to postulate a state of immunological tolerance to virus-induced antigens in the animals.

Evidence of tolerance is obtained only if adult animals naturally or artificially infected as newborns are incapable of responding to retreatment with the antigen or the antigen-inducing agent. There are now a number of data obtained by transplantation as well as by serological studies showing the nonresponsiveness following infection of newborns.

A. TOLERANCE TO GROSS VIRUS-INDUCED ANTIGENS

In the Gross leukemia system, Axelrad (1963, 1965) demonstrated by the spleen colony method that reinoculation of virus extract into 3-week-old neonatally infected C3H mice failed to immunize against Gross lymphoma cells. There was an increase in the number of colonies per spleen after lymphoma cell inoculation as compared with immunized and even untreated animals of the same age. Inhibition of colony formation in untreated animals is attributed to the unimpaired defense mechanism of the host. As a consequence, a great number of inoculated lymphoma cells is destroyed. If the animals had been artificially rendered tolerant by neonatal infection, the majority of cells would have proliferated and produced colonies.

Tolerance was also found to be the cause of immunological unresponsiveness against lymphoma cells in AKR mice (Bubeník et al., 1964; Axelrad, 1965; Pasternak and Hölzer, 1965; Wahren, 1966a). Animals of this strain transfer Gross virus vertically to the offspring. Since they harbor the virus from embryonic life, tolerance can naturally develop to virus-induced antigens. Application of Gross virus extract into animals infected in this way is comparable with retreatment in the case of tolerant C3H mice.

In experiments of Bubeník *et al.* (1964), irradiated lymphoma tissue, repeated subthreshold doses of viable cells, cells lysed by distilled water, and cells killed with alcohol or formol were, indeed, incapable of producing even partial transplantation resistance against syngeneic AKR lymphoma cells. However, Gross virus-induced antigens were demonstrated in the lymphoma cells by the cytotoxic test with absorbed C57BL/6 and DBA 1 immune sera and by the passive transfer of resistance.

Axelrad (1965) was able to show that, with regard to spleen colony formation following intravenous inoculation of lymphoma cells, AKR mice behaved like tolerant C3H mice. The number of colonies in normal adult AKR could not be reduced by pretreatment with Gross virus extract prepared from C3H lymphomas or with an extract from spontaneous AKR lymphomas. Evidence of natural tolerance to Gross virus-induced antigens in AKR was obtained by testing the colony-forming efficiency of C3H Gross lymphoma cells in (AKR × C3H)F$_1$ hybrids. Like AKR mice, these hybrids harbor the Gross virus and, at a lower frequency, develop spontaneous leukemia. The C3H Gross lymphoma cells yielded more than 10 times as many colonies in the spleens of untreated hybrids than in the spleens of C3H hosts. Moreover, treatment of the hybrids with Gross virus extract before challenge with C3H lymphoma cells did not reduce the number of colonies. The number of colonies was also unchanged in hybrids which had been neonatally injected with Gross virus extract. In contrast, proliferation of C3H lymphoma cells was inhibited in normal as well as immunized C3H mice. From these data the conclusion was drawn that AKR mice and (AKR × C3H)F$_1$ hybrids are naturally tolerant to Gross virus-induced foreign antigens.

Lack of transplantation resistance against Gross lymphoma cells in AKR and certain F$_1$ hybrids was further shown by Pasternak and Hölzer (1965) and Pasternak (1967b). In some experiments, AKR lymphoma cells even grew better in animals pretreated with X-ray-killed lymphoma cells or subthreshold cell doses than in untreated controls. Immunological reactivity of the animals to Graffi virus-induced antigens, however, was normal and did not differ from that of other strains. Hence, syngeneic inocula of Graffi leukemia cells were rejected in Graffi-resistant AKR mice. Resistant animals also contained high amounts of Graffi-specific antibodies in their sera.

Absence of severe immunological deficiencies in AKR mice was also reported by Metcalf and Moulds (1967). They found a nearly normal hemaglutinin response in preleukemic AKR mice after immunization with sheep red cells. A general immunological depression is, therefore, not a prerequisite of leukemogenesis. On the other hand, passage lines of Gross virus may cause a defect in humoral and cellular immunity. Peterson *et al.* (1963) and Dent *et al.* (1965) have shown that 6-week-old C3H mice infected neonatally with Gross virus had a reduced antibody-forming capacity to T_2 bacteriophage and were unable to reject skin grafts across a weak histocompatibility barrier. The effects are apparently produced by an impairment of thymic function.

In our experiments, antigenicity of the AKR Gross lymphoma cells was detected by the passive transfer of resistance. After immunization of allogeneic recipients with Gross leukemia cells, immune sera could be obtained which after absorption of the H-2 activity *in vivo* produced a prolongation of the survival of AKR mice, which had been inoculated with Gross leukemia cells. Furthermore, the immunofluorescence test with C3H Gross immune sera demonstrated the presence of virus-induced surface antigens in AKR lymphoma cells.

Although the data are suggestive of immunological tolerance to Gross antigens in AKR mice, we do not know whether tolerance alone may also explain the unresponsiveness of the hybrids used. The female parents were from strains XVII and C57BL. Assuming the transmission of Gross virus by males is of minor importance, the hybrids could not have developed tolerance. The absence of significant amounts of virus is indicated by the fact that such animals have a very low incidence of spontaneous leukemia. Other virus assays have to be used, however, to verify the absence of virus in these hybrids. From this, it is not ruled out that genetic factors may determine the reactivity to Gross virus-induced antigens in AKR and AKR hybrids, also. It is interesting in this context that Aoki *et al.* (1966a) detected Gross-specific natural antibodies in the sera of (C57BL/6 × AKR)F_1 hybrids by the immunofluorescence technique.

Normal immunological reactivity of AKR mice to Graffi virus-induced leukemias, even of AKR origin, is evidence that Graffi and Gross antigens are different. However, it is thus far not known whether Graffi leukemias induced in AKR mice simultaneously contain Gross-specific antigens. In general, immunological tolerance is abrogated by adaptive immunization, i.e., by inoculation of immune cells into tolerant recipients. On the analogy of this finding, Spärck and Volkert (1965) tested the effect of immune cells on C3H mice neonatally infected with Gross virus. Immune cells were derived from spleens and lymph nodes of adult C3H mice which had been pretreated with leukemic extracts from AKA mice. For adoptive immunization, doses of 10^8 cells were injected into 1-month-old C3H mice injected at birth with the same AKA leukemic extract. Controls had received the leukemic extract at birth alone. In both groups, leukemic deaths occurred within 11 to 18 months after infection. However, the frequency of leukemia among treated mice was found to be less than one-eighth of the frequency among untreated mice. The data indicate that adoptive immunity can be established in the leukemia system. It would be of interest to know whether the activity of immune cells is directed against the virions or against antigens present in the membrane of infected cells.

Findings of Wahren (1966b) support the theory that adoptive immunity is possible in the mouse leukemia system. After injection of immunologically competent C3H lymph node cells every month into C3H mice which had received Gross virus at birth, the frequency of primary leukemias was found to decrease from 65 to 23%.

Wahren (for review, 1966c), furthermore, studied the state of immunological tolerance to Gross virus-induced antigens by serological methods. Thus, cytotoxic antibodies were occasionally detected in mice more than 1 year old, which had been neonatally infected with Gross virus (Wahren, 1964). Even preleukemic AKR mice were found to develop cytotoxic antibodies against Gross antigens (Wahren, 1966b). Antibodies did not appear until 2 months after birth. Activity of the sera was generally low when tested with sensitive target cells, but 25–28% of the animals had antibodies in their sera. The proportion of antibody-producing AKR mice could not be increased by repeated inoculations of tissues containing the G antigen.

As measured by the cytotoxic index, there was only a slight rise in antibody activity in positive mice. Cytotoxic antibodies were not detected in sera of AKR and C3H mice with manifest leukemia.

Most interesting is the fact that all animals ultimately developed leukemias, irrespective of whether cytotoxic antibodies had been found or not. Apparently, the amount of antigen in leukemic mice is so high that the relatively low immune response is overwhelmed.

With regard to the temporal presence of antibodies in infected mice it is suggested that there may be a state in which the amount of antigen is insufficient to maintain complete tolerance. Another possibility is that complete tolerance will not be obtained in every host, owing to biological variations in the sensitive age for tolerance induction (Wahren, 1966c). The latter explanation seems to be less likely.

In contrast to these findings Aoki et al. (1966a) did not detect antibodies in mice of strains with a high incidence of leukemia (G+ strains) by the immunofluorescence technique. However, normal serum antibody with specificity for the Gross antigen was found in some mice of strains with a low incidence of spontaneous leukemia. For example, older normal C57BL/6 and C57BL/6 hybrid mice frequently contained antibodies in their sera.

It is suggested on the basis of antibody distribution among mouse strains that the capacity to produce G antibody is important for the resistance of mice of certain genotypes to leukemia induction by naturally transmitted Gross virus. In mice of susceptible genotype, Gross virus replicates rapidly and, thus, it may induce immunological tolerance. Particularly, the H-2^{kk} genotype is known to be associated with high susceptibility to leukemia induction by Gross virus.

Presence of G antibody in mice of H-2^{bb} and H-2^{kb} genotypes, but not in mice of H-2^{kk}, is taken as indication that the differences in susceptibility to Gross viral leukemogenesis in relation to H-2 type have an immunological basis (Aoki et al., 1966a).

In summary, the majority of C3H mice neonatally infected with Gross virus is tolerant to Gross virus-induced antigens. Reinfection of adult mice failed to produce transplantation resistance against Gross lymphoma cells. Tolerance was also found to be the cause of immunological unresponsiveness against Gross lymphoma cells in AKR mice. The animals did not develop transplantation resistance. In general, mice of strains with a high incidence of leukemia do not contain Gross-specific antibodies in their sera, whereas antibodies are frequently present in mice of low-incidence strains. Immunological tolerance can be abolished by adoptive immunization.

B. Tolerance to Moloney Virus-Induced Antigens

By studying the antibody response in mice neonatally infected with Moloney virus, Klein and Klein (1965) found a high individual variation with regard to antibody appearance as compared with mice infected as adults which reacted promptly. Immunofluorescence tests between sera from individual mice and Moloney target cells were completely negative in some cases and, in others, the antibody response against Moloney antigens was considerably delayed.

Mice responding with high antibody levels showed a longer survival than poor antibody producers which developed leukemia earlier. In the latter, proliferation of cells is nearly uninhibited, whereas in the antibody-producing mice leukemia only develops after breakdown of the defense mechanism. The data indicate that the immunological state of the primary host influences the outgrowth and generalization of antigenic leukemia cells.

Antibody response of neonatally infected mice was also measured after a second virus challenge (Klein and Klein, 1966). All the nonreactive mice reinfected with Moloney virus failed to respond with detectable antibody formation as measured by the immunofluorescence test with Moloney target cells. There was a parallel lack of virus-neutralizing antibodies. The sera did not reduce the antibody-inducing capacity of standard virus-containing homogenates (positive MAP test), whereas Moloney immune sera neutralized this activity.

Neonatally infected mice lacking humoral antibodies did not reject small inocula of Moloney lymphomas. However, the grafts were rejected when the animals had antibodies at the time of tumor challenge.

The nonresponsiveness of neonatally infected mice after a second virus challenge is evidence of tolerance to Moloney virus-induced antigens. Immunological reactivity against unrelated antigens was not impaired as was shown by immunization with sheep red cells.

C. Tolerance to Graffi Virus-Induced Antigens

Immunizing treatment with an extract containing Graffi virus, although effective in control animals, failed to produce tumor-specific transplantation resistance in mice that had been infected with Graffi virus early in the postnatal period (Chieco-Bianchi et al., 1967). This result demonstrates that immunological tolerance plays a role in the Graffi leukemia system, too.

In relation to this problem the authors further tested the age-dependency of susceptibility to viral leukemogenesis. It is known that with increasing age mice are less susceptible to leukemia induction by Graffi virus (Graffi et al., 1956). Chieco-Bianchi et al. (1967) found that injection of virus on the first day after birth produced leukemia in 96% of the animals. Leukemia incidence decreased to about 12% after the virus had been injected into 15- or 20-day-old animals. If animals injected with virus at various ages between 1 and 37 days were inoculated with 1 million syngeneic leukemia cells at 45 days, only those mice that had received Graffi virus within the first week developed about 100% positive takes. With increasing age at virus injection, the percentage of positive takes decreased and reached almost zero in animals injected with virus after the third week of life. Development of tolerance or immunity to virus-induced antigens, in each case depending on the time of virus injection indicates that the age-dependency of susceptibility to viral leukemogenesis is an immunological phenomenon.

In the experiments of Chieco-Bianchi et al. (1967) the transfer of pre-immunized or normal spleen cells prevented or abolished tolerance to Graffi virus-induced antigens. Adoptive immunization was achieved after inoculation of 40 million spleen cells into 3- to 7-day-old mice infected with virus at birth. Challenge inoculation with leukemia cells at 6 to 8 weeks of age reduced the incidence of takes to 25% when the animals had received immune cells, and to 44% when the animals had been inoculated with immunologically competent normal cells.

In adult mice the incidence of primary Graffi leukemia is increased after X-irradiation (Graffi and Krischke, 1956). Apparently, the nonspecific suppression of immunological reactivity which is caused by this treatment favors the outgrowth of antigenic cells transformed to malignancy. Immunosuppressive drugs, although they show considerable differences with regard to the site of action, might have a similar influence on the development of leukemia. In addition to the nonspecific immunosuppression, tolerance could also be a promoting factor in viral leukemogenesis in adults.

Tolerance in adult rabbits after immunosuppressive drugs, simultaneously given with a protein antigen, has been reported by Schwarz (1966). It is assumed that the presence of antigen during regeneration of the drug-damaged lymphatic system is an important prerequisite to tolerance induction in adults.

In a first attempt to study the influence of immunosuppressive drugs on the immune response to virus-induced leukemia antigens, cyclophosphamide was given to mice inoculated as adults with Graffi virus-containing preparations (Pasternak, 1967e). The immune response to virus-induced antigens was measured by the graft rejection and by formation of antibodies reacting with the surface of leukemia cells (MAP test). Table XIII shows that Graffi leukemia cells grew progressively in untreated mice and in mice that had received an immunizing pretreatment in the presence of

TABLE XIII

INFLUENCE OF CYCLOPHOSPHAMIDE ON THE IMMUNE RESPONSE TO GRAFFI VIRUS-INDUCED ANTIGENS—SUPPRESSION OF GRAFFI VIRUS-INDUCED TRANSPLANTATION RESISTANCE

| | Growth of Graffi leukemia cells[c] | |
Immunizing pretreatment[a]	In cyclophosphamide-treated animals[b]	In immunized controls
X-ray-killed leukemic tissue preparation diluted 1:4 (0.3 ml. subcutaneously per animal)	5/5	1/5
Subthreshold dose of leukemia cells (10^7 cells subcutaneously)	5/5 15/15	0/5 3/15
Cell-free leukemia filtrate (0.1 ml. of 1:100 diluted filtrate intraperitoneally)	5/5	2/5
Untreated control	10/10	

[a] Graffi virus-containing preparations were inoculated 1 hour after the first injection with cyclophosphamide.

[b] Cyclophosphamide was injected intravenously in doses of 1.0 mg. per animal for 5 successive days. Four days after the final injection with cyclophosphamide the animals were subcutaneously challenged with 10^3 cells of Graffi leukemia L184/3a.

[c] Animals with progressively growing grafts per total number inoculated.

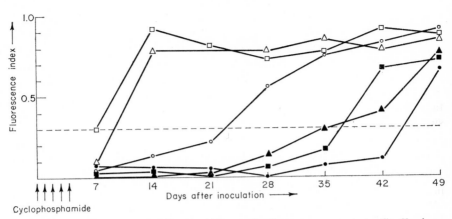

FIG. 4. Influence of cyclophosphamide on the immune response to Graffi virus-induced antigens. Delay of antibody appearance as measured by the mouse antibody production test. Antibody response after X-ray-killed leukemic tissue (filled triangles = cyclophosphamide, empty triangles = control group), subthreshold dose of leukemia cells (filled squares = cyclophosphamide, empty squares = control group), and cell-free leukemia filtrate (filled circles = cyclophosphamide, empty circles = control group). For dose and mode of inoculation, see Table XIII.

cyclophosphamide. In this experiment the drug was injected intravenously in doses of 1.0 mg. per animal for 5 successive days (total amount: 250 mg./kg. body weight). For mice of strain XVII this dose represents the upper limit of tolerance. Immediately after the first injection of cyclophosphamide, Graffi virus-containing preparations were given to the animals. By the ninth day the animals were challenged with 10^3 cells of Graffi leukemia L184/3a. In contrast to the cyclophosphamide-treated group, animals of the group injected with Graffi virus-containing preparations alone revealed a clear-cut resistance effect.

Data of the humoral antibody response of animal groups treated in the same way are presented in Fig. 4. Treatment with cyclophosphamide was found to produce a significant delay in antibody formation as measured by the immunofluorescence test. Whereas immunized controls had produced detectable antibodies at the latest 28 days after inoculation, the cyclophosphamide-treated groups were negative until the thirty-fifth day. Delay of antibody appearance is also demonstrable if cyclophosphamide is given 8 days after the immunizing injections. Thus, cyclophosphamide is active in the inductive as well as in the early productive phase of antibody formation. Although antibodies appeared with considerable delay, the mice were not tolerant to virus-induced antigens.

In summary, immunological tolerance to virus-induced antigens is a promoting factor in the leukemogenesis induced by certain viruses. Tolerance favors the outgrowth and generalization of malignant cells. This is applicable to the Gross, Moloney, and Graffi leukemias developing after infection of newborn mice. There are no indications, as yet, whether tolerance also plays a role in the leukemogenesis induced by Friend and Rauscher viruses which produce the disease in adult mice after short latency periods.

XI. Problems of Differentiation between Viral and New Cellular Antigens in Leukemia Cells

The hypothesis that virus-induced surface antigens of leukemia cells consist of both viral and new cellular antigens is based on the following facts: (1) Cells of primary and transplanted leukemias are continuously producing virus by budding it from the cell surface. During this process, viral antigens may represent an integral part of the membrane. (2) For a number of tumors induced by viruses other than leukemia viruses, evidence was obtained that the specific surface antigens of their cells are new cellular antigens unrelated to viral antigens. The tumors include those induced in mammalian species by Rous sarcoma virus which, like the murine leukemia viruses, contains RNA as genetic material. The general occurrence of new cellular antigens in a variety of viral neoplasms is suggestive of the presence of such antigens in virus-induced leukemia, too. It is hardly conceivable that leukemias occupy an exceptional position.

Persistence of virus in leukemia cells, however, renders the differentiation between these antigenic specificities more difficult. After immunization of mice with virus-containing leukemic preparations, anticellular as well as antiviral activities are demonstrable in the sera. Whereas antiviral activity that is measured by neutralization characterizes the antigen concerned, anticellular activity as measured by graft rejection, immunofluorescence, or cytotoxicity does not allow conclusions with regard to the nature of antigens participating in the reactions. Theoretically there are several chances to differentiate between these antigenic specificities at the surface of leukemia cells. (1) Immunization of mice with inactivated, but antigenically active, pure preparations of virus—inactivation would prevent infection of cells and thus induction of a new cellular antigen; then resulting antiviral antibodies could be tested for anticellular activities. Demonstration of viral antigens at the surface of leukemia cells, however, would not rule out the possibility that new cellular antigens are simultaneously present. (2) Immunization of mice with a virus-free viral leukemia—immune sera lacking virus-neutralizing antibodies but having anticellular activities would be applicable for the detection of new cellular antigens in infected cells. (3) Absorption of immune sera containing antiviral and anticellular activities with cells which contain viral antigens only—after removal of antiviral antibodies the serum could be tested for remaining anticellular activities. By separate measurement of viral and new cellular antigens the question might be answered whether the techniques hitherto used for the detection of virus-induced surface antigens measure the same or distinct antigenic specificities.

Antibody formation after administration of active and formalin-treated preparations of Graffi virus was tested by Pasternak (1965). Virus was isolated by fractionated centrifugation from the plasma of infected CBA mice. The sediment from the last centrifugation was suspended 10:1, corresponding to the starting amount of blood, in 0.05 M sodium citrate buffer, to attain a high virus concentration. Of this material, 0.1 ml. was injected intraperitoneally into C57BL mice. Other samples were treated with formalin at a final concentration of 1:500. After storage for 3 weeks at 2°C., 0.1 ml. of the material was injected intraperitoneally. Eight days after the injection of active virus, antibodies reacting with Graffi target cells in the immunofluorescence test were demonstrated in the serum. Formalin-treated material also induced formation of antibodies, but these were not demonstrable until the fifteenth day after injection. Moreover the fluorescence index was not as high as in the group that was inoculated with active virus. The data suggest that antigens present in the virion are located at the surface of leukemia cells, also. Apparently they are not antigens of the normal cell membrane since the immune sera contained no antibodies against spleen and lymph node cells of CBA mice which were used as virus donors. Therefore, the concentration, at least of H-2 substances present as contaminants in the virus preparations or as an integral part of the virus particle, seems to be below the concentration still capable of exerting an antigenic activity.

Absence of host cell components incorporated into the coat of the virus particles is also indicated by experiments of Klein and Klein (1964b). There was no detectable neutralizing effect after treatment of a Moloney virus homogenate with H-2 isoimmune serum against the virus–donor cell genotype. If normal host cell components are actually present in the virions, they certainly do not play a significant role in the neutralization reaction.

Sera that have been obtained after immunization of mice with formalin-treated Graffi virus and that react with leukemia cells seem to confirm the hypothesis that viral antigens appear at the cell membrane. However, it is not entirely ruled out that the immune response was caused by some active virus particles still capable of infecting the cells after incomplete formalin action. Here, the antibodies formed would be directed against antigens developing under the influence of virus infection.

In similar experiments, Wahren (1966c) studied the effects of serum from mice immunized with formalin-inactivated Friend plasma virus. The immune sera were found to be cytotoxic for Friend leukemia cells but not for lymph node cells of normal donors. In addition to this effect, virus-neutralizing activity was demonstrable. The sera prevented the development of Friend leukemia in newborn as well as in adult mice. Cytotoxic and neutralizing activity, however, was relatively low as compared with immune sera obtained by inoculation of animals with viable Friend cells. Both activities are assumed to be exerted by the same antibody. The fact that Friend virus pellets used for absorption reduced the cytotoxic activity to Friend cells whereas a plasma pellet from normal mice was ineffective is in line with this hypothesis. In accordance with the experiments with Graffi virus, it is not excluded that the immunizing effect of the formalin-treated material could have been caused by the presence of a few active virus particles. Another difficulty connected with virus immunization is the isolation of highly purified leukemia virus in sufficient quantity. After preparation of virus-containing fractions from tissue homogenates, cellular material is certainly present as a contaminant. Even after density gradient centrifugation of the material which accumulates the virus at a certain density, it is not possible to rule out the presence of some cellular material in the virus fraction (Wahren, 1966d). On the other hand, enrichment of virus from the plasma generally yields only low quantities. Inactivated fractions of tissue- or plasma-derived virus obtained by density gradient centrifugation have not yet been tested in immunological experiments. Considering the possibility that membrane antigens may be included in the virus envelope, it appears to be impossible to differentiate viral and new cellular antigens in leukemia cells in this way.

Immunization of mice with a virus-free viral leukemia would be another method to distinguish viral from cellular antigens, provided the cells are not capable of synthesizing antigens of the viral envelope. Most investigators failed to isolate such leukemia lines and, thus, they studied the problem by indirect methods. Klein et al. (1966b) were able to show that there is a rough parallelism between immunosensitivity of Moloney lymphoma cells in vivo and in vitro. As measured by immunofluorescence and absorption, immunosensitivity appeared to be related to the concentration of surface antigen. Contrary to this, the amount of infectious virus released from the lymphomas was independent of this surface concentration. Lymphomas, for example, having the same surface antigen concentration were found to release different amounts of virus. Although this indicates the presence of distinct antigens at the surface of leukemia cells, the authors conclude that the results do not critically distinguish between the possibility that cellular antigenicity is due to virus release or, alternatively, that a new cellular antigen appears independently of virus maturation. However, cellular antigenicity could be well explained by viral specificities if the quantity of membrane-bound viral antigens was unrelated to the amount of virus released.

Establishment of a nonvirus-producing Friend leukemia cell line, containing no demonstrable viral antigen, was reported by Oboshi *et al.* (1967). This line was obtained by serial transplantation of the cells into mice immunized with formalin-inactivated Friend virus. Absence of virus and viral antigens was concluded from the fact that inoculation of lysate of 2×10^7 cells per mouse failed to produce the disease and did not induce detectable neutralizing antibodies against Friend virus. Although cells of the virus-containing original Friend line were rejected in mice preimmunized with formalin-inactivated virus, the virus-free subline grew progressively in immunized as well as in control animals.

The data indicate that graft rejection against the original Friend line was caused by an antiviral immune response of the host and that cells of this line, therefore, contain viral antigens at their surface. Only cells lacking such antigens might grow in antivirus immune mice. The virus-free Friend subline apparently belongs to this cell type.

Although the mice immunized with virus-free Friend cells did not produce virus-neutralizing antibodies, they were resistant to Friend virus infection. Infected mice did not develop Friend leukemia. The authors interpret the findings by assuming the existence of a new cellular antigen unrelated to viral antigens in the virus-free Friend leukemia cells. Inhibition of the development of Friend disease is supposed to be due to the immune response against the new cellular antigens. Thus, all infected cells forming the antigen are immediately eliminated by the anticellular immune response without simultaneous presence of antiviral activities. It would be most important to know whether mice immunized with virus-free cells are also resistant to inoculation with virus-free Friend cells.

In virus-free Friend leukemia obtained by passage in virus immune mice the production of virus appears to be only temporarily suppressed. When serially transplanted into normal mice the cells began to produce virus again. The mechanism of viral suppression exerted by antiviral immunity is as yet unknown.

With regard to the presence of both viral and new cellular antigens the findings of Oboshi *et al.* (1967) are consistent with those published at the same time by Pasternak (1967d), although distinction of the antigenic specificities was obtained by different experimental conditions. In the Graffi leukemia system the possibility of distinguishing between viral and new cellular antigens was based on the hypothesis that certain cell types infected with the leukemia virus might produce virus or viral antigens but would be incapable of expressing the new cellular antigens. Antigens of the latter type were expected to occur preferably in leukemic cells and in cells of the hematopoietic system which are known to be sensitive to malignant transformation. If certain cells are carrying only viral antigens they could be used for the absorption of immune sera containing both antiviral and

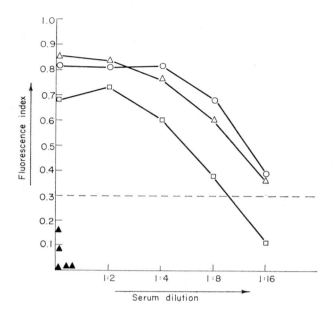

Fig. 5. Titration of a Graffi immune serum pool using L 414/2a Graffi chloroleukemia cells as targets. Results of the indirect fluorescent antibody test. Graffi immune serum pool: circles = unabsorbed; empty triangles = absorbed with normal spleen and lymph node cells; squares = absorbed with Landschütz sarcoma I cells; filled triangles = absorbed with L 414/2a leukemia cells (Pasternak, 1967d).

anticellular activities. To verify the independence of both antigenic specificities, anticellular activity must still be present in absorbed sera.

Landschütz sarcoma I cells, which naturally harbor the Graffi virus, were found to be resistant to the specific rejection response of Graffi-resistant animals *in vivo* and to cytotoxic antibodies *in vitro*. These cells, however, reveal a weak but distinct membrane fluorescence in the immuno-fluorescence test with Graffi hyperimmune sera. Provided the positive fluorescence reaction with sarcoma cells is solely the result of the presence of virus or viral antigens on the cell surface, then absorption with the cells would eliminate antiviral antibodies from Graffi immune sera.

For absorption, usually 0.1-ml. samples of Graffi immune serum were added to cell pellets containing 80 million living cells. The mixture was then incubated for 60 minutes at 37°C. After centrifugation the supernatant serum was again absorbed with another pellet of sarcoma cells. This serum was then tested against Graffi target cells using the immunofluorescence test. Its virus-neutralizing capacity was subjected to the MAP test.

Figure 5 shows that the titer of the immune serum, as measured by the

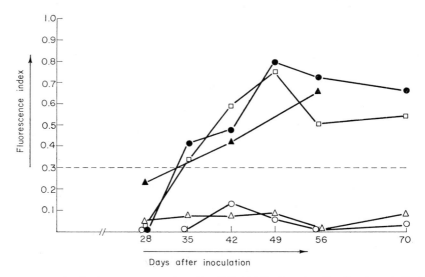

Fig. 6. Antibody response against Graffi L 414/2a target cells after inoculation of adult XVII/Bln mice with a cell-free Graffi leukemia filtrate incubated with absorbed and unabsorbed Graffi immune serum *in vitro*. Antibody response after inoculation of filtrate plus unabsorbed Graffi immune serum (empty circles); plus Graffi immune serum absorbed with normal spleen and lymph node cells (empty triangles); plus Graffi immune serum absorbed with Landschütz sarcoma I cells (empty squares); plus Graffi immune serum absorbed with L 414/2a leukemia cells (filled triangles); plus normal mouse serum (filled circles) (Pasternak, 1967d).

FI, did not decrease after two control absorptions with normal spleen and lymph node cells and decreased only slightly after absorption with Sarcoma I cells. Antibodies were completely eliminated, however, after absorption with Graffi leukemia cells.

The results of the virus neutralization test are shown in Fig. 6. Absorbed and unabsorbed serum samples to be tested for virus-neutralizing antibodies were mixed at a ratio of 10:1 with a cell-free Graffi leukemia filtrate diluted 1:100 (w/v). After 60 minutes incubation at 37°C., 0.2-ml. samples of the mixtures, containing cell-free filtrate at a final dilution of 1:1000, were injected intraperitoneally into adult mice. Humoral antibody response was controlled weekly by the immunofluorescence test. It was found that the serum absorbed with Sarcoma I cells had lost its virus-neutralizing activity although antibodies against surface antigens of leukemia cells were still present. However, the leukemia cells absorbed both virus-neutralizing and anticellular antibodies. The conclusion was drawn that virus-induced surface antigens of leukemia cells appear to consist of viral and new cellular antigens, whereas Sarcoma I cells only contain virus or viral antigens.

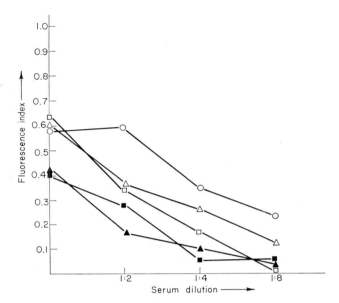

Fig. 7. Titration of a Graffi immune serum pool by use of the indirect immuno-fluorescence test. Absorbed and unabsorbed serum samples were tested for the presence of antibodies reacting with the surface of Graffi leukemia cells. Symbols: empty circles = unabsorbed; empty squares = absorbed with homogenate from sarcoma UV 14306; empty triangles = absorbed with homogenate from sarcoma MC 11504; filled squares = absorbed with Graffi virus-infected sarcoma UVGr 14306; filled triangles = absorbed with Graffi virus-infected sarcoma MCGr 11504.

The finding that certain cells may contain viral antigen only was confirmed by another series of experiments using sarcomas artificially infected with Graffi virus (L. Pasternak and G. Pasternak, 1968b). Unlike previous absorptions, however, the sediments of tissue homogenates served as material for absorption. Results of the experiments are presented in Figs. 7 and 8. Although antibodies reacting with Graffi leukemia cells were still present in immune sera absorbed with the Graffi virus-infected UV and methylcholanthrene-induced (MC) sarcomas, the sera no longer neutralized the antibody inducing capacity of a cell-free Graffi leukemia filtrate. Antibodies appeared even earlier than in the animal group inoculated with leukemia filtrate plus normal serum, indicating a higher amount of virus in the former groups. This is probably due to residual virus present in those serum samples that were absorbed with virus-containing tissue sediment. In other words, centrifugation to eliminate the tissue sediment was not sufficient for the complete removal of virus. After addition of the cell-free filtrate, virus concentration was thus higher in such samples than in the sample containing cell-free filtrate plus normal serum. Homogenates

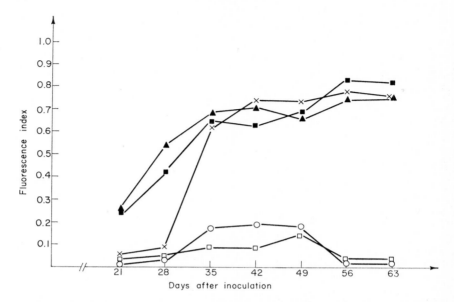

FIG. 8. Antibody response against Graffi target cells after inoculation of mice with a cell-free Graffi leukemia filtrate incubated with absorbed and unabsorbed Graffi immune serum *in vitro*. Antibody response after inoculation of filtrate plus unabsorbed Graffi immune serum (empty circles); plus Graffi immune serum absorbed with homogenate from sarcoma UV 14306 (empty squares); plus Graffi immune serum absorbed with homogenate from Graffi virus-infected sarcoma UVGr 14306 (filled squares); plus Graffi immune serum absorbed with homogenate from Graffi virus-infected sarcoma MCGr 11504 (filled triangles); plus normal mouse serum (crosses).

prepared from the uninfected UV sarcoma did not remove antibodies from the Graffi immune serum.

Differentiation between viral and new cellular surface antigens inducible by leukemia viruses is a prerequisite for their quantitative determination and for the elucidation of the problem whether the variety of *in vivo* and *in vitro* techniques used for the demonstration of virus-induced surface antigens measures the same or different antigenic specificities. Experiments are in progress to examine these possibilities.

More information is required with regard to qualitative and quantitative differences in the synthesis of virus and virus-induced antigens in various cell types including those superinfected with an unrelated leukemia virus. Investigations in this field are most important to the understanding of the process of viral leukemogenesis. The murine leukemia system is finally considered a model for the elaboration of tests applicable to the search for antigens in human leukemia. First findings obtained with the Burkitt lymphoma are encouraging. It remains to be seen whether a similar phenomenon may be detected in other types of human leukemia.

REFERENCES

Aoki, T., Boyse, E. A., and Old, L. J. 1966a. *Cancer Res.* **26**, 1415–1419.
Aoki, T., Old, L. J., and Boyse, E. A. 1966b. *Natl. Cancer Inst. Monograph* **22**, 449–457.
Axelrad, A. A. 1963. *Nature* **199**, 80–83.
Axelrad, A. A. 1965. *Progr. Exptl. Tumor Res.* **6**, 30–83.
Axelrad, A. A., and Steeves, R. A. 1964. *Virology* **24**, 513–518.
Barski, G., and Youn, J. K. 1965. *Science* **149**, 751–752.
Barski, G., and Youn, J. K. 1966. *Natl. Cancer Inst. Monograph* **22**, 659–669.
Bauer, H., and Schäfer, W. 1966. *Virology* **29**, 494–496.
Bianco, A. R., Glynn, J. P., and Goldin, A. 1966. *Cancer Res.* **26**, 1722–1728.
Boyse, E. A., Old, L. J., and Stockert, E. 1962. *Ann. N. Y. Acad. Sci.* **99**, 574–587.
Boyse, E. A., Old, L. J., and Luell, S. 1963. *J. Natl. Cancer Inst.* **31**, 987–995.
Boyse, E. A., Old, L. J., and Luell, S. 1964. *Nature* **201**, 779.
Boyse, E. A., Old, L. J., and Stockert, E. 1966. *Immunopathol., 4th Intern. Symp. Monte Carlo, 1965.* pp. 23–40.
Breyere, E. J., and Williams, L. B. 1964. *Science* **146**, 1055–1056.
Breyere, E. J., Moloney, J. B., and Jordan, W. P. 1966. *J. Natl. Cancer Inst.* **37**, 699–705.
Brown, E. R., Buinauskas, P., and Schwartz, S. O. 1966a. *J. Bacteriol.* **92**, 978–982.
Brown, E. R., Buinauskas, P., and Schwartz, S. O. 1966b. *Experientia* **22**, 687.
Bruce, W. R., and van der Gaag, H. 1963. *Nature* **199**, 79–80.
Bryan, W. R. 1957. *Ann. N. Y. Acad. Sci.* **69**, 698–728.
Bubeník, J., and Koldovský, P. 1964. *Folia Biol. (Prague)* **10**, 427–442.
Bubeník, J., and Koldovský, P. 1965. *Folia Biol. (Prague)* **11**, 258–265.
Bubeník, J., Adamcová, B., and Koldovský, P. 1964. *Folia Biol. (Prague)* **10**, 293–300.
Buffett, R. F., Grace, J. T., and Mirand, E. A. 1963. *Proc. Am. Assoc. Cancer Res.* **4**, 8.
Celada, F., and Rotman, B. 1967. *Proc. Natl. Acad. Sci. U.S.* **57**, 630–636.
Chieco-Bianchi, L., Fiore-Donati, L., Tridente, G., and Pennelli, N. 1967. *Nature* **214**, 1227–1228.
Dalton, A. J. 1966. *Natl. Cancer Inst. Monograph* **22**, 143–167.
Davies, D. A. L., Boyse, E. A., Old, L. J., and Stockert, E. 1967. *J. Exptl. Med.* **125**, 549–558.
Defendi, V. 1963. *Proc. Soc. Exptl. Biol. Med.* **113**, 12–16.
Dent, P. B., Peterson, R. D. A., and Good, R. A. 1965. *Proc. Soc. Exptl. Biol. Med.* **119**, 869–871.
Dirlugyan, R. P., and Stepina, V. N. 1966. *Vestn. Akad. Med. Nauk SSSR* **9**, 7–12.
Dirlugyan, R. P., and Stepina, V. N. 1967. *Folia Biol. (Prague)* **13**, 136–142.
Dougherty, R. M. 1964. *In "Techniques in Experimental Virology"* (R. J. C. Harris, ed.), pp. 169–223. Academic Press, New York.
Duc-Nguyen, H., Rosenblum, E. N., and Zeigel, R. F. 1966. *J. Bacteriol.* **92**, 1133–1140.
Duesberg, P. H., and Robinson, W. S. 1966. *Proc. Natl. Acad. Sci. U.S.* **55**, 219–227.
Ellem, K. A. O. 1958. *Cancer Res.* **18**, 1179–1185.
Fefer, A., McCoy, J. L., and Glynn, J. P. 1967a. *Cancer Res.* **27**, 962–967.
Fefer, A., McCoy, J. L., and Glynn, J. P. 1967b. *Cancer Res.* **27**, 1626–1631.
Fefer, A., McCoy, J. L., and Glynn, J. P. 1967c. *Intern. J. Cancer* **2**, 647–650.
Fey, F., and Graffi, A. 1958. *Naturwissenschaften* **45**, 471.
Fieldsteel, A. H., Dawson, P. J., and Bostick, W. L. 1961. *Proc. Soc. Exptl. Biol. Med.* **108**, 826–829.
Fieldsteel, A. H., Dawson, P. J., and Scholler, J. 1966. *J. Natl. Cancer Inst.* **36**, 71–80.
Fink, M. A., and Cowles, C. A. 1965. *Science* **150**, 1723–1725.
Fink, M. A., and Malmgren, R. A. 1963. *J. Natl. Cancer Inst.* **31**, 1111–1121.

96 G. PASTERNAK

Fink, M. A., and Rauscher, F. J. 1964. *J. Natl. Cancer Inst.* **32**, 1075–1082.
Fink, M. A., Malmgren, R. A., Rauscher, F. J., Orr, H. C., and Karon, M. 1964. *J. Natl. Cancer Inst.* **33**, 581–588.
Fink, M. A., Karon, M., Rauscher, F. J., Malmgren, R. A., and Orr, H. C. 1965. *Cancer* **18**, 1317–1321.
Fink, M. A., Cowles, C. A., and Chirigos, M. A. 1966. *Natl. Cancer Inst. Monograph* **22**, 439–447.
Friend, C. 1956. *Proc. Am. Assoc. Cancer Res.* **2**, 106.
Friend, C. 1957. *J. Exptl. Med.* **105**, 307–318.
Friend, C. 1959. *J. Exptl. Med.* **109**, 217–228.
Galibert, F., Bernard, C., Chenaille, P., and Boiron, M. 1966. *Nature* **209**, 680–682.
Geering, G., Old, L. J., and Boyse, E. A. 1966. *J. Exptl. Med.* **124**, 753–772.
Gerber, P., and Birch, S. M. 1967. *Proc. Natl. Acad. Sci. U.S.* **58**, 478–484.
Gerber, P., O'Connor, T. E., and Birch, S. M. 1966. *Science* **152**, 1074–1075.
Glynn, J. P., Bianco, A. R., and Goldin, A. 1964. *Cancer Res.* **24**, 502–508.
Goodman, H. S. 1961. *Nature* **190**, 269–270.
Gorer, P. A., and O'Gorman, P. 1956. *Transplant. Bull.* **3**, 142–143.
Graffi, A., and Fey, F. 1955. *Naturwissenschaften* **42**, 652.
Graffi, A., and Gimmy, J. 1958. *Z. Ges. Inn. Med. Ihre Grenzgebiete* **13**, 881–884.
Graffi, A., and Krischke, W. 1956. *Naturwissenschaften* **43**, 333.
Graffi, A., and Schramm, T. 1963. *Acta Biol. Med. Ger.* **11**, 929–933.
Graffi, A., Bielka, H., Fey, F., Scharsach, F., and Weiss, R. 1954. *Naturwissenschaften* **41**, 503–504.
Graffi, A., Bielka, H., and Fey, F. 1956. *Acta Haematol.* **15**, 145–174.
Graffi, A., Fey, F., Hoffmann, F., and Krischke, W. 1957. *Klin. Wochschr.* **35**, 465–468.
Graffi, A., Gimmy, J., and Fey, F. 1962. *Acta Biol. Med. Ger.* **9**, 280–292.
Gross, L. 1951. *Proc. Soc. Exptl. Biol. Med.* **76**, 27–32.
Gross, L. 1961. "Oncogenic Viruses." Macmillan (Pergamon), New York.
Habel, K. 1961. *Proc. Soc. Exptl. Biol. Med.* **106**, 722–725.
Habel, K., and Eddy, B. E. 1963. *Proc. Soc. Exptl. Biol. Med.* **113**, 1–4.
Haguenau, F. 1966. *Rev. Franc. Etudes Clin. Biol.* **11**, 969–986.
Hall, W. T., Andresen, W. F., Sanford, K. K., Evans, V. J., and Hartley, J. W. 1967. *Science* **156**, 85–88.
Hamburg, V. P., and Svet-Moldavsky, G. J. 1964. *Nature* **203**, 772–773.
Hartley, J. W., and Rowe, W. P. 1966. *Proc. Natl. Acad. Sci. U.S.* **55**, 780–786.
Hartley, J. W., Rowe, W. P., Capps, W. I., and Huebner, R. J. 1965. *Proc. Natl. Acad. Sci. U.S.* **53**, 931–938.
Harvey, J. J. 1964. *Nature* **204**, 1104–1105.
Haughton, G. 1965. *Science* **147**, 506–507.
Hellström, I. 1965. *Nature* **208**, 652–653.
Hellström, K. E., and Möller, G. 1965. *Progr. Allergy* **9**, 158–245.
Huebner, R. J., Hartley, J. W., Rowe, W. P., Lane, W. T., and Capps, W. I. 1966. *Proc. Natl. Acad. Sci. U.S.* **56**, 1164–1169.
Ichikawa, Y., and Notake, K. 1962. *Ann. Rept. Inst. Virus Res., Kyoto Univ.* **5**, 103–117.
Jakobsson, S., and Wahren, B. 1965. *Exptl. Cell Res.* **37**, 509–515.
Jenkins, V. K., and Upton, A. C. 1963. *Cancer Res.* **23**, 1748–1755.
Kaliss, N. 1965. *Federation Proc.* **24**, 1024–1029.
Klein, E., and Klein, G. 1964a. *J. Natl. Cancer Inst.* **32**, 547–568.
Klein, E., and Klein, G. 1964b. *Nature* **204**, 339–342.
Klein, E., and Klein, G. 1965. *Cancer Res.* **25**, 851–854.

Klein, E., and Klein, G. 1966. *Nature* **209**, 163–165.
Klein, G., and Klein, E. 1964. *Science* **145**, 1316–1317.
Klein, G. Sjögren, H. O., and Klein, E. 1962. *Cancer Res.* **22**, 955–961.
Klein, G., Clifford, P., Klein, E., and Stjernswärd, J. 1966a. *Proc. Natl. Acad. Sci. U.S.* **55**, 1628–1635.
Klein, G., Klein, E., and Haughton, G. 1966b. *J. Natl. Cancer Inst.* **36**, 607–621.
Kobayashi, H., and Takeda, K. 1967. *Gann* **58**, 25–30.
Kobayashi, H., Kodama, T., and Takeda, K. 1966. *Nature* **212**, 1260.
Kobayashi, H., Takeda, K., Kodama, T., and Itoh, T. 1967. *Z. Krebsforsch.* **69**, 10–18.
Koch, M. A., and Sabin, A. B. 1963. *Proc. Soc. Exptl. Biol. Med.* **113**, 4–12.
Koldovský, P., and Bubeník, J. 1964. *Folia Biol. (Prague)* **10**, 81–89.
Lieberman, M., and Kaplan, H. S. 1959. *Science* **130**, 387–388.
Maruyama, K., and Oboshi, S. 1967. *Gann* **58**, 89–93.
Mayyasi, S. A., Schidlovsky, G., and Bulfone, L. M. 1965. *Virology* **27**, 431–434.
Mayyasi, S. A., Schidlovsky, G., Bulfone, M., and Clifford, N. L. 1966. *Natl. Cancer Inst. Monograph* **22**, 379–387.
Mazurenko, N. P. 1960. *Vopr. Onkol.* **6**, 76–83.
Metcalf, D., and Moulds, R. 1967. *Intern. J. Cancer* **2**, 53–58.
Micheel, B., and Pasternak, G. 1968a. *Arch. Geschwulstforsch.* **31**, 123–132.
Micheel, B., and Pasternak, G. 1968b. *Intern. J. Cancer* **3**, 603–613.
Möller, G. 1961. *J. Exptl. Med.* **114**, 415–434.
Möller, G. 1965. *Nature* **204**, 846–847.
Moloney, J. B. 1959. *Proc. Am. Assoc. Cancer Res.* **3**, 44.
Moloney, J. B. 1960. *J. Natl. Cancer Inst.* **24**, 933–951.
Moloney, J. B. 1962. *Federation Proc.* **21**, 19–31.
Moloney, J. B. 1966. *Natl. Cancer Inst. Monograph* **22**, 139–141.
Mora, P. T., McFarland, V. W., and Luborsky, S. W. 1966. *Proc. Natl. Acad. Sci. U.S.* **55**, 438–445.
Nowinski, R. C., Old, L. J., Moore, D. H., Geering G., and Boyse, E. A. 1967. *Virology* **31**, 1–14.
Oboshi, S., Itakura, K., and Maruyama, K. 1967. *Gann* **58**, 367–376.
Old, L. J., and Boyse, E. A. 1964. *Ann. Rev. Med.* **15**, 167–186.
Old, L. J., and Boyse, E. A. 1965. *Federation Proc.* **24**, 1009–1017.
Old, L. J., Boyse, E. A., and Lilly, F. 1963a. *Cancer Res.* **23**, 1063–1068.
Old, L. J., Boyse, E. A., and Stockert, E. 1963b. *J. Natl. Cancer Inst.* **31**, 977–986.
Old, L. J., Boyse, E. A., and Stockert, E. 1964. *Nature* **201**, 777–779.
Old, L. J., Boyse, E. A., and Stockert, E. 1965. *Cancer Res.* **25**, 813–819.
Old, L. J., Boyse, E. A., Oettgen, H. F., de Harven, E., Geering, G., Williamson, B., and Clifford, P. 1966. *Proc. Natl. Acad. Sci. U.S.* **56**, 1699–1704.
Old, L. J., Stockert, E., Boyse, E. A., and Geering, G. 1967. *Proc. Soc. Exptl. Biol. Med.* **124**, 63–68.
Osato, T., Mirand, E. A., and Grace, J. T. 1965. *Proc. Soc. Exptl. Biol. Med.* **119**, 1187–1191.
Pasternak, G. 1965. *J. Natl. Cancer Inst.* **34**, 71–83.
Pasternak, G. 1966. *In* "Comparative Leukemia Research," Wenner-Gren Center Intern. Symp. Ser. (G. Winqvist, ed.), Vol. 6, pp. 157–160. Macmillan (Pergamon), New York.
Pasternak, G. 1967a. *Z. Versuchstierkunde* **9**, 114–123.
Pasternak, G. 1967b. *In* "Specific Tumour Antigens," UICC Monograph (R. J. C. Harris, ed.), Vol. 2, pp. 86–96. Munksgaard, Copenhagen.

Pasternak, G. 1967c. *Arch. Geschwulstforsch.* **29,** 113–141.
Pasternak, G. 1967d. *Nature* **214,** 1364–1365.
Pasternak, G. 1967e. *Proc. 5th Intern. Congr. Chemotherapy, Vienna* pp. 313–315.
Pasternak, G. 1969. *Folia Haematol.* **91,** 266–269.
Pasternak, G., and Graffi, A. 1963. *Brit. J. Cancer* **17,** 532–539.
Pasternak, G., and Hölzer, B. 1965. *Neoplasma* **12,** 339–355.
Pasternak, G., and Pasternak, L. 1967. *J. Natl. Cancer Inst.* **38,** 157–168.
Pasternak, G., and Pasternak, L. 1968. *Folia Biol. (Prague)* **14,** 43–47.
Pasternak, G., Horn, K.-H., and Graffi, A. 1962. *Acta Biol. Med. Ger.* **9,** 314–317.
Pasternak, G., Graffi, A., and Horn, K.-H. 1964. *Acta Biol. Med. Ger.* **13,** 276–279.
Pasternak, G., Fey, F., Pasternak, L., and Hölzer, B. 1967. *Z. Krebsforsch.* **69,** 297–306.
Pasternak, L., and Pasternak, G. 1968a. *Arch. Geschwulstforsch.* **31,** 243–251.
Pasternak, L., and Pasternak, G. 1968b. *Arch. Geschwulstforsch.* **32,** 301–308.
Peterson, R. D. A., Hendrickson, R., and Good, R. A. 1963. *Proc. Soc. Exptl. Biol. Med.* **114,** 517–520.
Pinkel, D., Yoshida, K., and Smith, K. 1966. *Natl. Cancer Inst. Monograph* **22,** 671–682.
Pluznik, D. H., and Sachs, L. 1964. *J. Natl. Cancer Inst.* **33,** 535–546.
Prigozhina, E. L. 1962. *Vopr. Onkol.* **7,** 19–26.
Prigozhina, E. L., and Stavrovskaja, A. A. 1964. *Nature* **201,** 934–936.
Rauscher, F. J. 1962. *J. Natl. Cancer Inst.* **29,** 515–543.
Rich, M. A. 1966. *Natl. Cancer Inst. Monograph* **22,** 425–437.
Rich, M. A., Geldner, J., Johns, L. W., Kalocsky, M., Meyers, P., Rothstein, E. L., Siegler, R., and Gershon-Cohen, J. 1963. *Trans. N. Y. Acad. Sci.* **25,** 580–589.
Rich, M. A., Geldner, J., and Meyers, P. 1965. *J. Natl. Cancer Inst.* **35,** 523–536.
Rowe, W. P., and Brodsky, I. 1959. *J. Natl. Cancer Inst.* **23,** 1239–1248.
Rowe, W. P., Hartley, J. W., and Capps, W. I. 1966. *Natl. Cancer Inst. Monograph* **22,** 15–19.
Sachs, L. 1962. *J. Natl. Cancer Inst.* **29,** 759–764.
Sarma, P. S., Turner, H. C., and Huebner, R. J. 1964. *Virology* **23,** 313–321.
Sarma, P. S., Cheong, M. P., Hartley, J. W., and Huebner, R. J. 1967. *Virology* **33,** 180–184.
Schoolman, H. M., Spurrier, W., Schwartz, S. O., and Szanto, P. B. 1957. *Blood* **12,** 694–700.
Schramm, T., and Graffi, A. 1963. *Acta Biol. Med. Ger.* **11,** 934–936.
Schwarz, R. S. 1966. *Federation Proc.* **25,** 165–168.
Shershulskaya, L. V., and Ievleva, E. S. 1964. *Vestn. Akad. Med. Nauk SSSR* **11,** 46–50.
Simons, P. J., Bassin, R. H., and Harvey, J. J. 1967. *Proc. Soc. Exptl. Biol. Med.* **125,** 1242–1246.
Sinkovics, J. G., Bertin, B. A., and Howe, C. D. 1966. *Natl. Cancer Inst. Monograph* **22,** 349–367.
Sinkovics, J. G., Pienta, R. J., Fiorentino, M. and Bertin, B. A. 1967. *Cancer Res.* **27,** 88–98.
Sjögren, H. O. 1961. *Virology* **15,** 214–219.
Sjögren, H. O. 1964a. *J. Natl. Cancer Inst.* **32,** 361–374.
Sjögren, H. O. 1964b. *J. Natl. Cancer Inst.* **32,** 645–659.
Sjögren, H. O. 1965. *Progr. Exptl. Tumor Res.* **6,** 289–322.
Sjögren, H. O. 1966. *Ann. Med. Exptl. Biol. Fenniae (Helsinki)* **44,** 227–231.
Sjögren, H. O., and Hellström, I. 1965. *Exptl. Cell Res.* **40,** 208–212.
Sjögren, H. O., and Hellström, I. 1967. *In* "Specific Tumour Antigens," UICC Monograph (R. J. C. Harris, ed.), Vol. 2, pp. 162–170. Munksgaard, Copenhagen.

Sjögren, H. O., and Jonsson, N. 1963. *Exptl. Cell Res.* **32**, 618–621.
Sjögren, H. O., Hellström, I., and Klein, G. 1961. *Exptl. Cell Res.* **23**, 204–208.
Sjögren, H. O., Minowada, J., and Ankerst, J. 1967. *J. Exptl. Med.* **125**, 689–701.
Slettenmark, B., and Klein, E. 1962. *Cancer Res.* **22**, 947–954.
Spärck, J. V., and Volkert, M. 1965. *Nature* **206**, 578–579.
Steeves, R. A., and Axelrad, A. A. 1967. *Intern. J. Cancer* **2**, 235–244.
Stepina, V. N., Mazurenko, N. P., and Zueva, Y. N. 1966. *Neoplasma* **13**, 353–360.
Stück, B., Old, L. J., and Boyse, E. A. 1964a. *Proc. Natl. Acad. Sci. U.S.* **52**, 950–958.
Stück, B., Old, L. J., and Boyse, E. A. 1964b. *Nature* **202**, 1016–1018.
Stück, B., Boyse, E. A., Old, L. J., and Carswell, E. A. 1964c. *Nature* **203**, 1033–1034.
Svet-Moldavsky, G. J., and Hamburg, V. P. 1964. *Nature* **202**, 303–304.
Svet-Moldavsky, G. J., Mkheidze, D. M., and Liozner, A. L. 1967. *J. Natl. Cancer Inst.* **38**, 933–938.
Tennant, J. R. 1962. *J. Natl. Cancer Inst.* **28**, 1291–1303.
Ting, R. C. 1966. *Virology* **28**, 783–785.
Trentin, J. J., and Bryan, E. 1966. *Proc. Soc. Exptl. Biol. Med.* **121**, 1216–1219.
Wahren, B. 1963. *J. Natl. Cancer Inst.* **31**, 411–423.
Wahren, B. 1964. *Cancer Res.* **24**, 906–914.
Wahren, B. 1965. *Nature* **205**, 409–410.
Wahren, B. 1966a. *Intern. J. Cancer* **1**, 41–50.
Wahren, B. 1966b. *Exptl. Cell Res.* **42**, 230–242.
Wahren, B. 1966c. Ph. D. Thesis, Karolinska Inst., Stockholm.
Wahren, B. 1966d. *Intern. J. Cancer* **1**, 161–168.
Wigzell, H. 1965. *Transplantation* **3**, 423–431.
Wright, B. S., and Lasfargues, J. C. 1965. *J. Natl. Cancer Inst.* **35**, 319–327.
Wright, B. S., and Lasfargues, J. C. 1966. *Natl. Cancer Inst. Monograph* **22**, 685–700.
Yumoto, T., Recher, L., Sykes, J. A., and Dmochowski, L. 1966. *Natl. Cancer Inst. Monograph* **22**, 107–141.
Zeigel, R. F., and Rauscher, F. J. 1964. *J. Natl. Cancer Inst.* **32**, 1277–1307.
Zueva, Y. N. 1964. *Vestn. Akad. Med. Nauk SSSR* **11**, 51–54.
Zueva, Y. N. 1967. *Folia Biol. (Prague)* **13**, 343–349.

IMMUNOLOGICAL ASPECTS OF CARCINOGENESIS BY DEOXYRIBONUCLEIC ACID TUMOR VIRUSES

G. I. Deichman

Institute of Experimental and Clinical Oncology, Academy of Medical Sciences,
Moscow, U.S.S.R.

I. Introduction

Specific immunization against tumors seems to be one of the most popular and stable ideas for the practical solution of the cancer problem. Sixty or seventy years ago this idea was based on vague associations between infectious and oncological diseases. Much later several ribonucleic acid (RNA)- and deoxyribonucleic acid (DNA)-containing viruses inducing cancer in animals were isolated, and some attempts to use virus-neutralizing sera or active immunization for the therapy of experimentally induced or spontaneous tumors were made without success. However, at the same time, studies of transplantation immunity and the use of inbred animals paved the way for the next essential step, when the existence of specific immunological defense of the organism against syngeneic or autochthonous

101

tumors induced by chemical carcinogens was revealed (Foley, 1953; Prehn and Main, 1957; Revesz, 1960; Klein *et al.*, 1960). Thus, the presence of tumor-specific transplantation antigens (TSTA), distinct from isoantigens and responsible for antitumor immunity, was established.

Ten years ago, discussing the problem of specific antigens in tumors of viral origin, Zilber (1958) emphasized the significance of some questions concerning the problem, such as the possible cell or viral nature of specific tumor antigens, and the time of their appearance in the course of carcinogenesis. Later, for tumors induced by DNA-containing viruses these antigens were found to be distinct from the structural viral proteins, though their specificity and synthesis were found to be determined by the corresponding oncogenic virus (Habel, 1961, 1962a; Sachs, 1961; Sjögren *et al.*, 1961; Sjögren, 1961). In contrast to the tumors induced by chemical carcinogens, the cells of virus-induced tumors contain apparently similar or identical TSTA in all cells transformed by the same virus, independent of the host species or histopathology of the tumor. When the presence of common specific antigens was established in virus-induced tumors, they were defined as "tumor-specific." At present, it is obvious that apparently indistinguishable antigens are also produced during the early stages of abortive or acute infection of cells with DNA tumor viruses. The significance of these data for epidemological and immunological studies in viral oncology can hardly be exaggerated.

The appearance of TSTA in cells infected by DNA tumor viruses can be analyzed in two ways. One aspect concerns the relationship between virus and cell and is connected with the following general question: What relationship exists between the appearance of TSTA in infected cells and viral-induced cell transformation? The other aspect concerns the conditions under which the growth of virus-transformed cells bearing TSTA becomes possible in the organism.

The first aspect is concerned with early events which occur after virus infection inside and on the surface of cells, and the second aspect deals with relationships between populations of tumor cells and cells responsible for recognition of "foreign" cells. The conditions under which TSTA appear firmly unite both aspects of the problem. For instance, if TSTA appear in the cells before any malignant transformation takes place and if this event is not followed by transformation in most infected cells, it will follow that the absence of tumors in adult animals inoculated with DNA tumor viruses and the almost complete absence of DNA virus-induced spontaneous tumors are, in a way, a direct consequence of a dissociation between antigenic conversion and transformation, although both are brought about by the same oncogenic virus.

In this review, data concerning both aspects of the problem and a survey of methods used for detection of surface antigens in DNA virus-induced tumors will be presented.

II. Methods Used for Indicating Surface Antigens in Cells of DNA Virus-Induced Tumors

It is generally assumed that TSTA, i.e., antigens responsible for anti-tumor immunity are located on the cell surface. The presence of TSTA in tumor cells is the basis for the following two essential characteristics of these cells; (1) immunogenicity in autologous and syngeneic systems and (2) immunosensitivity *in vivo* and *in vitro*.

Thus, there exist several indirect methods of detection of TSTA in live tumor cells. Some of these methods, such as the transplantation test or adoptive transfer, reveal the presence of TSTA by their functional activity, that is, immunogenic and sensitizing activity, or by the *in vivo* immunosensitivity of the tumor cells bearing the antigens. Some other methods, such as destruction of tumor cells *in vitro* in tissue culture (for instance, colony inhibition test) by immune lymphoid cells or cytotoxic antibodies, are apparently related to the transplantation test. A third group of methods, such as immunofluorescence or mixed agglutination, is concerned with localization of a specific antigen, but not with its function. The only direct evidence of the possible identity of specific surface antigens detectable by indirect methods must ultimately be isolation of the antigen in pure form and its immunochemical study. Unfortunately, purified TSTA, at least from DNA viral-induced tumors are still unavailable because of their apparent instability.

A. Transplantation Test

The transplantation test is one of the most useful methods for indication of TSTA in tumor cells, especially of viral origin (Sjögren, 1965). The presence of TSTA in DNA virus-induced tumors can be studied with the use of the three following modifications of the immunization procedure: (a) immunization of autochthonous, syngeneic, or allogeneic hosts by the cells of the tumor which is under investigation, and the subsequent challenge of animals with the cells of syngeneic standard test-tumor containing the corresponding TSTA; (b) immunization of animals with the cells of standard test-tumor, syngeneic or allogeneic, with subsequent challenge with the syngeneic tumor under study; (c) immunization of animals with the corresponding virus (viruses), with subsequent challenge of animals with the cells of the tumor under study.

All necessary positive and negative controls are to be included in any transplantation test.

Thus, two main specific characteristics of tumor cells, i.e., immunogenicity and immunosensitivity are confronted in the transplantation test. Unfortunately, correlation between these two functions of TSTA on the cell membrane may be absent. There are some data showing that immunosensitivity of tumor cells is a more labile quality than immunogenicity (Koldovsky and Svoboda, 1962; Globerson and Feldman, 1964).

Immunization of adult animals with some DNA oncogenic viruses against the TSTA carried in cells of the corresponding transplantable tumor may give clues in the study of specific immunity to DNA virus-induced tumors. Since an analogous effect can be obtained in animals immunized by the tumor cells, it has been suggested that the resistance, which appears as a result of any of these immunization procedures, is an immunological reaction of the organism directed against some new, virus-induced "foreign" antigen in tumor cells (Habel, 1961, 1962a,b,c; Sjögren et al., 1961; Sjögren, 1963, 1964a). The immunological character of the resistance phenomenon induced by the inoculation of adult animals with the virus was confirmed by adoptive transfer and irradiation experiments.

Tumor-specific transplantation antigens induced by DNA tumor viruses in the cells of different animal species were found to be common and specific for the inducing virus (Girardi, 1965). Inoculation of adult hamsters with polyoma virus controls the growth of transplantable polyoma-induced tumors but does not protect animals inoculated with SV40 tumor cells (Habel and Eddy, 1963; Koch and Sabin, 1963; Defendi, 1963). Spontaneous tumors as well as tumors induced by some chemical carcinogens grow equally well as a rule in the normal and polyoma virus-inoculated animals (Sachs, 1962, Sjögren, 1961, 1963). Specificity of the resistance was found to be independent of the presence or absence of the corresponding infectious virus in the tumor cells used for challenge (Habel, 1962a,b; Sjögren, 1963, 1964c). By the use of the transplantation test, a possible similarity between two apparently different oncogenic DNA viruses of the papova group, that is, SV40 and human warts virus, was demonstrated (Melnick and Rapp, 1965).

One inoculation of adult animals with a virus preparation with a high infectious titer is sufficient for induction of resistance, which will be retained for an indefinitely long time. For SV40 and polyoma virus, the immunizing dose of virus in adult Syrian hamsters is not less than $10^{5.0}$ TCID$_{50}$.* However, the immunizing effect is not connected with the action of infectious virus particles, as the same effect can be obtained in animals inoculated with hydroxylamine-inactivated virus preparation (Altstein et al., 1966).

The level of resistance induced in adult animals by inoculation of DNA

* 50% tissue culture infectious dose.

tumor virus or tumor cells is relatively low. Challenge of immunized animals with higher doses of tumor cells leads to the growth of transplanted tumor cells. But if standard test-tumor is used for simultaneous challenge in several groups of animals immunized by different preparations, one finds that some groups are protected against only 1 to 10 doses of tumor cells growing in normal animals, whereas others are resistant to 100 to 1000 or more doses of the same tumor cells.

Low levels of resistance induced by any of the known methods of specific antitumor immunization cause the necessity to challenge with 2 to 4 relatively small doses of tumor cells, usually with a tenfold difference between doses (Sjögren et al., 1961; Habel, 1962c).

Previously used methods of challenge of immunized animals by inoculation of a dense suspension of tumor cells, often without cell counting, could give positive results only if the level of immunity was high enough. Such a technique appears to be useless when the level of immunity is insufficient or when the results of experiments made at different times are to be compared. Challenge of animals with several tenfold doses of tumor cells and estimation of cell dose giving transplanted tumor growth in 50% of inoculated animals (TrD_{50}) (Melnick and Askenazi, 1963) made the transplantation test more sensitive. Further development of this technique employs the challenge of each normal and immune animal in the group with four different doses of tumor cells, transplanted subcutaneously into different parts of the body (Vassilieva and Altstein, 1964; Murka, 1965). This latter modification of the transplantation test permits not only the use of fewer animals in each experiment but, also, to obtain individual sensitivity characteristics of animals to transplanted tumor cells without the loss of precision.

The selection of standard test-tumor for the transplantation test is particularly essential. For such purposes tumor cells characterized by a high and stable level of immunosensitivity are to be used. With certain reservations, standard test-tumor can be used not only as a qualitative, but also as a quantitative equivalent of the tumor under study. From our experience with SV40-induced hamster tumors, we have an impression that nonimmunized animals in which the primary tumors grow in less than 20 days are the best source of stable and immunosensitive tumors. Use of standard test-tumors in challenge, estimation of TrD_{50} in normal and immune animals, and determination of the resistance index makes the results of the transplantation test highly reproducible. The following quantitative data have become available, owing to the improvement of transplantation tests: (a) the level of immunity (or sensitivity) of different groups of animals under study to transplantation of standard tumor cells and (b) sensitivity of the tumor cells under study to growth in immune and normal organisms. Determination of these parameters under standard conditions permits one to compare the results of experiments made at different times.

At present the transplantation test is a basic method for detection of antigens responsible for antitumor immunity. Being indirect, the method has some significant limitations, which require the search for other methods of TSTA detection. For instance, challenge of tumors in the transplantation test in animals inoculated with the corresponding virus or standard tumor cells, if positive, demonstrates the presence of TSTA in the cells. However, when the results of the same test are negative, they may be interpreted in two ways: (*1*) as a loss or a decrease of immunosensitivity, or (*2*) as a loss or a decrease of TSTA. *In vivo* study of the immunogenic activity of immunoresistant cells in syngeneic animals is one of the main approaches to the problem. Unfortunately, data concerning the relationships between immunogenicity and immunosensitivity in DNA virus-induced tumors are absent, as are data on the mechanism of the decrease (or increase) of their immunosensitivity. There are still no data on the possible loss of TSTA from tumor cells or from cells transformed by DNA oncogenic viruses, though this possibility cannot be excluded.

Thus, the main method of TSTA determination in tumor cells, the transplantation test, is inadequate when immunosensitivity of tumor cells is lost or decreased, owing to the selection of immunoresistant cell variants or to the loss of TSTA. It has been shown that such decrease and the loss of immunosensitivity is regularly seen during the growth of SV40-induced primary hamster tumors in immune organism and especially their metastases (Deichman and Kluchareva, 1966a).

B. Adoptive Transfer

Determination of TSTA by adoptive transfer of sensitized lymphoid cells is one of the very essential, though indirect methods for its detection. In contrast to the transplantation test, the use of adoptive transfer permits one to distinguish the role of cellular factors of antitumor immunity from humoral factors. Two main modifications of adoptive transfer experiments are used:

1. Immune and normal lymphocytes are mixed *in vitro* with the target cells of three kinds: (*a*) standard test-tumor containing TSTA (positive control), (*b*) tumor from the same species but which does not contain TSTA (negative control), and (*c*) tumor under study. After short contact at 37°C. the cell mixtures are transplanted in normal animals syngeneic with the tumor cells.

2. Immune and normal lymphocytes are immediately transplanted in normal animals with the subsequent inoculation of animals with the corresponding target cells [preceding paragraph, points (*a*), (*b*), and (*c*)]. In

contrast to the first modification, contact of lymphocytes and tumor cells take place only *in vivo*.

Inhibition of tumor cell growth *in vivo* after their contact *in vivo* or *in vitro* with sensitized lymphocytes and the absence of the same effect in negative control series, may indicate the presence of TSTA in the tumor cells under study. In experiments of this kind the possible involvement of nonimmunological cell interactions, such as allogeneic inhibition (Hellström, 1963, 1964), are to be kept in mind when the cell mixtures are prepared *in vitro*.

The effective relation between the number of lymphoid and tumor cells in adoptive transfer may vary from 1–10:1 to 1000 (or more): 1; usually it is equal to 10^2 to 10^3 lymphoid cells per tumor cell. As the number of tumor cells that comprise 1 TrD_{50} is, as a rule, 10^5–10^6 cells for the primary DNA viruses-induced tumors, and 10^3–10^4 for transplantable tumors, it means that very high doses of lymphoid cells are to be used for effective inhibition of tumor growth. The necessity of using such large quantities (usually not less than 10^8) of lymphoid cells limits to some extent the potentialities of adoptive transfer for a routine test of the presence of TSTA.

Nevertheless, adoptive transfer was successfully used by several investigators in attempts to prove the immunological character of resistance phenomena induced by DNA tumor viruses as well as for immunoprophylaxis of tumors (Defendi and Koprowski, 1959; Habel, 1962a; Sjögren, 1963, 1964c; Law *et al.*, 1967). When large quantities of lymphoid cells were used, an effective adoptive transfer was demonstrated in cases of primary tumors of rats and tumors induced by chemical carcinogens (Klein *et al.*, 1960; Delorme and Alexander, 1964; Mikulska *et al.*, 1965; Alexander *et al.*, 1966; Jeejeebhoy *et al.*, 1966). In some of these experiments xenogeneic lymphoid cells of sheep sensitized by rat tumor cells were used (Alexander *et al.*, 1966). The authors presented some evidence of the specificity of sensitized sheep lymphocyte action on rat tumor and consider the reaction as directed against TSTA. This interpretation connects the inhibiting effect of xenogeneic lymphoid cells on the primary rat tumor growth with a messenger that can stimulate the immune system of the host against autochthonous tumor cells. Possibility of transfer of specific information by xenogeneic sensitized cells may appear very important in further attempts to increase immunological destruction of tumors and, thus, for the detection of TSTA by the use of adoptive transfer.

C. Inhibition of Tumor Cell Growth *in Vitro* by Immune Lymphocytes and Humoral Antibodies

Destruction of target cells *in vitro*, resembling a cytopathogenic effect, after their contact with lymphocytes, sensitized *in vivo* by corresponding isoantigens, was demonstrated by several investigators (Govaerts, 1960;

Rosenau and Moon, 1961; Koprowski and Fernandes, 1962; Taylor and Culling, 1963; Wilson, 1963). Yoshida and Southam (1963) used the same method for detection of specific antigens in tumors induced by chemical carcinogens. Recently, the destruction of human tumor cells was demonstrated in monolayer tissue cultures treated with immune lymphocytes (Chu et al., 1967).

Though humoral antibodies apparently do not play a significant role in the specific immune reaction of organisms against the DNA virus-induced tumors, a cytotoxic action of humoral antibodies was demonstrated on the cells of some such tumors in vitro (Tevethia and Rapp, 1965). These data, thus, have shown that the same technique which was routinely exploited for several years in experiments with leukemia cells (Slettenmark and Klein, 1962; Pasternak and Graffi, 1963; Wahren, 1963; E. Klein and Klein, 1964; Old et al., 1964) can be used for the demonstration of the presence of specific antigens on the cell surface in some tumors induced by DNA viruses. The degree of sensitivity of solid tumor cells to the cytotoxic action of antibodies is apparently much less than in leukemia cells. In the latter, sensitivity was proportional to the concentration of isoantigen or to specific antigen on the cell surface (Winn, 1960; Möller and Möller, 1962; Klein et al., 1966b).

Very elegant combination of the two systems was developed by Sjögren and Hellström (1967a) when Moloney leukemia cells were superinfected with polyoma virus, and the appearance of polyoma-specific surface antigen (antigens?) was demonstrated by a modified cytotoxic test (Bases, 1963), as well as by the transplantation test. The modification of the cytotoxic technique involves plating of tumor cells for in vitro colony formation after their incubation with antibodies and complement. Determination of plating efficiency of tumor cells treated with immune sera and its comparison with the plating efficiency of the same cells treated with the control sera and complement revealed the specific inhibiting action of antibodies on the formation of tumor cell colonies in tissue culture. The colony inhibition technique (CI) was shown to be useful for determination of H-2 isoantigens and for specific polyoma tumor antigens as well (Hellström and Sjögren, 1965). Later the CI test was successfully used for demonstration of specific antigens in tumors induced by human adenoviruses and Rous sarcoma virus (Sjögren and Hellström, 1967b; Hellström and Sjögren, 1967).

Cross-reactivity was found between the cells of tumors induced by adenoviruses of type 12 and 7, but not with the type 5 in both tests, that is, in CI test in vitro and transplantation test in vivo. These data may be interpreted in favor of the identity of specific antigens revealed by these different tests. Other evidence of the possible identity of the antigens determined by transplantation and CI tests is that the specific antigens revealed are common for tumors induced by the same virus in different species of animals (Sjögren and Hellström, 1967b). These authors also modified the CI test for the demonstration of cell-bound immunity reactions against polyoma and adenovirus tumor-specific antigens (Hellström and Sjögren, 1967). This makes the supposed similarity between the antigenic target of these two *in vitro* and *in vivo* tests more likely. Though direct proof is still lacking, the identity of the antigens revealed by transplantation and CI tests appears to be quite possible. In any case, sensitivity of tumor cells to the cytotoxic action of humoral antibodies and lymphocytes *in vitro* extends the sphere of techniques useful for indication of specific tumor antigens on the cell membrane.

Among other approaches to the *in vitro* determination of surface antigens in tumor cells, the inhibition of migration activity of cells from the spleen fragment in the presence of cells bearing the corresponding TSTA should be mentioned. This technique was recently developed by Haškova *et al.* (1967) for determination of isoantigens and by Pekarek (1967) for TSTA determination. The method consists of the cultivation of spleen fragments from normal and immune animals on monolayers of target and control cells. In the presence of the corresponding transplantation antigen in the cells of the monolayer culture the inhibition of the migration zone surrounding the spleen fragments was demonstrated. Until now this technique was used for the demonstration of specific antigen in cells transformed by or infected with SV40 virus (Pekarek, 1967). Possible application of such technique for indication of surface antigens in the cells of tumors of different origin is to be studied.

D. Demonstration of the Presence of Specific Cell Membrane Antigens in DNA Virus-Induced Tumors

Presence of specific cell membrane antigens (SCMA) in tumor cells can be established after the treatment of the cells with labeled anti-SCMA antibodies. Immunofluorescence test (IF) and mixed agglutination techniques are at present the most useful methods for indication of SCMA. Recently, antibodies labeled with ^{125}I were used for the same purpose (Harder and McKhann, 1968).

Originally, the IF test was used for detection of H-2 isoantigens on the cell membrane (Möller, 1961); later it was adapted for determination of SCMA in tumors induced by chemical carcinogens (Möller, 1964; Lejneva *et al.*, 1965) and in the cells of Moloney virus-induced leukemia (G. Klein and Klein, 1964). Specific antigen reactive in the IF test was demonstrated on the surface of Burkitt lymphoma cells (G. Klein *et al.*, 1966a, 1967;

E. Klein *et al.*, 1967). The most reactive sera were obtained from patients with Burkitt lymphoma after complete regression of tumors.

In tumors induced by DNA tumor virus SV40, specific SCMA were discovered by Tevethia *et al.* (1965) in Syrian hamster tumor cells. Immune sera reactive with SCMA were obtained from hamsters immunized by inoculation of SV40 virus followed by transplantation of subthreshold doses of SV40 tumor cells. In subsequent experiments (Kluchareva *et al.*, 1967), two types of immune hamster sera were compared for demonstration of SCMA in SV40 hamster tumors. One type of sera was prepared according to Tevethia *et al.*; the other was obtained from hamsters in which the regression of primary tumors was induced by reinfection of animals with SV40 virus during the latent period (Deichman and Kluchareva, 1966b). Both types of immune sera behaved similarly in all positive and negative control series. However, the presence of isoantibodies against the weak hamster transplantation antigens could not be excluded in the first type of serum.

Cell membrane antigens specific to polyoma virus were also found by the use of the sera of mice immunized with allogeneic polyoma tumor, followed by challenge with syngeneic tumor cells (Irlin, 1967).

Thus, until now, immune sera, reactive in the IF test were obtained only by a few methods as follows:

1. Immunization of allogeneic animals with live SCMA-bearing tumor cells. In this case the rejection of tumor cells was connected with the reaction directed against both isoantigens and SCMA. Use of syngeneic tumor cells in combination with such immune sera permits one to ignore the presence of isoantibodies in the sera obtained.

2. Immunization of noninbred animals (only Syrian hamsters) with tumor cells of the same species. Though the isoantigenic differences among Syrian hamsters are weak, the use of such sera leaves doubts about the specificity of the reaction.

3. Immunization of animals by reinfection with the oncogenic virus during the latent period of viral carcinogenesis. The subsequent appearance and regression of autochthonous tumor leads in some cases to the appearance of antibodies reactive in the IF test with SCMA. Though such a procedure for immunization takes much time and is rather difficult for routine work, the specificity of the reaction is clearer. The regression of primary tumors can be induced sometimes by chemotherapy as it has been shown in African patients with Burkitt lymphoma. Sera from such patients were reactive with autochthonous as well as with allogeneic Burkitt lymphoma cells in the IF test (G. Klein *et al.*, 1966a, 1967; E. Klein *et al.*, 1967). The spontaneous regression of primary tumors, possibly connected with an efficient autoimmune reaction is characteristic for several

virus-induced tumors of mammals and birds (for example, Rous sarcoma virus-induced tumors of monkeys, quail, pigeons, and some other species or Shope virus- and polyoma virus-induced papillomas of rabbits). It is striking that an excellent potential source of immune sera such as animals with spontaneous regression of virus-induced tumors was not yet sufficiently studied in the IF or other serological tests.

All methods of immunization against SCMA include the destruction of live or minimally altered tumor cells bearing SCMA in the organism of immunologically competent animals. Growth of primary or transplanted tumor as a rule does not lead to accumulation of antibodies against SCMA. In contrast, the level of antibodies against specific complement-fixing tumor (T—)antigen of DNA virus-induced tumors increases as the tumor grows larger. The nuclear localization of T-antigen and its instability at 37°C. apparently create the conditions for accumulation of antibodies against T-antigen almost without any loss. Absence of antibodies against SCMA in the sera of animals with the growing tumors may be due to different reasons. Adsorption of antibodies on the surface of growing tumor cells is one possibility; the immunological paralysis of the host to SCMA of growing tumor cells is another.

Theoretically, there is still another way to obtain antisera against SCMA of DNA virus-induced tumors. This method does not use tumor cells for immunization of animals and is based on data showing that SCMA (as well as TSTA) appear in cells infected with the corresponding virus long before any signs of cell transformation take place. As shown by Kluchareva *et al.* (1967), SV40 *in vitro* infected, hamster embryo cells a few days after infection are immunogenic for adult hamsters and protect them against subsequent challenge with SV40 tumor cells, although they do not contain detectable amounts of virus nor of transformed cells. With the use of the IF test, the appearance of SCMA on the membrane of SV40- or polyoma virus-infected cells in tissue cultures was demonstrated a few hours after the treatment of the culture cells with high doses of the virus (Kluchareva *et al.*, 1967; Irlin, 1967). It is conceivable that immunization of animals with the virus-free syngeneic cells infected by DNA virus in tissue culture may permit one to obtain sera reactive in the IF test with the corresponding SCMA. The advantage of using infected, virus-free cells for immunization (in contrast to tumor cells) is the possibility to inoculate adult animals with an unlimited number of SCMA-bearing live cells. In this case risk of tumor growth, connected with the presence of a few already transformed cells in the inocula will be minimal.

Recently, the mixed agglutination test was used for detection of SCMA in the cells of tumors induced by DNA viruses, such as SV40 and polyoma. The presence of SCMA in the tumor cells was revealed by the fixation of two different antigen–antibody complexes, one of which was the same as in the IF test, i.e., SCMA on the tumor cell membrane and anti-SCMA antibody, whereas the other is an indicator system consisting of sheep red cells and antisera against it, obtained from animals homologous to the anti-SCMA serum donor. As a bridge between these two complexes, immune sera were used, directed against the globulins of the antiserum donor animals (Barth *et al.*, 1967; Metzgar and Oleinick, 1968). This rather cumbersome system was modified for the demonstration of SCMA, not only in tumor cell suspensions, but also in monolayer tissue cultures. The latter is the so-called mixed hemadsorption test. Originally, the technique of mixed hemadsorption was developed for the detection of viral antigens on the membrane of virus-infected monolayer culture cells (Fagreus and Espmark, 1961). The possibility to detect visually the presence of SCMA in the cells of unaltered monolayer cultures may be one of the most interesting advantages of this method which can permit, for instance, a study of the dynamics of SCMA appearance and its distribution during the *in vitro* infection and transformation process in the cell population.

III. Induced Synthesis of Tumor-Specific Transplantation Antigens and Other Functions of DNA Tumor Viruses in the Cell

Constant synthesis of TSTA in the cells transformed by DNA tumor viruses is only one of a number of changes that occur in virus-infected cells during carcinogenesis. In this section an attempt will be made to evaluate the relationship of TSTA synthesis to other changes of DNA virus-infected cells.

A. Defectiveness of DNA Tumor Viruses in Different Cell Systems and Transformation

As a result of DNA tumor virus interaction with different kinds of cells, the following types of reaction are noted: (*a*) acute lytic infection characterized by a cytopathogenic effect (CPE) and active production of viral protein (V-antigen) and of infectious viral progeny; (*b*) abortive infection characterized by an incomplete cycle of virus replication without production of infectious virions. This latter type of cell infection with DNA tumor viruses is apparently an essential part of the transformation process and, therefore, an object of particular interest. Many different kinds of evidence are available at present which show that replication of infectious tumor virus in cells is not necessary for transformation. Many years ago it was suggested by Zilber (1945) that induction of tumors by viruses is connected with the hereditary changes of infected cells and that growth of tumors does not need the presence of inducing virus. Possible integration of viral genetic material into the cell genome was latter discussed (Zilber and Abelev, 1962).

Different types of DNA tumor virus–cell interactions are apparently connected with the inability of the infectious particle under conditions of single infection to provide itself, in some types of cells, with the synthesis of all products necessary for maturation of viral progeny. Abortive infection of cells is one example of such virus–cell interaction and is a demonstration of the defectiveness of the virus in the given cell system.

The denomination "defective virus" has many meanings at present, including virions with incomplete or artificially inactivated genome and even particles without viral genome and empty capsids. The relative character of viral defectiveness, its dependence on the cell system and significance of the heterogeneity of viral populations were emphasized by Rowe (1967) who defined a defective virus particle as "one which under conditions of single infection in the cell system under study can initiate viral synthesis, but cannot carry out all the steps necessary for efficient production of new virus."

In trying to classify virus–cell interactions it must be noted that, on the level of single cell–virus interaction, any type of reaction can take place, the choice being dependent both on the cell and the virion. In viral carcinogenesis, *in vivo*, or *in vitro*, heterogeneous populations of cells and virions initiate the process. In relation to each cell type the proportion of defective virions and the character of their defectiveness may vary widely. As demonstrated by Michel *et al.* (1967), from 60 to 90% of the particles are noninfectious in some preparations of polyoma virus and contain not viral, but host DNA. Such particles can adsorb to the cell membrane and agglutinate red cells, the same as complete polyoma virus particles, but they are unable to induce the synthesis of viral hemagglutinins, cellular or viral DNA, and infectious progeny. Thus, in polyoma virus population, strange particles, defined by the authors as "pseudovirions," can appear.

A somewhat special type of viral defectiveness was demonstrated by the use of the hybrid virus, the so-called PARA (SV40)–adenovirus 7. Hybrid particles with a defective SV40 genome component and a capsid of adenovirus type induced SV40-specific T-antigen and transplantation antigen synthesis. No infectious SV40 progeny appeared in infected competent cells. Morphologically, the tumors induced by the hybrid virus were very similar to SV40 tumors. The defective SV40 genome included in the hybrid particles has, thus, retained determinants for the specific tumor antigens and apparently for the histopathological appearance of the tumor as well (Huebner *et al.*, 1964; Rowe and Baum, 1964, 1965; Rapp *et al.*, 1964, 1965b, 1967; Rowe, 1965; Rapp, 1967; Rapp and Melnick, 1966).

Defective virus particles were discovered in preparations of SV40 virus (Sauer *et al.*, 1967; Altstein *et al.*, 1967b) which were unable to induce V-antigen or infectious virus production in green monkey kidney cells but were capable of inducing an abortive infection characterized by the appearance of T-antigen. In green monkey kidney cultures, competent to support a lytic interaction, abortive infection can thus take place as well, depending on the competence of the infecting virions.

Susceptibility to virus infection is usually different in different tissues of the same species. In mouse kidney cultures, 80–90% of the cells are epithelial, the rest being spindle-shaped fibroblasts. After infection with polyoma virus, a complete cycle of virus replication and CPE can be observed in epithelial cells, whereas the fibroblastic cells show abortive infection, without the production of mature polyoma virus, but with subsequent morphological transformation (Weil *et al.*, 1967). In hamster embryo or kidney cells, infection with both SV40 or polyoma viruses results in abortive infection and transformation.

An incomplete virus replication cycle is apparently one essential prerequisite for transformation by DNA tumor viruses. However, it is evident that the number of abortively infected cells is larger than the number of transformed cells (Black, 1966). Abortively infected cells may thus frequently recover within infected cell populations.

Aging of cells in tissue culture is one of several factors promoting the transformation process induced by DNA tumor viruses. The SV40 infection of aging human fibroblast cultures was found to restore cell proliferation with rapid transformation as a result (Jensen *et al.*, 1963). Unfortunately, there are no quantitative data concerning the capacity of aging human cell populations to support abortive SV40 infection, in comparison with young cells.

In general, abortive infection may take place in the following two situations of single infection:

1. Infection with virions defective for the given cell system (e.g., hamster cells infected with SV40, polyoma, or adenoviruses). This type of defectiveness is related to the cell system and other fully competent cell systems can be found for the same viruses.

2. Infection of competent cells with noninfectious particles (e.g., green monkey kidney cells infected with SV40 particles containing an incomplete or inactivated viral genome). This type of defectiveness can be defined as absolute, being unrelated to cell type. Apparently, it cannot be compensated by single infection of any known kind of cells free from antigenically related or distinct helper viruses or their genomes.

Theoretically, this means that any DNA tumor virus can induce an abortive infection in at least part of the cells in any cell system and that absolutely or relatively defective particles may be responsible for this. In practice, abortive infection and transformation induced by the same DNA tumor virus have been found to occur in different cell systems, including cells competent to support virus multiplication (for example, mouse embryo or kidney cells infected with polyoma virus or green monkey cells infected with SV40).

At present there is no direct proof that absolutely defective virus particles can be responsible for transformation of competent cells, although this possibility has been suggested (Defendi and Jensen, 1967; Sauer *et al.*, 1967).

B. EARLY EVENTS IN DNA TUMOR VIRUS-INFECTED CELLS

Although the final results of the DNA tumor virus–cell interaction may be distinct, the order of the early events is very similar in the abortively and the lytically infected cell.

The sequence of events is approximately the following: (*1*) appearance of SCMA (possibly identical to TSTA); (*2*) appearance of T-antigen and increased production of enzymes necessary for DNA synthesis; (*3*) increased production of cellular and viral DNA and RNA hybridizing with viral DNA; (*4*) appearance of viral coat protein (V-antigen) and mature virions. V-antigen and virion production are late events characteristic for lytic infection and a nonintegrated virus–cell relationship. In contrast, the synthesis of early products is characteristically retained in abortive infection and in transformed cells. A full infectious cycle in the single cell needs about 72 hours, with only few hours between the early and the late events. It was suggested that the fate of the cell is determined during these few hours (Habel, 1967). The process can develop in different directions. Early events can be followed by the late ones with cell death and CPE as a result. A blocking of late events by some unknown mechanism may either lead to the recovery of the abortively infected cell, or more rarely, to transformation and the appearance of potentially immortal cells.

The appearance of specific antigens on the cell surface seems to be one of the earliest changes during viral transformation, demonstrated to occur during the first 6 hours after SV40 and polyoma infection of normal cells (Kluchareva *et al.*, 1967; Irlin, 1967). Recently, Malmgren *et al.* (1968) demonstrated SCMA in polyoma-infected cells 20 hours after infection, but not at 4 hours. It is not clear if SCMA is identical with TSTA. Possible identity of SCMA and TSTA is supported by the early appearance of both in SV40-infected hamster cells (Kluchareva *et al.*, 1967).

Another early product of DNA tumor virus infection localized in the cell nuclei, T-antigen, is distinct from TSTA (Habel, 1965; Defendi and Taguchi, 1966). Though, T-antigens, as well as SCMA, or TSTA, apparently do not represent structural viral proteins, their antigenic specificity is determined by the inducing virus. Each of them seem to be shared by cells of different species. Specific tumor antigens appear in infected cells a few hours after infection and their synthesis remains constant indefinitely after transformation. These antigenic markers are present in all virus-transformed cells and were referred to as viral "fingerprints" (Habel, 1966).

There are yet no data concerning the source of the DNA information initiating the synthesis of SCMA and TSTA in infected cells. The early appearance of SCMA in most infected cells and its virus-dependent specificity suggests that viral DNA contains sufficient information for the induction of specific surface antigens in infected cells. Results of viral nucleic acid inactivation experiments, discussed in more detail later, have shown that the part of viral DNA responsible for TSTA in hamster cells that are SV40-infected *in vivo* is less than half of the whole target (Altstein *et al.*, 1966).

There are no data on a possible connection between T-antigen appearance and surface antigen production as suggested by Sachs (1965). The appearance of SCMA apparently precedes the appearance of T-antigen, at least in SV40- and polyoma-infected cells; furthermore, SCMA can be demonstrated in a much larger proportion of abortively infected cells than T-antigen. Thus, the relationship between T-antigen and SCMA-inducing functions of DNA tumor viruses is not yet clear.

Information necessary for T-antigen synthesis in infected cells is most probably provided by viral DNA. The inhibitors of DNA synthesis, such as FUDR (5'-fluorodeoxyuridine), cytosine arabinoside and low doses of actinomycin D do not stop or prevent T-antigen synthesis in the cells infected with SV40 and polyoma in contrast to V-antigen production. Inhibitors of protein synthesis, such as puromycin and cycloheximide, and of DNA dependent RNA, such as high doses of actinomycin D, inhibit T-antigen and some early enzymes as well as V-antigen synthesis during acute lytic infection with SV40 and polyoma (Sabin and Koch, 1964; Butel and Rapp, 1965; Habel *et al.*, 1965; Hoggan *et al.*, 1965; Gilden *et al.*, 1965; Rapp *et al.*, 1965a,b,c; Carp and Gilden, 1966; Defendi *et al.*, 1966; Gilden and Carp, 1966; Sabin, 1966; Habel, 1967).

Almost simultaneously with the appearance of T-antigen in SV40-infected green monkey kidney cells the production of some enzymes required for cellular DNA metabolism increases 3–10 times, as compared with normal cells.

The insensitivity of the production of one of these enzymes (dT kinase) to inhibitors of cellular DNA synthesis, such as mytomycin C and the inactivation of this function by ultraviolet irradiation suggests that the production of dT kinase is controlled by the viral genome, similarly to T-antigen (Kit, 1967). It has been also shown that cytosine arabinoside added to cells 2 hours after SV40 infection did not inhibit dT kinase, DNA polymerase, and FH_2 reductase activities (Frearson *et al.*, 1966; Kit, 1967).

However, T-antigen is apparently distinct from most of the enzymes that participate in cellular DNA metabolism, and its characteristics resemble only one of them, DNA polymerase. Some data that raise doubts about the identity of T-antigen and DNA polymerase have been presented (Kit, 1967). They do not exclude that T-antigen may have enzymic activity of an as yet unknown type.

Deoxyribonucleic acid tumor virus infection is followed by an early increase of cell DNA synthesis (Dulbecco et al., 1965; Weil et al., 1965; Gershon et al., 1966; Hatanaka and Dulbecco, 1966). In polyoma-infected cells undergoing a full lytic infection, this increase was related to the appearance of V-antigen and mature virus, i.e., with rather late viral functions (Weil et al., 1967). In hamster kidney cells abortively infected with polyoma virus, the process was blocked at a stage that precedes the increase of cellular and viral DNA. Sauer and Defendi (1966) demonstrated an increase in DNA synthesis in human diploid cells abortively infected with SV40. Adenovirus DNA was also shown to increase during the abortive infection of green monkey cells without the subsequent synthesis of virus protein (Rapp, 1967).

In the process of acute lytic infection induced by polyoma virus in mouse kidney tissue culture cells a virus-specific RNA fraction appears (Benjamin, 1966, 1967; Weil et al., 1967). Hybridization experiments have shown that this fraction combines specifically with polyoma DNA. Its synthesis coincides with the production of viral DNA during acute infection. Virus-specific RNA was discovered by the same author in polyoma- and SV40-transformed, nonvirus-yielding mouse cells, in amounts corresponding to about 1% of the virus-specific RNA found in productively infected cells. A small fraction of virus-specific RNA was found in adenovirus-transformed cells (Fuginaga and Green, 1966; Green and Fuginaga, 1967). It was not clear whether the virus-specific RNA of the transformed cells hybridizes with the same parts of the viral DNA as the RNA of productively infected cells.

The late products of DNA tumor virus infection, i.e., V-antigen and infectious virions, are not produced by tumor cells as a rule. This is reminiscent of lysogenic conversion in bacteria (Luria, 1959). Information necessary for the production of mature virions is retained in some DNA virus-transformed cells, however, as in lysogenic bacteria, virus production can be activated in a number of ways.

C. Virus-Specific Tumor Antigens and Transformation Process

It has been pointed out frequently that the term "transformation" includes a variety of phenomena and its use requires a clear definition. This problem has been discussed in detail by Koprowski et al. (1966).

It seems reasonable to separate the events at the cell level, i.e., cell "conversion," from the events at the population level, i.e., "transformation." Both cell conversion and transformation are dynamic processes that may lead to an endless series of sequential developments. The beginning of each process is a much debated question. Some investigators localize the beginning of transformation to the loss of contact inhibition or the appearance of morphologically altered foci in monolayer cultures. Others regard as an objective sign of transformation the ability of cells to form colonies in semisolid agar or to grow *in vivo* as a transplantable tumor. It has been demonstrated (Vogt and Dulbecco, 1963; Todaro *et al.*, 1963) that the morphological transformation of cells by oncogenic DNA viruses *in vitro* can be registered much earlier than their transplantability *in vivo*.

It seems logical to assume that an integration between viral and cellular genomes initiates a series of qualitative cellular changes that renders them different from simply infected cells. This change may occur very early in cells infected with oncogenic DNA viruses and its fixation requires apparently only one cell division (Todaro and Green, 1966). Constant synthesis of early proteins without the production of V-antigen and infectious particles may be a symptom of integration. Unfortunately, it is difficult to reveal this symptom at the level of the infected cell population, where the infection process is asynchronous and its products cannot be distinguished from the same ones of integration process.

The early events initiating the conversion process seem to be very complex and the meaning of the term "integration" is not clear. Experiments on the induction of virus production from SV40- and polyoma-transformed cells demonstrated that the viral genome may be integrated with the cell genome to different degrees. It may be characterized as "reactivatable" in cases where infectious virus production can be induced and as "not reactivatable" where this is not the case, as in many polyoma-transformed cells (Watkins and Dulbecco, 1967). The state of integration may obviously differ in different cells of the same population as well. Retained ability of some tumor cells to produce mature virus particles, retained susceptibility of some tumor cells to superinfection with the same oncogenic virus, and the presence of reactivatable and nonreactivatable viral genomes in different tumor cells may all reflect different states of integration.

Methods are still lacking to establish the integrated state of the viral genome at the earliest possible stage. An indirect approach would be a test for early virus-determined protein synthesis, distinct from the mere presence of such proteins. A possible example, still the only one of its kind, is the T-antigen, which is apparently identical in cells during early lytic infection and in transformed cells. However, the information for T-antigen synthesis is probably translated in different ways in these two systems (Oxman and Black, 1966; Oxman *et al.*, 1967). Synthesis of T-antigen during productive infection with SV40 virus is inhibited by interferon, added before or immediately after infection. Interferon has no effect on T-antigen synthesis in transformed cells. It is suggested that in the transformed cell, "hybrid" mRNA molecules are carrying the viral and cellular information formed, from the integrated genome to the ribosomes. Such "hybrid" molecules may not be recognized by the intracellular protein induced by interferon, in contrast to viral mRNA. Although the authors do not exclude other interpretations, the use of interferon may distinguish between the same type of synthetic processes in cells characterized by an integrated and a nonintegrative cell–virus relationship.

As already mentioned, the presence of virus-specific tumor antigens in transformed cells is a convincing, although indirect, argument in favor of an integration between viral genetic material and the cell genome. Direct proof of integration was presented by the discovery of virus-specific RNA in virus-free cells transformed by SV40, polyoma, or adenoviruses (Benjamin, 1966, 1967; Fuginaga and Green, 1966; Green and Fuginage, 1967). A demonstration of a virus-specific RNA fraction characteristic for the integrated state of the viral genome and distinct from the RNA's found in productively infected cells may be one of approaches toward an early identification of viral integration in infected cells.

Another possibility may be connected with the isolation of molecules of viral DNA from the abortively infected cells. Recently it was demonstrated that molecules of viral DNA in the virus-free cells transformed by polyoma or SV40 could be discovered. The number of viral DNA equivalents per cell varied from 5 to 60 in different cell lines. No free viral DNA of the size similar to that present in virions could be recovered from SV40-transformed cells. Viral DNA in transformed cells was integrated with the cell DNA and the existence of alkali-stable covalent linkages between them was established (Westphal and Dulbecco, 1968; Sambrook *et al.*, 1968).

Since abortive infection with DNA tumor virus does not lead to transformation in most cells, the question arises whether some of the early products, T-antigen, SCMA, and TSTA in particular, are really necessary for transformation. It has been suggested that T-antigen functions in transformed cells as an activator of DNA synthesis (Weil *et al.*, 1967) and is necessary for the replication of the viral genome (Rapp and Melnick, 1966). Unfortunately, nothing definite is known about the possible role of TSTA and SCMA during cell transformation, nor is there any information about their biochemical nature and mechanism of synthesis and function in infected and transformed cells. Thus, the early appearance of

SCMA and TSTA in infected cells, long before morphological transformation occurs, and their role in transformation is an area of pure speculation. One of the hypotheses in this field is that antigenic conversion of the cell membrane may lead to immunological and nonimmunological changes in the relationships of such cells with their neighbors. If cells with an altered cell membrane become less susceptible to the signals inhibiting their growth, a cell population may appear that has lost contact inhibition. This tempting concept is contradicted, however, by the following considerations:

1. Synthesis of SCMA (and possibly TSTA) takes place in a large number of infected cells, but only a very small proportion lose contact inhibition and become transformed.

2. In infected cells, SCMA and TSTA appear at an early stage, whereas loss of contact inhibition becomes evident much later.

3. There seems to be no correlation between the transforming (oncogenic) activity of a virus and its ability to induce TSTA synthesis *in vivo*, the latter judged by the graft rejection test (Hare and Morgan, 1963; Hare, 1964a,b, 1966; Hare and Godal, 1965).

4. There are no data to indicate a possible direct relationship between the antigenic changes of the cell membrane and the changes in the social behavior of the cells. It is conceivable that the latter may be induced by a central alteration of some growth-controlling mechanism, directly or indirectly connected with the functioning of the viral genome.

These comments do not exclude a possible major role of antigenic changes in carcinogenesis, but at present there are no experimental data in favor of this theory.

Another explanation of the role of specific membrane antigens in transformed cells may be derived from quite the opposite approach to the problem. It may be suggested that SCMA and TSTA have no relation to the transformation process. They would be present in transformed cells only as an expression of early viral functions, linked with the part of the viral genome responsible for transformation. This rather extreme position may become stronger if it will be established that nononcogenic DNA viruses can induce the same type of SCMA or TSTA synthesis as oncogenic DNA viruses. If so, induction of specific antigens of the transplantation type may not be an exclusive feature of tumor viruses. Some data on the induction of transplantation-type antigens in the tumor cells infected with DNA infectious viruses, such as herpes simplex virus, were presented by Hamburg and Svet-Moldavsky (1964). Recently Rapp and co-workers (1968) have shown that transcapcidation of genetic material of PARA to some human nononcogenic adenoviruses results in the appearance of new PARA viral populations which were capable to induce transplantation immunity against SV40 tumor cells as well as SV40 T-antigen synthesis, though some of such PARA viral populations were nononcogenic. Direct proof could be obtained if a mutant DNA tumor virus would be found that has lost the TSTA-inducing function with retained transforming activity or if differential inactivation of the viral genome would permit the separation of the two viral functions.

D. DIFFERENTIAL INACTIVATION OF DNA TUMOR VIRUS FUNCTIONS IN THE CELL

One of the methods for the study of different virally determined functions is partial inactivation of the viral genome. Ultraviolet (UV) irradiation, ^{60}Co irradiation, nitrous acid, hydroxylamine, and some other agents are known to damage predominantly viral nucleic acids, but not viral protein. The comparative study of the dynamics of the inactivation of various viral functions and the establishment of dose–response curves may reveal the target size within the viral genome responsible for a given function. It is generally assumed that a more rapid inactivation rate corresponds to a larger target size for the corresponding function; a slower rate of inactivation corresponds to a smaller target size. During the last few years it has been demonstrated that some functions of DNA tumor viruses, expressed in the target cell, are 2 to 5 times more resistant to the inactivating action of agents damaging viral nucelic acids than infectivity (Basilico and diMayorca, 1965; Benjamin, 1965, 1966; Carp and Gilden, 1965; Carp et al., 1966; Gershon et al., 1965; Altstein et al., 1966, 1967a; Defendi et al., 1966; Kit 1967; Latarjet et al., 1967).

Since the target sizes of the different functions were determined only very approximately even in experiments where the same virus and inactivator were used, it is not possible at present to compare the target sizes of all viral functions. Such a comparison could be possible if all functions were determined in an experiment with the same virus preparation and if precise quantitative methods would be available to establish the activity of all viral functions. There is no doubt, however, that all early functions are significantly more resistant to inactivation than infectivity. The latter apparently represents a function of the total unaltered viral genome. There is a rather strong impression that *in vivo* oncogenic and TSTA-inducing activities of at least one DNA tumor virus, SV40, are more resistant to hydroxylamine inactivation than both infectivity and T-antigen-inducing activity *in vitro* (Altstein et al., 1966, 1967a). These functions were studied by using the same inactivated virus preparation. One unexplained finding was, however, that cells of the tumors which appeared in hamsters inoculated with hydroxylamine-inactivated SV40 contained T-antigen, although the same virus preparation did not induce T-antigen synthesis *in vitro* in the most competent cell system, namely, green monkey kidney cultures. The discussion of this finding is difficult since the function of T-antigens remains unknown (Defendi, 1966; Takemoto *et al.*, 1966).

Increased tumor and leukemia frequently were found in animals inoculated with irradiated preparations of RNA tumor viruses such as milk agent and Friend leukemia (Ardashnikov and Spasskaya, 1949; Ardashnikov *et al.*, 1955; Latarjet and Chamaillard, 1962). Defendi and Jensen (1967) registered a definite increase in the oncogenic activity of SV40, polyoma, and LLE46 (hybrid of adeno 7 and SV40) in animals inoculated with UV- or ^{60}Co-irradiated virus preparations. Here again, cells of tumors induced by irradiated virus preparations were synthesizing complement-fixing T-antigen, although inactivation of the T-antigen-inducing function *in vitro* was much more rapid and did not coincide with the inactivation of the oncogenic activity *in vivo*. Data on the increase in the tumorigenic activity of irradiated SV40, polyoma, and LLE46 virus preparations *in vivo* do not correlate with the decrease of the *in vitro* transforming activity of polyoma virus after the irradiation of virus preparations with increasing doses of radiation (Basilico and diMayorca, 1965; Benjamin, 1965).

Experiments on differential inactivation of DNA tumor virus-induced cell functions have, thus, demonstrated that *in vivo* and *in vitro* expressions of the same viral functions may differ significantly. Another conclusion from inactivation experiments is that the targets of *in vivo* transforming and TSTA-inducing functions have apparently similar sizes. It is not clear whether the same part of the viral genome is responsible for both viral functions. Such an assumption seems contradictory to the absence of any correlation between oncogenic and TSTA-inducing activities in a comparison between different strains of polyoma virus (Hare and Morgan, 1963; Hare, 1964a,b, 1966; Hare and Godal, 1965).

If TSTA-inducing and transforming functions represent activities of different parts of the viral genome, these functions should be theoretically separable from each other. The possible conditions for dissociating the two functions might be as follows: (*1*) at the level of the infected cell population, the two functions may not coincide in the same cell with regard to time and expression; (*2*) a mutant or hybrid virus variant could be found lacking the part of the viral genome responsible for TSTA synthesis; (*3*) differential inactivation of the TSTA-inducing capacity of the viral genome, without damage to its transforming activity.

The immunogenicity of hamster cells infected *in vitro* with SV40 and free of infectious virus or of transformed cells may be interpreted as indirect evidence that these two functions of SV40 virus are dissociated at the level of cell population, at least in time.

The possible significance of the dissociation of TSTA-inducing and transforming functions of DNA tumor viruses *in vivo* in animals infected when newborn, or adult, will be discussed in the next section.

IV. Specific Antitumor Immunity and Induction of Primary Tumors by DNA Tumor Viruses

An immunological study of DNA virus-induced carcinogenesis reveals that appearance of primary tumors is an exception to the general rule, which prohibits the growth of TSTA-bearing tumor cells in the organism. Primary tumors can only appear under the following special conditions:

1. If the presence of TSTA in the tumor cells is not recognized by the organism or is recognized too late. Failure of recognition may occur for different reasons. Acquired immunological tolerance to TSTA, natural decrease of immunological competence in the aging organism, various types of immunosuppression, weakness of the antigenic differences between normal and tumor tissues, masking of specific antigens on the cell membrane by antibodies and the enhancement phenomenon—all these factors may be impediments against the immunological recognition of primary tumor growth.

2. The TSTA-containing tumor may change its immunosensitivity during growth in an immunologically competent (immune) organism. This may be due to the immunoselection of less antigenic, or nonantigenic (?) variants of tumor cells or to an adaptive modification with continued synthesis of TSTA, but together with cellular immunoresistance.

In this section some quantitative and qualitative aspects of the immunological relationships between the primary tumor and its host will be reviewed.

A. Immunological Status of the Host and Primary Tumor Appearance

The current ideas on the role of immunological factors in the induction of primary tumors by DNA tumor viruses are based on the resistance phenomenon discovered in 1961–1962 by Sjögren *et al.*, Habel, and Sachs. Previously it was demonstrated that within the same species newborn animals are more susceptible than adults, as a rule, to the tumorigenic action of DNA tumor viruses (Stewart *et al.*, 1958; Eddy *et al.*, 1962). As shown in 1961 by Sjögren *et al.*, Habel (1961), and Sachs (1961), polyoma virus-inoculated adult mice acquire specific resistance to subsequent transplantation of polyoma induced tumor cells. It was suggested that the specific antitumor resistance is due to the reaction of the organism against common foreign antigens, induced in virus-transformed cells. According to a hypothesis of Habel (1962a,b,c) such virus-transformed cells appear in virus-inoculated adult animals as well as in newborns. Immunologically competent adult animals recognize the appearance of TSTA, however, and reject transformed antigenic cells. Thus, the immunological reaction of adult animals inhibits tumor induction. In contrast to adults, immunologically immature newborn animals inoculated with tumor virus acquire tolerance to the TSTA of virus-transformed cells and thus multiplication of tumor cells may take place without immunological control.

Habel's hypothesis explained almost all experimental data obtained in the study of resistance phenomenon. However, the following three proposals lack experimental proof: (a) appearance of immunological tolerance to TSTA in animals infected with DNA tumor virus when newborn; (b) the role of immunological tolerance in viral carcinogenesis; and (c) the connection between the appearance of TSTA and cell transformation in DNA tumor virus-infected cells.

Although no direct proof was available, some data favor the possible development of immunological tolerance in polyoma virus-inoculated newborn animals (Habel, 1961a, 1962b,c). Resistance to challenge with live polyoma tumor cells developed later in animals inoculated with polyoma virus as newborns than in animals inoculated as adults. It has also been demonstrated that polyoma tumors *can* be induced in adults if immunological reactivity is decreased as a result of total-body irradiation (Law and Dawe, 1960) or thymectomy (Law and Ting, 1965).

In Syrian hamsters, SV40-infected when newborn, it was demonstrated that, however, at any time during the latency period, infected animals do not differ from noninfected animals of the same age with regard to their sensitivity to challenge with different doses of SV40 tumor cells (Deichman and Kluchareva, 1964b, 1965). Furthermore, when SV40-infected newborn hamsters are reinfected with SV40 after they have become immunologically mature, they are capable of acquiring specific antitumor resistance, similarly to normal animals of the same age. These experiments show that animals infected with SV40 during the first few hours of their life do not become tolerant, nor are they resistant to the TSTA of SV40-induced tumors. Appearance of specific resistance in SV40-infected hamsters was first observed 15 to 20 days after primary tumor nodules became palpable.

Since SV40-infected hamsters are immunologically competent during the latent period, it must be assumed that continuous contact of the organism with a certain number of TSTA-bearing cells during a long period of time is insufficient for the induction of a state of antitumor immunity. As with any contact of competent hosts with foreign antigens, a definite threshold antigen quantity is required for efficient recognition. In the case of SV40-induced tumors this is attained soon after the appearance of palpable tumors. If a rejection process, connected with an immunological or nonimmunological recognition of the most antigenic tumor cell variants is really taking place during the latent period, this process is apparently not pronounced during SV40-oncogenesis, since it failed to increase the level of resistance or to induce antibodies against specific T- or surface antigens (Black et al., 1963; Deichman and Kluchareva, 1964b, 1966b). It is also well known that inoculation of adult animals with 10^5 to 10^6 tumor cells is often insufficient for the induction of specific antitumor resistance.

It seems possible that in the process of carcinogenesis there is a moment when the situation becomes critical. This is the time when the number of tumor cells (or perhaps more precisely, the concentration of TSTA) attains the threshold level and the presence of foreign antigens is recognized. The level of immune reactivity, expressed by the number of tumor cells that can be rejected during a given time unit, the number of tumor cells, and the rate of their doubling, determines the outcome of this conflict situation which was referred to, regarding successful tumor appearance, as the "sneaking through" of the tumor (Alexander, 1965; Mikulska et al., 1965).

It is not clear whether there is a similar situation during the latent period of chemical carcinogenesis with retained immunological competence but lack of recognition toward the antigenically distinct cells. In DNA viral oncogenesis, there is clearly a state of immunological nonreactivity which resembles acquired tolerance, but is also quite distinct from it. The essential difference is demonstrated by the fact that an immune response can be readily induced in such animals, capable of preventing primary tumor appearance or of the growth of tumor grafts bearing the same TSTA (Deichman and Kluchareva, 1964a,b; Eddy et al., 1964). It was demonstrated that tumors can be induced even in adult SV40-infected hamsters, although in a much lower percentage and after prolonged latent period (Allison et al., 1967).

Thus, the following postulates can be put forward:

1. Infection of newborn animals with DNA tumor viruses does not necessarily lead to induction of immunological tolerance to the TSTA of corresponding tumor cells.

2. A state of immunological tolerance is not a necessary condition for tumor induction in neonatally infected animals.

3. The absence of an immunological reaction in animals infected with some DNA tumor viruses when newborn together with their inability to recognize subthreshold quantities of TSTA-bearing cells promotes the development of primary tumors.

Could this be true for RNA virus-induced tumors and leukemias as well? It is generally assumed, that immunological tolerance is characteristic for spontaneous leukemias and mammary tumors in mice, caused by vertically transmitted RNA viruses. However, it seems very doubtful that immunological tolerance is a necessary condition for the induction of such neoplasms.

Inoculation of adult mice with leukemia viruses leads to the induction of resistance against the transplantation of syngeneic leukemia cells. Animals that were resistant against challenge with syngeneic leukemia cells may develop primary virus-induced leukemia later (Prigogina and Stavroskaya, personal communication).

It follows that mouse leukemia may appear not only in immunologically tolerant animals, but in immune animals as well. A state of immunological tolerance to virally induced mammary tumors in mice may not prevail in all infected animals (Morton, 1964), even under conditions of vertical transmission (Blair, 1966; Blair et al., 1966). Moreover, in some primary mammary tumor-bearing animals a state of immunoligical resistance can be demonstrated against the transplantation of autochthonous tumor cells (Weiss and Attia, 1964; Weiss et al., 1964).

In mice inoculated with polyoma virus when newborn, a state of specific resistance against transplantation of polyoma tumor cells was demonstrated during the latent period. This state apparently did not impede primary polyoma tumor induction (Habel, 1962a). In this case the antitumor resistance may have been induced by the continuing replication of infectious polyoma virus beginning in the newborn and continuing for some time after immunological maturation of the animals. The appearance of polyoma hemagglutination-inhibiting antibodies in newborn infected mice (Habel, 1962c) may serve as evidence in favor of this explanation.

In mice infected with Rous sarcoma virus when newborn, specific antitumor resistance was demonstrated in those animals in which tumors did not appear (Sjögren and Jonsson, 1963; Jonsson and Sjögren, 1965a,b; Jonsson, 1966). Since the same state of resistance could not be induced in Rous virus-inoculated adults, it was suggested that immunization with virus-transformed cells is involved in the case of infected newborn animals.

Thus, appearance of primary tumors induced by DNA or RNA tumor viruses is possible not only in immunologically tolerant or nonreactive organisms, but sometimes under conditions of acquired antitumor immunity as well.

B. QUANTITATIVE ASPECTS OF THE IMMUNOLOGICAL
   RELATIONSHIP BETWEEN THE HOST AND DNA TUMOR
   VIRUS-INFECTED OR TRANSFORMED CELLS

It has been noted that virus-induced primary tumors can appear in hosts with widely different immunological status. Since both the tumorigenic and the resistance-inducing functions of the DNA tumor viruses are involved in tumor induction in vivo, the quantitative relationships of these functions in time, and particularly during the latent period, is apparently a factor of decisive significance. In other words, if the virus-induced conversion of a certain number of normal cells into tumor cells requires a smaller dose of virus and less time than is necessary for the induction of a resistance level sufficient for the rejection of all transformed cells, a tumor may appear. Such "positive" balance favoring oncogenic action is usually observed after DNA tumor virus infection of newborn, immunologically immature animals. A similar situation may prevail in animals infected as adults, under one of the following conditions: (1) if a relatively large number of cells is involved in transformation; (2) if the virus is immunodepressive; and (3) if the multiplication rate of the transformed cells is high. For example, Rous sarcoma virus induces tumors in adult fowls apparently owing to condition (1), and maybe (3), whereas mouse leukemia may be more related to conditions (1) and (2).

As already discussed in Section III, the resistance-inducing and oncogenic activities of a DNA tumor virus *in vivo* may reflect two different viral functions in the cell. It has not yet been excluded that it may become possible to separate these functions at the virus–cell interaction level by using partly inactivated or defective viral genomes. The consequences of the two functions at the level of the organism infected with the DNA tumor virus are apparently separable in time. In other words, if tumor virus infection leads to a large number of cells synthesizing TSTA, sufficient for the induction of antitumor immunity, and the number of transformed cells does not exceed the critical level that can be rejected by the same immune organism, specific resistance to challenge with established tumor cells may be the only obvious result of tumor virus infection. Such a positive balance in favor of antitumor immunity apparently occurs after the inoculation of adult animals with some DNA tumor viruses. There are no data showing the appearance of even small numbers of transformed cells in adult DNA virus-infected animals, however. Resistance is induced very rapidly and is demonstrable a few days after virus inoculation (Habel, 1962c; Deichman and Kluchareva, 1965). It seems doubtful that transformed cells have enough time to appear before the resistant state becomes established. We, therefore, favor the explanation that the two functions of DNA tumor viruses in the cell, i.e., TSTA synthesis and transformation, are separate. This would explain the resistance phenomenon observed in DNA tumor virus-infected adult animals.

It should be mentioned that a similar interpretation of the resistance phenomenon induced by polyoma virus in adult mice was presented in 1961 by S. E. Luria in discussing the original experimental data of Sjögren, Hellström, and Klein. It was speculated that polyoma virus can induce new cellular antigens in infected, although nontransformed cells; these would correspond to the tumor-specific antigens responsible for immunity (Sjögren *et al.*, 1961).

If one assumes that TSTA synthesis can be induced early in the process of abortive cell infection with DNA tumor viruses and that this is the cause of the resistance of adult virus-inoculated animals to challenge with tumor cells, the absence of such resistance in immunologically competent animals infected with the same virus when newborn (Deichman and Kluchareva, 1964b) must be reconsidered. The following explanation may be suggested: TSTA synthesis is induced in infected cells of newborn animals as well as in the cells of adult animals. For unknown reasons, this antigen disappears from the majority of the infected cells, however, before the recognition mechanisms of immunologically mature animals may begin their work. During the first 8 days of life the weight of newborn hamsters increases 2.5 to 3-fold. Rapid cell division in newborn animals is one of the possible reasons for the disappearance of virus-induced antigens from cells where their synthesis has not been fixed by the integration of the viral genome. In this case the remaining and probably small number of cells undergoing virus-induced transformation would not be sufficient to be recognized as foreign.

This suggestion is indirectly confirmed by experiments on the immunization of adult hamsters with SV40-infected, nontransformed and virus-free hamster embryo tissue culture cells. The specific immunogenicity of 10^8 such cells is comparable to the effect of about 10^6 to 10^7 $TCID_{50}$ doses of live virus (Kluchareva et al., 1967). These experiments were performed with stationary cultures, and it is not known whether the same result could be obtained after immunization of animals with the cells of infected cultures undergoing serial passage.

Obviously, some other alternatives cannot be excluded at present, although they require additional assumptions regarding the antigenic behavior of DNA tumor virus-infected and -transformed cells. A different explanation is apparently required for the behavior of some RNA tumor virus-infected cells. No tumor-specific resistance phenomenon could be demonstrated in adult mammals infected with the Rous sarcoma virus (RSV), although these animals could be readily immunized against the grafting of Rous virus-induced mouse sarcoma, by inoculating virus-free syngeneic or allogeneic tumor cells of the same origin (Sjögren and Jonsson, 1963; Jonsson and Sjögren, 1965a,b; Jonsson, 1966). Animals infected with RSV as newborns and which remained free from induced tumors appeared to be resistant against challenge with corresponding tumor cells. Attempts to immunize adult mice with mouse embryo tissue culture cells infected with RSV *in vitro* not only failed to protect against tumor cell inoculation, but lead, on the contrary, to RSV tumor induction (Kryukova and Obuch, 1968).

These data can be interpreted to indicate that the Rous virus induces

TSTA synthesis only in cells that become transformed, whereas in DNA virus-infected cells TSTA appears in the majority of the infected cells, presumably long before transformation, as discussed above. On the other hand, viral structural proteins, which appear during virus maturation on the membrane of virogenic cells transformed by some RNA tumor viruses seem to render the cells vulnerable to antiviral antibodies. It is not clear whether the resistance phenomenon induced by mouse leukemia viruses and the cytotoxic effect of the sera from resistant animals (Klein *et al.*, 1962; Sachs, 1962; Wahren, 1963; Pasternak and Graffi, 1963; Prigogina and Stavrovskaya, 1964) can be fully explained by the action of antiviral antibodies. Absence of correlation between Moloney leukemia virus release from leukemic cells and cellular immunosensitivity *in vitro* led to the suggestion that TSTA, distinct from viral coat protein, could be responsible for the immunosensitivity of mouse leukemia cells (G. Klein and Klein, 1964).

The suggested basic difference between the synthesis of TSTA in DNA and in RNA tumor virus-infected cells explains some differences in the oncogenic expression of the two virus groups in nature. The following three examples show that in spite of widespread contamination of certain human and animal populations with some potentially oncogenic DNA viruses, there is no corresponding appearance of spontaneous tumors: (*1*) polyoma virus dissemination among laboratory and wild mice; (*2*) SV40 among some species of monkeys; (*3*) adenoviruses among humans and monkeys. Conceivably, the absence of spontaneous tumors induced by these agents in the natural host may be explained as being not only due to protection by antiviral antibodies or to infection with too low, nononcogenic virus doses, but also due to the development of antitumor resistance in naturally infected animals. In nature, human wart virus and the Shope papilloma virus are the only known tumor inducers that belong to the DNA papova tumor virus group. In contrast, many RNA tumor viruses are known, capable of inducing spontaneous tumors and leukemia in different animal species.

It is tentatively concluded that the quantitative and time relationships between the transforming and TSTA-inducing activities of a tumor virus at the level of the infected cell population is the most essential factor in determining the outcome of a potentially oncogenic virus–cell interaction, with regard to DNA and RNA viruses, in newborn and adult animals as well.

C. Qualitative Changes of Tumor Cells during Their *in Vivo* Growth in the Primary Host

Induction of primary tumors in animals infected when newborn with some DNA tumor viruses (SV40 and adeno 12) can be prevented by reinfection with the same virus during the latent period (Deichman and

Kluchareva, 1964a; Eddy *et al.*, 1964) or by the inoculation of live cells transformed by the same virus (Girardi, 1965). A decreased tumor incidence was noted in hamsters inoculated with irradiated homologous SV40 tumor cells during the latent period (Goldner *et al.*, 1964). A single second inoculation of SV40 virus 3.5 months before the termination of the latent period was sufficient for tumor prevention in all infected animals (Deichman and Kluchareva, 1964a). The efficiency of prophylactic immunization against primary SV40 tumors decreases gradually if reinfection with the virus is performed at later stages, and falls to zero 2 weeks prior to the termination of the minimum latent period. Thus, the selection of the most appropriate time for prophylactic immunization against primary tumors depends not only on the time that has passed from the beginning of the process, but also on the time remaining until tumor appearance. Although there are no data on the rate of tumor cell growth during the latent period, immunization experiments indicate that there is apparently some relationship between the quantity of tumor cells present in the organism and the efficiency of tumor prevention. The finding of antibodies against T-antigen and SCMA in some animals immunized during the latent period and the absence of such antibodies in infected nonimmunized animals until tumors appear, indicates that reinfection during the latent period leads to the destruction of tumor cells (Deichman and Kluchareva, 1966b).

However, qualitative tumor cell changes akin to tumor progression (Foulds, 1954, 1958) during the latent period and expressed as a decrease of cellular immunosensitivity cannot be excluded. Published data of Sjögren (1964b) and our observations show that passage of DNA virus-induced tumors in normal or virus-inoculated animals does not lead to any significant changes in their immunosensitivity.

The quantitative approach to the problems of antitumor immunization is an attempt to simplify the situation and so far it seems that it may hold true for the initial stages of carcinogenesis. After termination of the latent period, as the primary tumor grows, the immunological situation becomes more complicated and specific and qualitative tumor cell changes appear to be further involved in the process. The graft rejection test has demonstrated a decrease in the immunosensitivity of SV40 hamster tumor cells during primary tumor growth in an immune organism (Deichman and Kluchareva, 1966a). A direct correlation was found between the duration of tumor growth in the immune organism and the loss of immunosensitivity. Immunoresistant cells appeared earlier and more frequently in metastases than in primary tumor nodules. In general, appearance of lung metastases of SV40 hamster tumors coincided with the beginning of the decline in immunosensitivity. This may lead to the paradoxical situation where the cells of the primary tumor are still immunosensitive, whereas the metastases are immunoresistant, all in the same animal. This may be interpreted as indicating the selection of immunoresistant tumor cell variants in the metastases. In rare instances, lung metastases appeared subsequent to the regression of palpable subcutaneous primary SV40-induced tumors in hamsters immunized during the late stages of the latent period (Deichman, Prigogina, and Kluchareva, 1967 unpublished data). It is not surprising that attempts to immunize animals against the metastases of the primary tumor failed. Qualitative changes and selection of immunoresistant cells, thus, probably take place even during the early stage of carcinogenesis, before the appearance of palpable tumors. These changes in immuno-sensitivity were not stable and attempts to select immunoresistant tumor cell lines, stable in subsequent passages, failed, although more than thirty lines of SV40-induced tumors and metastases were assayed in transplantation tests. Thus, the loss of TSTA by immunoresistant variants, an explanation that appeared to us most probable previously (Deichman and Kluchareva, 1966a), seems to be doubtful, although not completely excluded, at present.

Loss of immunosensitivity by cells of DNA virus-induced tumors is not observed as a rule during the *in vivo* transplantation of tumor cells in normal or resistant animals (Sjögren, 1964b). A study of the role played by the prolonged action of humoral antibodies on the TSTA of growing tumor cells is one of the possible approaches to this problem.

In conclusion, it may be emphasized that in spite of common antigens in virus-induced tumors, potentially capable of eliciting immunity, there are some other factors connected both with the tumor and the organism, that inhibit the potential immunological destruction of the tumor to a significant degree. The most important factors appear to be the following:

1. The level of antitumor immunity that can be induced is relatively low and may be inefficient if a large number of tumor cells is present.

2. Tumor cells may undergo specific qualitative changes during their growth in an immune organism and immunoresistant cell variants may appear.

3. In certain instances, there may be a state of immunological non-reactivity or tolerance to the TSTA of the tumor cells.

4. The immunological competence of the organism may decrease for various reasons.

Thus, the numerous negative results obtained in attempts to mobilize immunity for the therapy of primary tumors or their metastases is probably not accidental. From this point of view, the elucidation of *in vivo* factors capable of inhibiting effective immunological rejection of tumor cells can be considered as a token of definite progress in tumor immunology in recent years.

In addition to specificity, immunological reactions against tumor cells, although limited by quantitative and qualitative factors, have an exceptionally important advantage in their capacity to recognize and reject minimal numbers of antigenically foreign tumor cells at almost any site in the organism. Realization of this advantage is an easy task when relatively small numbers of tumor cells are present in an immunologically competent host at the time of immunization, and if all tumor cells are immunosensitive. During experimental carcinogenesis induced by some DNA tumor viruses this situation prevails only during the latent period. It is possible that the same situation may apply, or be created, in some cases of spontaneous carcinogenesis. However, this optimism is based on the study of rather artificial models of DNA virus-induced tumors which probably do not have exact copies in nature.

REFERENCES

Alexander, P. 1965. *In* "Scientific Basis of Surgery" (W. T. Irvine, ed.), pp. 478–495. Churchill, London.

Alexander, P., Delorme, E., and Hall, J. 1966. *Lancet* **I** (N7448), 1186–1189.

Allison, A. C., Chesterman, F. C., and Baron, S. 1967. *J. Natl. Cancer Inst.* **38**, 567–572.

Altstein, A. D., Deichman, G. I., and Dodonova, N. N. 1966. *Virology* **30**, 747–749.

Altstein, A. D., Deichman, G. I., Saricheva, O. F., Dodonova, N. N., Zeitlin, E. M., and Vassilieva, N. N. 1967a. *Virology* **33**, 747–748.

Altstein, A. D., Saricheva, O. F., and Dodonova, N. N. 1967b. *Virology* **33**, 744–746.

Ardashnikov, S. N., and Spasskaya, I. G. 1949. *Zh. Mikrobiol. Epidemiol. i Immunobiol.* **9**, 44–48.

Ardashnikov, S. N., Prigogina, E. L., and Spasskaya, I. G. 1955. *Vopr. Onkol.* **6**, 71–74.

Barth, R. F., Espmark, Y. A., and Fagreus, A. 1967. *J. Immunol.* **98**, 888–892.

Bases, R. 1963. *Cancer Res.* **23**, 811–817.

Basilico, C., and diMayorca, G. 1965. *Proc. Natl. Acad. Sci. U.S.* **54**, 125–127.

Benjamin, T. L. 1965. *Proc. Natl. Acad. Sci. U.S.* **54**, 121–124.

Benjamin, T. L. 1966. *J. Mol. Biol.* **16**, 359–373.

Benjamin, T. L. 1967. *In* "Subviral Carcinogenesis," 1st Intern. Symp. Tumor Viruses (Y. Ito. ed.), pp. 62–81. Nissha, Kyoto.

Black, P. H. 1966. *Virology* **28**, 760–763.

Black, P. H., Rowe, W. P., Turner, H. C., and Huebner, R. J. 1963. *Proc. Natl. Acad. Sci. U.S.* **50**, 1148–1156.

Blair, P. B. 1966. *In* "Viruses Inducing Cancer, Implications for Therapy" (W. J. Burdette, ed.), pp. 288–304. Univ. of Utah Press, Salt Lake City, Utah.

Blair, P. B., Lavrin, D. H., Dezfulian, M., and Weiss, D. W. 1966. *Cancer Res.* **26**, 647–651.

Butel, J. S., and Rapp, F. 1965. *Virology* **27**, 490–495.

Carp, R. I., and Gilden, R. V. 1965. *Virology* **27**, 639–641.

Carp, R. I., and Gilden, R. V. 1966. *Virology* **28**, 150–162.

Carp, R. I., Kit, S., and Melnick, J. L. 1966. *Virology* **29**, 503–509.

Chu, E. H. Y., Stjernswärd, J., Clifford, P., and Klein, G. 1967. *J. Natl. Cancer Inst.* **39**, 595–617.

Defendi, V. 1963. *Proc. Soc. Exptl. Biol. Med.* **113**, 12–16.

Defendi, V. 1966. *Progr. Exptl. Tumor Res.* **8,** 125–188.

Defendi, V., and Jensen, F. 1967. *Science* **157,** 703–705.

Defendi, V., and Koprowski, H. 1959. *Nature* **184,** 1579–1580.

Defendi, V., and Taguchi, F. 1966. *Ann. Med. Exptl. Biol. Fenniae (Helsinki)* **44,** 232–241.

Defendi, V., Carp, R. I., and Gilden, R. V. 1966. *In* "Viruses Inducing Cancer, Implications for Therapy" (W. J. Burdette, ed.), pp. 269–287. Univ. of Utah Press, Salt Lake City, Utah.

Deichman, G. I., and Kluchareva, T. E. 1964a. *Nature* **204,** 1126–1128.

Deichman, G. I., and Kluchareva, T. E. 1964b. *Virology* **24,** 131–137.

Deichman, G. I., and Kluchareva, T. E. 1965. *In* "Viruses, Cancer and Immunity," pp. 270–278. Medicina, Moscow. In Russian.

Deichman, G. I., and Kluchareva, T. E. 1966a. *J. Natl. Cancer Inst.* **36,** 647–655.

Deichman, G. I., and Kluchareva, T. E. 1966b. *Vestn. Akad. Med. Nauk SSSR* **9,** 12–19.

Delorme, E. J., and Alexander, P. 1964. *Lancet* **II** (W7351), 117–120.

Dulbecco, R., Hartwell, L. H., and Vogt, M. 1965. *Proc. Natl. Acad. Sci. U.S.* **53,** 403–410.

Eddy, B., Borman, G., Grubbs, G., and Young, R. 1962. *Virology* **17,** 65–75.

Eddy, B., Grubbs, G., and Young, R. 1964. *Proc. Soc. Exptl. Biol. Med.* **117,** 575–579.

Fagreus, A., and Espmark, Y. A. 1961. *Nature* **190,** 370–371.

Foley, E. J. 1953. *Cancer Res.* **13,** 835–837.

Foulds, L. 1954. *Cancer Res.* **14,** 327–339.

Foulds, L. 1958. *J. Chronic Diseases* **8,** 2–37.

Frearson, P. M., Kit, S., and Dubbs, D. R. 1966. *Cancer Res.* **26,** 1654–1660.

Fuginaga, K., and Green, M. 1966. *Proc. Natl. Acad. Sci. U.S.* **55,** 1567–1574.

Gershon, D., Hausen, P., Sachs, L., and Winocour, E. 1965. *Proc. Natl. Acad. Sci. U.S.* **54,** 1584–1592.

Gershon, D., Sachs, L., and Winocour, E. 1966. *Proc. Natl. Acad. Sci. U.S.* **56,** 918–925.

Gilden, R. V., and Carp, R. I. 1966. *J. Bacteriol.* **91,** 1295–1297.

Gilden, R. V., Carp, R. I., Taguchi, F., and Defendi, V. 1965. *Proc. Natl. Acad. Sci. U.S.* **53,** 684–694.

Girardi, A. J. 1965. *Proc. Natl. Acad. Sci. U.S.* **54,** 445–451.

Globerson, A., and Feldman, M. 1964. *J. Natl. Cancer Inst.* **32,** 1229–1243.

Goldner, H., Girardi, A. J., Larson, V. M., and Hilleman, M. R. 1964. *Proc. Soc. Exptl. Biol. Med.* **117,** 851–857.

Govaerts, A. 1960. *J. Immunol.* **85,** 516–522.

Green, M., and Fuginaga, K. 1967. *In* "Subviral Carcinogenesis," 1st Intern. Symp. Tumor Viruses (Y. Ito, ed.), pp. 82–95. Nissha, Kyoto.

Habel, K. 1961. *Proc. Soc. Exptl. Biol. Med.* **106,** 722–725.

Habel, K. 1962a. *J. Exptl. Med.* **115,** 181–193.

Habel, K. 1962b. *Virology* **18,** 553–558.

Habel, K. 1962c. *Ann. N. Y. Acad. Sci.* **101,** 173–179.

Habel, K. 1965. *Virology* **25,** 55–61.

Habel, K. 1966. *Cancer Res.* **26,** 2018–2024.

Habel, K. 1967. *In* "Subviral Carcinogenesis," 1st Intern. Symp. Tumor Viruses (Y. Ito, ed.), pp. 195–206. Nissha, Kyoto.

Habel, K., and Eddy, B. 1963. *Proc. Soc. Exptl. Biol. Med.* **113,** 1–4.

Habel, K. Jensen, F., Pagano, J. S., and Koprowski, H. 1965. *Proc. Soc. Exptl. Biol. Med.* **118,** 4–9.

Hamburg, V. P., and Svet-Moldavsky, G. I. 1964. *Nature* **203,** 772–773.

Harder, F. H., and McKhann, C. F. 1968. *J. Natl. Cancer Inst.* **40,** 231–242.

Hare, J. D. 1964a. *Proc. Soc. Exptl. Biol. Med.* **115**, 805–810.

Hare, J. D. 1964b. *Proc. Soc. Exptl. Biol. Med.* **117**, 598–603.

Hare, J. D. 1966. *Proc. 9th Intern. Cancer Congr., Tokyo* p. 299. Abstr. SO515.

Hare, J. D., and Godal, T. 1965. *Proc. Soc. Exptl. Biol. Med.* **118**, 632–636.

Hare, J. D., and Morgan, H. R. 1963. *Proc. Am. Assoc. Cancer Res.* **4**, 26.

Haškova, V., Svejcar, J., Pekarek, J., Johanovsky, J., and Hilbert, J. 1967. *Folia Biol. (Prague)* **13**, 293–298.

Hatanaka, M., and Dulbecco, R. 1966. *Proc. Natl. Acad. Sci. U.S.* **56**, 736–740.

Hellström, J., and Sjögren, H. O. 1965. *Exptl. Cell Res.* **40**, 212–215.

Hellström, J., and Sjögren, H. O. 1967. *J. Exptl. Med.* **125**, 1105–1118.

Hellström, K. E. 1963. *Nature* **199**, 614.

Hellström, K. E. 1964. *Science* **143**, 477.

Hoggan, M. D., Rowe, W. P., Black, P. H., and Huebner, R. J. 1965. *Proc. Natl. Acad. Sci. U.S.* **53**, 12–19.

Huebner, R. J., Chanock, R. M., Rubin, B. A., and Casey, M. I. 1964. *Proc. Natl. Acad. Sci. U.S.* **52**, 1333–1340.

Irlin, J. S. 1967. *Virology* **32**, 725–728.

Jeejeebhoy, H. F., Delorme, E. J., and Alexander, P. 1966. *Transplantation* **4**, 397–403.

Jensen, F., Koprowski, H., and Ponten, J. A. 1963. *Proc. Natl. Acad. Sci. U.S.* **50**, 343–348.

Jonsson, N. 1966. *Proc. 9th Intern. Cancer Congr., Tokyo* p. 306. Abstr. SO529.

Jonsson, N., and Sjögren, H. O. 1965a. *J. Exptl. Med.* **122**, 403–421.

Jonsson, N., and Sjögren, H. O. 1965b. *Exptl. Cell Res.* **40**, 159–162.

Kit, S. 1967. *In* "Subviral Carcinogenesis," 1st Intern. Symp. Tumor Viruses (Y. Ito, ed.), pp. 116–143. Nissha, Kyoto.

Klein, E., and Klein, G. 1964. *J. Natl. Cancer Inst.* **32**, 547–568.

Klein, E., Clifford, P., Klein, G., and Hamberger, C. A. 1967. *Intern. J. Cancer* **2**, 27–36.

Klein, G., and Klein, E. 1964. *Science* **145**, 1316–1317.

Klein, G., Sjögren, H. O., Klein, E., and Hellström, K. E. 1960. *Cancer Res.* **20**, 1561–1572.

Klein, G., Sjögren, H. O., and Klein, E. 1962. *Cancer Res.* **22**, 955–961.

Klein, G., Clifford, P., Klein, E., and Sternswärd, J. 1966a. *Proc. Natl. Acad. Sci. U.S.* **55**, 1628–1635.

Klein, G., Klein, E., and Haughton, G. 1966b. *J. Natl. Cancer Inst.* **36**, 607–621.

Klein, G., Clifford, P., Klein, E., Smith, R. T., Minowada, J., Kourilsky, F. M., and Burchenal, J. H. 1967. *J. Natl. Cancer Inst.* **39**, 1027–1044.

Kluchareva, T. E., Shachanina, K. L., Belova, S., Chibisova, V., and Deichman, G. I. 1967. *J. Natl. Cancer Inst.* **39**, 825–832.

Koch, M. A., and Sabin, A. B. 1963. *Proc. Soc. Exptl. Biol. Med.* **113**, 4–12.

Koldovsky, P., and Svoboda, J. 1962. *Folia Biol. (Prague)* **8**, 95–100.

Koprowski, H., and Fernandes, M. V. 1962. *J. Exptl. Med.* **116**, 467–476.

Koprowski, H., Jensen, F., Girardi, A., and Koprowska, J. 1966. *Cancer Res.* **26**, 1980–1993.

Kryukova, J. N., and Obuch, I. B. 1968. *Nature* **219**, 174–177.

Latarjet, R., and Chamaillard, L. 1962. *Bull. Cancer* **49**, 382–389.

Latarjet, R., Cramer, R., and Montagnier, L. 1967. *Virology* **33**, 104–111.

Law, L. W., and Dawe, C. I. 1960. *Proc. Soc. Exptl. Biol. Med.* **105**, 414–419.

Law, L. W., and Ting, R. C. 1965. *Proc. Soc. Exptl. Biol. Med.* **119**, 823–830.

Law, L. W., Ting, R. C., and Leckband, E. 1967. *Proc. Natl. Acad. Sci. U.S.* **57**, 1068–1075.

Lejneva, O. M., Zilber, L. A., and Jevleva, E. S. 1965. *Nature* **206**, 1163–1164.
Luria, S. E. 1959. *Can. Cancer Conf.* **3**, 261–270.
Malmgrem, R. A., Takemoto, K. K., and Carney, R. G. 1968. *J. Natl. Cancer Inst.* **40**, 263–268.
Melnick, J. L., and Askenazi, A. 1963. *Federation Proc.* **22**, 438.
Melnick, J. L., and Rapp, F. 1965. *J. Natl. Cancer Inst.* **34**, 529–534.
Metzgar, R. S., and Oleinick, S. R. 1968. *Cancer Res.* **28**, 1366–1371.
Michel, M. R., Hirt, B., and Weil, R. 1967. *Proc. Natl. Acad. Sci. U.S.* **58**, 1381–1388.
Mikulska, L. B., Smith, C., and Alexander, P. 1965. *J. Natl. Cancer Inst.* **36**, 29–35.
Möller, E., and Möller, G. 1962. *J. Exptl. Med.* **115**, 527–552.
Möller, G. 1961. *J. Exptl. Med.* **114**, 415–434.
Möller, G. 1964. *Nature* **204**, 846–847.
Morton, D. L. 1964. *Proc. Am. Assoc. Cancer Res.* **5**, 46.
Murka, L. M. 1965. *Bul. Eksperim. Biol. i Med.* **12**, 111–112.
Old, L., Boyse, P. A., and Stockert, E. 1964. *Nature* **201**, 777–779.
Oxman, M. N., and Black, P. H. 1966. *Proc. Natl. Acad. Sci. U.S.* **55**, 1133–1140.
Oxman, M. N., Baron, S., Black, P. H., Takemoto, K. K., Habel, K., and Rowe, W. P. 1967. *Virology* **32**, 122–127.
Pasternak, G., and Graffi, A. 1963. *Brit. J. Cancer* **17**, 532–539.
Pekarek, J. 1967. *Meeting European Tumor Virus Group, 4th, Sorrento, Italy.*
Prehn, R. T., and Main, J. M. 1957. *J. Natl. Cancer Inst.* **18**, 769–778.
Prigogina, E. L., and Stavrovskaya, A. A. 1964. *Nature* **201**, 934–936.
Rapp, F. 1967. *In* "Subviral Carcinogenesis," 1st Intern. Symp. Tumor Viruses (Y. Ito, ed.), pp. 311–325. Nissha, Kyoto.
Rapp, F., and Melnick, J. L. 1966. *Progr. Med. Virol.* **8**, 349–399.
Rapp, F., Melnick, J. L., Butel, J. S., and Kitahara, T. 1964. *Proc. Natl. Acad. Sci. U.S.* **52**, 1348–1352.
Rapp, F., Butel, J. S., Feldman, L. A., Kitahara, T., and Melnick, J. L. 1965a. *J. Exptl. Med.* **121**, 935–944.
Rapp, F., Butel, J. S., and Melnick, J. L. 1965b. *Proc. Natl. Acad. Sci. U.S.* **54**, 717–724.
Rapp, F., Melnick, J. L., and Kitahara, T. 1965c. *Science* **147**, 625–627.
Rapp, F., Melnick, J. L., and Levy, B. 1967. *Am. J. Pathol.* **50**, 849–860.
Rapp, F., Jerkofsky, M., Melnick, J. L., and Levy, B. 1968. *J. Exptl. Med.* **127**, 77–90.
Revesz, L. 1960. *Cancer Res.* **20**, 443–451.
Rosenau, W., and Moon, H. D. 1961. *J. Natl. Cancer Inst.* **27**, 471–483.
Rowe, W. P. 1965. *Proc. Natl. Acad. Sci. U.S.* **54**, 711–717.
Rowe, W. P. 1967. *Perspectives Virol.* **5**, 123–146.
Rowe, W. P., and Baum, S. G. 1964. *Proc. Natl. Acad. Sci. U.S.* **52**, 1340–1347.
Rowe, W. P., and Baum, S. G. 1965. *J. Exptl. Med.* **122**, 955–966.
Sabin, A. B. 1966. *Proc. Natl. Acad. Sci. U.S.* **55**, 1141–1148.
Sabin, A. B., and Koch, M. A. 1964. *Proc. Natl. Acad. Sci. U.S.* **52**, 1131–1138.
Sachs, L. 1961. *Exptl. Cell Res.* **24**, 185–188.
Sachs, L. 1962. *J. Natl. Cancer Inst.* **29**, 759–764.
Sachs, L. 1965. *Nature* **207**, 1272–1274.
Sambrook, J., Westphal, H., Srinivasan, P. R., and Dulbecco, R. 1968. *Proc. Natl. Acad. Sci. U.S.* **60**, 1288–1295.
Sauer, G., and Defendi, V. 1966. *Proc. Natl. Acad. Sci. U.S.* **56**, 452–457.
Sauer, G., Koprowski, H., and Defendi, V. 1967. *Proc. Natl. Acad. Sci. U.S.* **58**, 599–606.
Sjögren, H. O. 1961. *Virology* **15**, 214–219.
Sjögren, H. O. 1963. *Can. Cancer Conf.* **5**, 377–386.

Sjögren, H. O. 1964a. *J. Natl. Cancer Inst.* **32,** 361–374.
Sjögren, H. O. 1964b. *J. Natl. Cancer Inst.* **32,** 661–666.
Sjögren, H. O. 1964c. *J. Natl. Cancer Inst.* **32,** 375–393.
Sjögren, H. O. 1965. *Progr. Exptl. Tumor Res.* **6,** 289–322.
Sjögren, H. O., and Hellström, J. 1967a. *In* "Specific Tumor Antigens," Intern. Symp. Sukhumi, SSSR, 1965 (R. J. S. Harris, ed.), pp. 162–171. Munksgaard, Copenhagen.
Sjögren, H. O., and Hellström, J. 1967b. *In* "Subviral Carcinogenesis," 1st Intern. Symp. Tumor Viruses (Y. Ito, ed.), pp. 207–219. Nissha, Kyoto.
Sjögren, H. O., and Jonsson, N. 1963. *Exptl. Cell Res.* **32,** 618–621.
Sjögren, H. O., Hellström, J., and Klein, G. 1961. *Exptl. Cell Res.* **23,** 204–208.
Slettenmark, B., and Klein, E. 1962. *Cancer Res.* **22,** 947–954.
Stewart, S. E., Eddy, B. E., Stanton, M. F., and Berkeley, W. H. 1958. *Proc. Am. Assoc. Cancer Res.* **2,** 348.
Takemoto, K. K., Malmgren, R. A., and Habel, K. 1966. *Virology* **28,** 485–488.
Taylor, H. E., and Culling, C. F. 1963. *Lab. Invest.* **12,** 884–894.
Tevethia, S. S., and Rapp, F. 1965. *Proc. Soc. Exptl. Biol. Med.* **120,** 455–458.
Tevethia, S. S., Kats, M., and Rapp, F. 1965. *Proc. Soc. Exptl. Biol. Med.* **119,** 896–901.
Todaro, G. I., and Green, H. 1966. *Proc. Natl. Acad. Sci. U.S.* **55,** 302–308.
Todaro, G. I., Nilausen, K., and Green, H. 1963. *Cancer Res.* **23,** 825–835.
Vassilieva, N. N., and Altstein, A. D. 1964. *In* "Memorial Tarasevitch Conference" (I. Michailow *et al.*, ed.), pp. 178–179. State Control Inst., Moscow. In Russian.
Vogt, M., and Dulbecco, R. 1963. *Proc. Natl. Acad. Sci. U.S.* **49,** 171–179.
Wahren, B. 1963. *J. Natl. Cancer Inst.* **31,** 411–423.
Watkins, J. F., and Dulbecco, R. 1967. *Proc. Natl. Acad. Sci. U.S.* **58,** 1396–1403.
Weil, R., Michel, M. R., and Ruschman, G. K. 1965. *Proc. Natl. Acad. Sci. U.S.* **53,** 1468–1477.
Weil, R., Petursson, G., Kara, J., and Diggelman, H. 1967. *In* "The Molecular Biology of Viruses" (S. J. Colter and W. Paranchych, eds.), pp. 593–626. Academic Press, New York.
Weiss, D. W., and Attia, M. A. 1964. *Proc. Am. Assoc. Cancer Res.* **5,** 67.
Weiss, D. W., Faulkin, L. I., and DeOme, K. B. 1964. *Cancer Res.* **24,** 732–741.
Westphal, H., and Dulbecco, R. 1968. *Proc. Natl. Acad. Sci. U.S.* **59,** 1158–1165.
Wilson, D. B. 1963. *J. Cellular Comp. Physiol.* **62,** 273–285.
Winn, H. J. 1960. *J. Immunol.* **84,** 530–538.
Yoshida, T. O., and Southam, C. M. 1963. *Proc. Am. Assoc. Cancer Res.* **4,** 74.
Zilber, L. A. 1945. *J. Mikrobiol. Epidemiol. i Immunol.* **45,** 16.
Zilber, L. A. 1958. *Advan. Cancer Res.* **5,** 291–329.
Zilber, L. A., and Abelev, G. I. 1962. "Virology and Immunology of Cancer," pp. 121–139. Medgiz, Moscow. In Russian.

REPLICATION OF ONCOGENIC VIRUSES IN VIRUS-INDUCED TUMOR CELLS—THEIR PERSISTENCE AND INTERACTION WITH OTHER VIRUSES*

H. Hanafusa

Department of Viral Oncology, The Public Health Research Institute of The City of New York, Inc., New York, New York

I. Introduction

Infection of cells with ordinary animal viruses generally results in lysis of host cells with a concomitant release of virus progeny. It is almost self-evident, however, that such a lytic interaction does not take place in virus-induced tumor cells. Instead of the destruction of cells, the tumor viruses induce the violent growth of infected cells which is characteristic of malignant tumors. In the history of tumor virus research, the fate of the virus in these proliferating cells has repeatedly come into question. It has been known that high titers of infectious virus are recoverable from certain tumor tissues, such as Rous sarcoma and mouse mammary tumors, and from the plasma of leukemic animals infected with avian or murine leukemia viruses. On the other hand, no infectious virus has been detected in rabbit carcinomas induced by papilloma virus, a phenomenon originally described as "masking" of virus in tumor cells (Shope, 1950).

In the last decade some important progress relevant to this problem has been made in the field of tumor virology, namely the isolation of a number of new tumor viruses in experimental animals, and the development

* Supported by Public Health Service Research Grant No. CA-08747 from the National Cancer Institute.

of an accurate quantitative assay of tumor viruses by *in vitro* transformation. Thus, the problem of virus persistence has been recently examined in more detail at the cellular level with a variety of viruses. Recognition of the fact that infectious virus eventually disappears in cultures of transformed cells induced by most DNA-containing tumor viruses was one important outcome of these studies. This calls attention to a possible analogy with the lysogenic bacteriophages in virus–cell interaction. In fact, several lines of evidence indicate that at least a portion of the genome of tumor viruses does exist in transformed cells, although nothing is yet known about how it exists in the cells.

On the other hand, chicken cells transformed *in vitro* by the RNA-containing Rous sarcoma virus (RSV) release infectious virus continuously. Rous sarcoma virus reproduction is complicated, however, by its consistent association with leukosis viruses. Analysis of interaction between these viruses led to the notion that some strains of RSV are dependent on the associated leucosis virus in reproduction, and the RSV was, therefore, assumed to be defective. More recent studies have disproved this assumption by showing that the transformed cells do produce RSV of which the host range is very limited. The role of the associated virus appears to be in extending the host range of RSV by modifying its outer structure. This, however, is not the case with mammalian cells transformed by RSV and infectious RSV can be recovered only when these cells are cultured in the presence of normal chicken cells.

Mutual interaction of tumor viruses has also been observed in other systems. The relationship between murine sarcoma virus and leukemia viruses is in many respects very similar to that between RSV and avian leukosis viruses. In deoxyribonucleic acid (DNA) viruses, a unique hybrid of adenovirus and simian virus 40 was discovered. This hybrid virus is defective and requires the assistance of adenovirus for its replication. These examples demonstrate the importance of the interaction between viruses in expression of oncogenic potentials and propagation in host cells.

The fate of virus in infected cells is not only a fundamental subject in the study of virus replication but also has important implications for the basic mechanism of virus carcinogenesis. Absence of complete virus in some transformed cells immediately suggests that the function of the whole virus genome may not be required for cellular transformation. If the presence of only a segment of the virus genome is responsible for the continued expression of the malignant character of cells, the analysis of the functions of that virus genome is of prime importance in understanding cellular malignancy. From a practical point of view, knowledge about the state of known viruses in transformed cells should serve as a valuable model for further research on virus etiology in cancers.

This article will present a summary of the present knowledge about replication of viruses in virus-induced tumor cells and the interaction of tumor viruses.

II. Rous Sarcoma Virus

A. Original Observations on Apparently Nonvirus-Producing Rous Cells

General properties of RSV and earlier observations made on the absence of detectable RSV in transformed cells have been reviewed by several authors (Rubin, 1964; Purchase, 1965; Vogt, 1965b; Hanafusa, 1968). The original findings on nonvirus production by RSV-infected cells (Hanafusa *et al.*, 1963) may be summarized as follows: (*1*) All stocks of the Bryan high-titer strain of RSV contain two viruses—RSV and at least one avian leukosis virus termed Rous-associated virus (RAV). These two viruses differ only in their pathogenicity for host cells: RSV produces sarcoma in chickens and transforms chick embryo fibroblasts into malignant sarcoma cells, whereas RAV produces leukosis in chickens and causes no morphologically recognizable alteration in chick embryo fibroblasts. Although these two viruses are indistinguishable for other biological and physical properties, the concentration of RAV is generally higher than RSV, so that RAV can be isolated simply by diluting the RSV/RAV mixture. (*2*) When monolayers of chick embryo cells are infected with very high dilutions of the mixture to assure the single infection of RSV, the RSV-infected cells become transformed. Most clones of these transformed cells produce no infectious RSV detectable by transforming activity in chick embryo cells. Some clones do produce RSV, but when this occurs RAV is also produced. (*3*) The nonvirus-producing transformed cells (NP cells) retain their characteristic morphology indefinitely. Rous sarcoma virus production can be elicited from every NP cell at any time by superinfection with RAV, but cannot be achieved by UV- or X-irradiation of the NP cells. In addition to RAV, all viruses that belong to the avian leukosis virus group are effective as helper viruses, but NDV and influenza viruses are not, even though they are close to RSV in virus particle ultrastructure. No single case was observed in which cells produced RSV in the absence of the leukosis virus.

These observations led to the conclusion that RSV is a defective virus in reproduction of infectious progeny. The defective function of the RSV genome present in every transformed cell is complemented by RAV, which, therefore, was designated as "helper virus" (Hanafusa *et al.*, 1963).

It should be noted here that the detection of RSV was made by measuring its ability to transform chick embryo cells of C/O type, according to the classification of chick embryo phenotypes described below (Section II, B, 3 and Table I). These C/O embryos are the most commonly available genetic type and are known to be susceptible to virtually all strains of leukosis viruses so far isolated. Therefore they were considered the most suitable cells for detection of any infectious RSV.

These studies were all made with Bryan high-titer strain of RSV. Some other strains, such as Bryan standard strain and Fujinami sarcoma virus are also apparently defective (Temin, 1962; Vogt, 1965b). However, the defective characteristic of RSV is not general to all other strains. The Schmidt-Ruppin strain of RSV was most extensively investigated and proved to be actively reproducing in transformed cells without any assistance of helper virus (Dougherty and Rasmussen, 1964; Hanafusa, 1964; Goldé, 1966; Hanafusa and Hanafusa, 1966a,b). Since this strain produced a relatively low titer of virus from transformed cells and the virus yield was increased by superinfection of transformed cells with helper virus, consideration was given for defectiveness of a quantitative rather than a qualitative nature. Later it was shown that this low infectivity is mainly attributable to its poor capacity to be adsorbed on host cells and not directly related to the quantitative yield of virus (Hanafusa and Hanafusa, 1967). It was concluded that the apparent defectiveness is a specific property of certain strains and that virus reproduction and cell transformation can coexist in transformed cells originally infected by a nondefective strain of RSV.

B. ROLE OF HELPER VIRUS

1. *Antigenicity of Rous Sarcoma Virus*

Further studies were made on the role of associated leukosis virus in production of RSV. Two observations suggested that NP cells do not contain virus-specific coat antigen for RSV (Hanafusa *et al.*, 1964a). First, the extract of NP cells has no capacity to absorb antibody for RAV and RSV. Second, chickens bearing tumors produced by transplantation of NP cells do not produce any neutralizing antibody for RSV and remain fully susceptible to challenge infection by another RSV. These results suggest that RSV lacks the ability to make viral surface antigen in infected cells, and probably this is the function provided by the helper virus. Supporting this conclusion is the fact that the antigenicity of RSV is determined strictly by the strain of helper virus used in production of RSV from NP cells and is identical to that of the helper virus (Hanafusa *et al.*, 1964a; Hanafusa, 1965; Vogt, 1965a). There is no cross-neutralization between RSV's activated by two distantly related helper viruses. Since the neutralizing antigens most likely localize in the outer coat of virus, it is reasonable to assume that RSV uses the components of virus coat made by the helper virus. Basically this phenomenon is the same as phenotypic mixing between two viruses grown in the same host cells (Novick and Szilard, 1951; Hirst and Gotlieb, 1953). Here antigenic components made by the two viruses are withdrawn in a random fashion by two types of virus genomes at the time of virus assembly.

Although NP cells lack viral coat antigens, they contain another virus-specific antigen. This antigen, detectable by complement fixation tests, is supposed to be an inner viral component common to all avian leukosis-sarcoma virus (Huebner et al., 1964a; Vogt et al., 1965; Payne et al., 1966; Bauer and Schäfer, 1966; Kelloff and Vogt, 1966).

In addition to antigenicity, some other RSV properties are also determined by the helper virus. These helper-dependent properties of RSV are presumably determined by the nature of the viral coat, which plays an essential role in some early steps of virus infection. Two of these properties will be discussed in the following sections, since they are relevant to the later development of studies.

2. Sensitivity to Interference

Rubin (1960) showed that multiplication of avian leukosis viruses in chick embryo cells rendered these cells resistant to infection by RSV. The degree of interference can be visualized by a marked reduction in the number of foci formed by the challenging RSV. Unlike the rather non-specific interference mediated by interferon, this interference by leukosis viruses is very specific for RSV and does not affect the multiplication of any other virus (Rubin, 1960; Hanafusa et al., 1964b). By the use of RSV activated by the different helper viruses, it was demonstrated that interference is also specific among certain combinations of leukosis virus and RSV (T. Hanafusa et al., 1964; Hanafusa, 1965; Vogt, 1965a). In general, RSV activated by one strain of helper virus was interfered with most strongly by that strain of helper virus.

Vogt and Ishizaki (1966) studied the interfering relationship among various strains of avian leukosis viruses and RSV. It was shown that the leukosis viruses belonging to one subgroup classification (based on host range specificity, see below) interfere with RSV activated by the same subgroup of leukosis viruses but not with those of other subgroups. Since the helper virus appears to determine some components in the viral coat of RSV, interference or blockage of RSV infection in the resistant cells probably occurs in some early steps of infection where the viral coat is involved. Steck and Rubin (1966a,b) identified penetration as a crucial step in this interference.

3. Host Range Specificity

It has been observed that different strains of chickens have different susceptibility to avian tumor viruses. Some reports indicate that this difference is a heritable characteristic of chicken strains (Waters and Fontes, 1960). Crittenden et al. (1963) demonstrated that the resistance found in animals can also be exhibited in tissue culture and, therefore, is a property of individual cells.

In the course of study of the interfering relationship, a heterogeneity in both embryos and virus preparations was discovered (T. Hanafusa et al., 1964). This led to the isolation of two different leukosis viruses from RSV stocks and recognition of the presence of embryos resistant to one of them (Hanafusa, 1965; Vogt, 1965a). A certain proportion of embryos obtained from commercial suppliers are resistant to RAV-2 and, thus, to RAV-2-activated RSV [designated RSV(RAV-2)], which has the same host range, but not to RAV-1 or its cognate RSV(RAV-1) whereas a majority of them are susceptible to both viruses. In the resistant cultures, virus growth as well as focus formation is inhibited. These characteristics of embryos are a property of cells and not due to the presence of helper virus in the embryos. Later, embryos having the reverse susceptibility, i.e., sensitive to RAV-2 but resistant to RAV-1, and embryos resistant to both viruses were found (Vogt and Ishizaki, 1965). Classification of these host cells and host range of RAV-1 and RAV-2 made by Vogt and Ishizaki (1965) are shown in Table I. Genetic studies on the resistance indicated that chickens have two independent genes for susceptibility to two types of viruses, RAV-1 and RAV-2. In each case the susceptibility is dominant over resistance (Rubin, 1965; Payne and Biggs, 1964; Crittenden and Okazaki, 1965; Crittenden et al., 1967).

Based on the host range character of many viruses examined, Vogt and Ishizaki (1965) proposed a classification of avian leukosis and sarcoma viruses in three subgroups, shown in Table I. There are certain viruses that do not fall into the two well-characterized A and B groups and are now classified in subgroup C (Vogt et al., 1966). It is noteworthy to point out that the specificity of the host range of avian leukosis viruses and their cognate RSV's is very profound. With purified preparations of RSV(RAV-1) or RSV(RAV-2) the ratio of the number of foci on sensitive cells to that on insensitive cells is greater than 10^5.

The determination of RSV host range by helper virus suggests that the cell resistance is due to a block at an early phase of infection (Hanafusa, 1965). Piraino (1967) showed that adsorption of virus takes place at the same rate in both resistant cells and susceptible cells, but the virus remains outside the resistant cells in a form accessible to the action of virus-neutral-

TABLE I
GENETIC CELLULAR RESISTANCE TO AVIAN TUMOR VIRUSES

Cell type	Avian tumor virus subgroup[a]		
	A	B	C
C/O	S[b]	S	S
C/A	R[b]	S	S
C/B	S	R	S
C/AB	R	R	S[c]

[a] The subgroup A includes RAV-1, RAV-3, RAV-4, RAV-5, avian myeloblastosis virus type 1, Fujinami associated virus type 1, Schmidt-Ruppin strain of RSV type 1, resistance-inducing factor type 1, lymphomatosis virus strain RPL-12, and Mill Hill strain of RSV. The subgroup B includes RAV-2, avian myeloblastosis virus type 2, Schmidt-Ruppin strain of RSV type 2, resistance-inducing factor type 2, and Harris strain of RSV. The subgroup C includes Carr-Zilber strain of RSV, Prague strain of RSV, and RAV-50.

[b] R—resistant; S—susceptible.

[c] C/AB type cells are partially resistant to Carr-Zilber and Prague strains of RSV.

izing antibody. It, therefore, appears that the block in the resistant cells is also in the penetration process. It is conceivable that chicken cells have a reaction site which is involved in the penetration of avian tumor viruses. At least two cellular genes, responsible for receptor sites for subgroups A and B, would determine the susceptibility or resistance of cells to these viruses. This hypothesis explains virus-induced RSV interference as well (Steck and Rubin, 1966a). When the receptors are occupied by preinfected leukosis virus, challenging RSV activated by the same leukosis virus cannot react with these sites and, therefore, fails to penetrate the cells. But RSV activated by other leukosis viruses is not affected by this interference because it reacts with different cell receptors.

The studies on the antigenicity of viruses (neutralization antigen) showed that the classification by host range coincides with the classification by antigenicity (Ishizaki and Vogt, 1966). Viruses that have the same host range are antigenically closely related. Thus the structural component contributed by the helper virus may determine the specificity of three characteristics of RSV—surface antigen(s), host range, and interfering capacity. The nature of the component(s) has not been established.

A recent study suggests that efficiency of adsorption of RSV is also determined by helper virus. Some RSV belonging to subgroups B and C are only poorly adsorbed to host cells, and the efficiency is greatly enhanced when they infect cells preinfected with RAV-1 or normal cells treated with diethylaminoethyl (DEAE)–dextran (Hanafusa and Hanafusa, 1967; Vogt, 1967b).

C. Reproduction of RSV in Transformed Cells

1. *Presence of Virus Particles in RSV-Transformed Cells*

In an extensive study of the ultrastructure of RSV-infected cells, Dougherty and Di Stefano (1965) revealed the presence of virus particles indistinguishable from those of the avian leukosis–sarcoma group on the surface of NP cells. No such virus particles were found on control non-infected chick embryo cells. In the culture fluids of these NP cells, neither detectable transforming virus nor avian leukosis virus was found. Although the average number of particles on the NP cells was smaller than that usually found on RSV-producing cells (on the average about 50 particles per NP cell compared to about 500 to 5000 particles per producing cell), there was no single NP line free of them. This finding was later confirmed by other investigators (Courington and Vogt, 1967; Haguenau and Hanafusa, 1968).

Robinson (1967) confirmed the presence of virus particles in NP cultures by another physical method. She found that when NP cells were cultured in the presence of tritiated uridine, labeled virus particles which sedimented at the same rate as infectious RSV were released into the culture fluid. Ribonucleic acid (RNA) extracted from the particles was indistinguishable in its sedimentation rate and base ratio from RNA obtained from an infectious RSV and RAV mixture. The number of labeled particles from NP cells sometimes reached about 50% of that from RSV-producing cells.

Further, these particles were demonstrated to be infectious. In repeated assays of the culture fluid of a number of NP lines, Weiss (1967) occasionally found distinct focus-forming virus. The titer was usually very low, but sometimes contained more than 10^3 focus-forming units (FFU) per milliliter. This finding first seemed strange since it obviously contradicts previous observations made by many investigators of the absence of focus-forming virus in NP cells. The contradiction was soon solved when Vogt (1967a) found that RSV produced from NP cells has a peculiar host range. Since there is no detectable helper virus in these NP cells, he designated the RSV as RSV(o), indicating its helper-independent production. His investigations showed that, unlike any RSV variants so far studied, RSV(o) is noninfectious for over 90% of the cells derived from C/O and for all C/B- and C/AB-type chick embryos. It is infectious, however, for chick embryo cells derived from a large proportion of C/A type, as well as a small proportion of C/O type embryos. The most susceptible host is the Japanese quail embryo cell, which is known to resemble the C/B type of chick embryo cell in susceptibility to known avian tumor viruses belonging to subgroups A and B. The unique host range of RSV spontaneously produced from NP cells was confirmed by Hanafusa and Hanafusa (1968).

Obviously RSV(o) does not belong to any subgroup classified by host range specificity of known avian tumor viruses. None of these viruses is restricted in its infection to C/O type chick embryo cells. Moreover, about 10% of embryos of C/O or C/A type are susceptible to RSV(o). Since the cells derived from a single embryo are always identical in susceptibility or resistance to RSV(o), it seems likely that this cellular characteristic is under the control of another different cellular gene.

The yield of RSV(o) from NP cells is relatively low—on the order of 10^4 to 10^5 FFU per 10^6 transformed cells. However, the infectivity of RSV(o) can be enhanced by the presence of certain agents which are active in enhancement of adsorption of RSV(RAV-2) and SR-RSV, so that the amount of virus actually produced from NP cells is of the same order as that produced by RSV in the presence of helper virus (Hanafusa and Hanafusa, 1968). Replication of RSV(o) does not require helper virus. In sensitive quail or chick embryo cells, RSV(o) can multiply and produce progeny RSV having the same host range as the parental virus (Hanafusa and Hanafusa, unpublished observations).

The possibility of the presence of an unrecognized helper virus in the NP cultures was considered and proved to be unlikely (Vogt, 1967a; Hanafusa and Hanafusa, 1968). The helper virus determines the host range of RSV in helper-assisted RSV production. Hence, the noninfectiousness of RSV(o) for C/O cells indicates the absence of helper virus able to infect the C/O cells which were used to produce NP cells. Indeed, no helper virus was isolated from RSV(o) preparations using sensitive C/A and quail cells. The possibility of the presence of another unknown type of helper virus was also eliminated (Hanafusa and Hanafusa, 1968).

The description of RSV as a defective virus was based on the notion that it was unable to form its own coat and that it relied on a helper virus for this function. The term "defectiveness" is given to a virus that lacks an essential virus function. It is now clear that RSV does produce a substantial amount of virus particles which are infectious for certain host cells without the aid of a helper virus and, therefore, is not lacking any vital function. The role of helper virus is to extend the limited host range of RSV by adding its determinant(s) to the outer structure of the RSV particle. Therefore the concept of defectiveness is not applicable to RSV. The failure of RSV to infect certain host cells must be explained in terms of its limited host range, and the failure to detect RSV coat antigen in earlier studies of NP cells must have been produced by the use of antibodies made by RAV-1 or RSV which chiefly contain RAV-1 and RSV(RAV-1). The now inappropriate term, NP cells, for the cells transformed by RSV has been replaced by "leukosis virus negative Rous cells" (L-R cells) (Hanafusa and Hanafusa, 1968).

There is no critical difference between Bryan strain RSV and other strains so far differentiated by their "defectiveness." Phenotypic mixing or, more properly, genomic masking of RSV by helper virus is found with all of these strains. Thus various strains of RSV may be considered as a series of host range variants.

2. *Variants of Bryan RSV*

Although most L-R cells (NP cells) release RSV infectious for C/A chick or quail embryo cells, some of them do not release this type of RSV (Hanafusa and Hanafusa, 1968). Among a number of clones of L-R cells made by infecting C/O cells with ordinary stocks of RSV(RAV-1), about 90% of the clones produced RSV(o), the virus with the host range described in the previous section. However, the other 10% of the clones produced no RSV detectable by infectivity on any available host cells, even in the presence of the enhancing agent. When this latter type of transformed cell was labeled with ³H-uridine, RSV particles were found having the same sedimentation rate in sucrose gradient as infectious RSV. The RSV infectious for quails was designated RSVβ, and the noninfectious RSVα. The L-R cells were also designated L-Rβ and L-Rα, depending on what type of RSV they released. Either type of L-R cell released only one type of RSV over an extended period of cultivation, indicating that if these viruses are variants they are genetically stable in transformed cells. When super-infected with RAV-1, both types of L-R cells produced almost the same amount of RSV(RAV-1). Reisolation of clones from C/O cells infected with RSV(RAV-1) derived from the two types of L-R cells indicated that the existence of the two virus types is primarily of viral origin. All L-R cells induced by RSV(RAV-1) derived from L-Rβ cells were β in type, and about 80% of the cells transformed by virus derived from L-Rα cells were α in type on reisolation. Since the same host cells were used throughout the reisolation studies of the two types of L-R cells, the contribution of host cells seems unlikely. However, about 20% of the RSV genomes derived from α-type L-R cells were β type on reisolation. Since no β-type RSV(o) is produced from L-Rα cells cultured for long periods, this result suggests the participation of RAV-1 in the conversion of α-type RSV to β type. The possible role of RAV in this conversion has not been determined.

These studies indicate that at least two variants of RSV are present in Bryan RSV stocks. The nature of the noninfectiousness of RSVα(o) is unknown, but it could be another host range variant having susceptible host cells which so far have remained unrecognized. More recently it was shown that RSVβ could be converted to RSVα by treatment with some mutagenic agents (T. Hanafusa, unpublished observations). This finding, together with the fact that α virus can also be converted to β by mixed growth with RAV-1, suggests that RSVα could be more deficient in the gene function of synthesizing virus coat efficient for penetration.

Besides these variants, various forms of RSV may exist in nature. Using X-irradiation, Goldé and Latarjet (1966) showed that the transforming capacity of the Schmidt-Ruppin strain of RSV is more radioresistant than its infectivity. The irradiated virus can transform chicken cells which do not produce infectious virus even after superinfection with leukosis viruses. Similarly, Vogt (1967a) described that, on rare occasions, cells transformed by Bryan RSV produce a very limited amount of RSV upon superinfection with RAV. These RSV's may well be a different type of variant, the repressed function of which cannot be complemented by leukosis virus.

3. *Rous Sarcoma Virus Reproduction in Mammalian Hosts*

Svet-Moldavsky (1957) and Zilber and Kryukova (1957) demonstrated that RSV can produce tumors even in rats and mice. This finding was followed by a number of reports of tumor production by RSV in various species of mammals (Vogt, 1965b). The tumors appeared either as hemorrhagic cysts or as sarcoma which, in their histological appearance, resemble those produced in chickens. However, the tumors in mammals differ from those in chickens in some basic aspects. (*1*) Although the tumors are transplantable into the same species of animal, they cannot be passaged by a cell-free tumor homogenate. These tumor homogenates are noninfectious even for chickens. (*2*) However, injection of the living tumor cells into chickens produces typical chicken sarcoma from which RSV is recoverable. (*3*) The tumor-bearing animals develop complement-fixing antibodies and graft rejection reaction, but no neutralizing antibody against RSV. (*4*) Certain strains of RSV are unable to produce tumors in mammals.

Most of the work on mammalian tumor production by RSV has been done with RSV strains maintained in the European laboratories, such as Schmidt-Ruppin, Carr-Zilber, and Engelbreth-Holm (Prague). The history of these viruses is not entirely clear, but they induce sarcomas in chickens which are similar to those induced by the Bryan strain of RSV, and are assumed to originate from the same virus isolated by Rous. On the other hand, many efforts to induce tumors in mammals with the Bryan and Harris strains have failed, and it was thought that there might be a distinct difference between these two groups of RSV strains (Ahlström and Jonsson, 1962; Klement and Svoboda, 1963; Harris and Chesterman, 1963; Munroe and Southam, 1964). However, recent studies with Bryan RSV showed that under certain conditions this strain is also capable of producing tumors in mammals (Febvre et al., 1964; Rabotti et al., 1965). More precise studies on the strain difference indicated that the nature of the virus coat may play a determining role in the ability of virus to infect mammals, and, therefore, this ability can be discussed on the same basis as host range specificity in chick embryo cells (Hanafusa and Hanafusa, 1966a). For example, the Schmidt-Ruppin strain of RSV is able to produce sarcomas in newborn hamsters but it becomes inactive when the virus is coated with RAV-1. Bryan RSV, which is usually noninfectious for hamsters in the form of RSV(RAV-1) or RSV(RAV-2), becomes infectious in the form of RSV(RAV-50). Tumors induced by the Bryan strain are similar in most characteristics to those induced by other strains. Therefore there seems to be no critical difference between strains of RSV in the ability to transform and replicate in mammalian cells.

Absence of infectious RSV in the induced tumors has been demonstrated with a wide variety of mammals and *in vitro* with transformed rat and hamster cells (Vogt, 1965b). The only exceptions to this rule were hamster sarcoma cells infected with Prague strain of RSV (Svoboda and Klement, 1963) and rat cells infected with a field isolate of avian sarcoma virus B77 (Thurzo et al., 1963; Hlavayova et al., 1964). Infectivity was, however, mainly tested by inoculating chickens or tissue cultures of chick embryo cells. The question arose as to whether these tumors, like the chicken transformed cells described earlier, release virus particles infectious only for certain types of host cells. This, however, seems to be unlikely, since virus is absent in mammalian cells transformed by Schmidt-Ruppin and Prague strains of RSV which can replicate in every chicken cell type in the absence of leukosis virus (Section II, A; Goldé and Vigier, 1966). The production of a noninfectious form of virus particle in mammalian tumors remains to be studied. Electron-microscopic studies on the glioma cells of dogs induced by Bryan RSV showed particles resembling avian tumor viruses (Rabotti et al., 1966). Such particles have so far not been found in tumors induced in other animals.

Svoboda (1960, 1961, 1962) found that when RSV-infected rat tumor cells are transplanted into chickens, sarcomas are produced which have chromosomes characteristic of chicken cells. Furthermore, infectious RSV can be recovered from these chicken tumors. No such tumors are induced by cell-free homogenates of the rat tumors. This phenomenon was also demonstrated *in vitro* when a mixed culture of rat tumor cells with normal chick embryo cells resulted in formation of chicken transformed cells which produced infectious RSV (Simkovic et al., 1963). This finding was confirmed with tumors induced by different strains of RSV in various species of animals (Ahlström and Forsby, 1962; Hanafusa and Hanafusa, 1966a; Sarma et al., 1966; Vigier and Svoboda, 1965). It was shown that the physical contact of tumor cells with living chicken cells is essential for virus production. Such a phenomenon has a close resemblance to the situation in the SV40 hamster system, and it was suggested that rescue of both viruses takes place by the same mechanism. Formation of giant cells by fusion can very frequently be seen with aged transformed cells, and RSV may be replicated in the heterokaryons formed by mammalian tumor cells and chicken cells. Indeed, the induction of RSV is enhanced when the mixed cultures are treated with UV-inactivated Sendai virus, which causes fusion of adjacent heterologous cells (Vigier and Montagnier, 1966). The same mechanism is proposed for rescue of SV40 from hamster cells cultured with monkey cells (Section IV).

The success in recovery of infectious RSV from cloned tumor cells by cell contact strongly suggests that the entire viral genome is present in every tumor cell (Simkovic et al., 1963). The reason why RSV fails to replicate in mammalian cells is not known. The presence of virus genome and absence of neutralizing antigen in tumor cells suggest that the block is in some late step before production of virus coat.

III. Murine Sarcoma Virus

Murine leukemia viruses are very similar to avian leukosis viruses in many physical and biological characteristics. Both viruses mature at the cell surface, and they are similar in size and ultrastructure (Rich and Moloney, 1966; Rich and Siegler, 1967). Relatively large RNA's were extracted from purified particles of both classes of virus (Robinson et al., 1965; Duesberg and Robinson, 1966; Baluda, 1966), and the replication of both is inhibited by the presence of actinomycin D (Temin, 1963; Bader, 1964; Duesberg and Robinson, 1967; Bases and King, 1967).

The absence of host cells supporting the growth of the virus in tissue culture and the lack of an accurate assay system were two major difficulties encountered in the early studies of murine leukemia virus. These problems have been solved to some extent in recent studies, especially following the discovery of murine sarcoma virus. The newly isolated murine sarcoma virus resembles avian sarcoma virus in its interaction with leukosis virus, as well as many other biological properties. Therefore, the knowledge obtained from avian sarcoma–leukosis virus studies can be successfully applied to these murine viruses.

Harvey (1964) and Moloney (1966) independently found a sarcoma-inducing virus in the stocks of Moloney leukemia virus. In mice and rats the sarcoma virus induces a fibrosarcoma which yields a mixture of sarcoma virus together with Moloney leukemia virus (MLV). On the other hand, hamster tumors induced by this sarcoma–leukemia mixture do not release infectious progeny.

A tissue culture system was soon developed for this murine sarcoma virus (MSV) (Hartley and Rowe, 1966; Ting, 1966). On a cell monolayer of mouse or rat embryo, MSV causes characteristic transformation, and the transformed cells grow into countable foci. Moloney leukemia virus also grows in the cultured cells, but causes no cytopathic changes. The presence of excess MLV in the stock of MSV was shown by production of MLV beyond the dilution end point of MSV. In dose–response experiments the number of foci decrease proportionately to the square of the dilution of inoculated virus (a mixture of MSV and MLV) (Hartley and Rowe, 1966). When excess MLV was added to the inoculum, a one-hit response curve was obtained. These results indicate that focus formation by MSV depends on simultaneous infection with MLV and, perhaps, takes place only when the initially infected cells release progeny virus which is infectious for surrounding cells. In this respect MSV differs from RSV, because the latter does not require leukosis virus for cellular transformation.

Recently O'Connor and Fischinger (1968) presented evidence suggesting that the MSV preparation may contain two kinds of MSV particles, one called "defective" which requires MLV for focus formation and another called "competent" which does not require MLV. This hypothesis is based on the dose response of focus formation by virus stocks obtained from infected cells of different ages. Virus produced in the early days after infection was rich in the defective form, whereas that produced later was rich in the competent form. However, the assay method for MSV used in these studies does not include an agar overlay of infected cultures. In such assay cultures the transformed cells loosely attached to the plate might be lost in a subsequent medium change, or the virus produced from the originally infected cells might spread far beyond the surrounding cells, resulting in either a lower or higher evaluation, respectively, of the number of FFU. Thus, more precise analysis seems to be required for the *in vitro* assay of MSV.

Mouse cells infected with the MSV–MLV mixture always produce progeny virus. Nonvirus-producing cells have not been isolated, probably because of the difficulty of isolating cells singly infected with MSV which always exists with a large excess of MLV (ratio of MLV to MSV is estimated to be about 1000). On the other hand, hamster cells do not release a detectable amount of infectious MSV. The presence of the virus genome in the hamster tumors was demonstrated by the method used for RSV-infected hamster tumors. When the hamster tumor cells were inoculated into mice carrying leukemia virus or cultured *in vitro* with mouse embryo cells in the presence of leukemia virus, mouse transformed cells appeared and produced MSV (Huebner *et al.*, 1966). In the absence of leukemia virus, no virus production was recorded. Using this technique with various strains of mouse leukemia virus, Huebner *et al.* (1966) were able to produce various pseudotypes of MSV, namely MSV having the antigenic specificity (coat) of leukemia virus strains Rausher, Friend, Gross, and Moloney. This virus reconstruction seems to be entirely the same as that seen with RSV and a number of avian leukosis viruses. Indeed, a relationship between MSV and MLV can be seen in antigenicity (Huebner *et al.*, 1966), host range (Huebner, 1967b), and interference (Sarma *et al.*, 1967). These artificially produced MSV pseudotypes will facilitate many important studies on murine leukemia virus by providing systems more easily controlled at the quantitative level.

So far no infectious MSV has been recovered from MSV-induced hamster cells. Considering the recent developments with RSV, it seems conceivable that these hamster tumor cells release MSV of which the host range is restricted in the mouse strain thus far used. There is an indication of the presence of genetically determined resistance among mouse strains. If, indeed, it is ultimately shown that they do not produce infectious virus, the MSV-hamster system may be equivalent to the RSV-hamster system.

The term "defectiveness" is used for MSV in a similar sense to that used for RSV before. At the moment it may be difficult to prove or disprove its adequacy, because that would depend on the existence of host cells with different virus susceptibility. In this connection it would be informative if one could isolate MSV-infected mouse or rat cells in the absence of MLV and examine their virus production.

The striking similarity between avian and murine sarcoma–leukosis viruses suggests that such a relationship may be present in other species of animals. It is needless to mention the significance of these models in studies of sarcoma and leukemia in the human being. The genesis of sarcoma and leucosis virus is also of interest in view of the relatedness shown in their profound mutual interaction. Most likely these two viruses could have originated by mutation from a common ancestor, though so far no induced mutation has been observed between them.

IV. Polyoma, SV40, and Adenoviruses

It has been recognized that some DNA-containing viruses can produce tumors by inoculation into certain species of animals, and the resultant tumors often do not contain infectious virus (see reviews by Dulbecco, 1963; Negroni, 1963; Rapp and Melnick, 1966). From *in vitro* studies with a variety of host cells, it is known that infection of cells with these DNA viruses results in three different types of interaction. (*1*) In certain cells the virus causes a *lytic* interaction—the virus multiplies with a cytocidal change in the cells. In this system the virus may be assayed by its plaque-forming ability. When these sensitive cells are in the growing stage, sometimes the lytic interaction is limited to only a small proportion of the cells. (*2*) In the majority of cells the virus causes an *abortive* interaction which results in formation of virus-specific antigens, but no complete virus. (3) A "proliferative" reaction which corresponds to tumor formation in vivo— the infected cells transform into morphologically altered cells which unrestrictedly continue their multiplication.

In the last type of interaction, cells may release small amounts of virus in the early stage of transformation, but this virus disappears eventually in cloned cells maintained with antiserum. In some cultures transformed by SV40, continuous shedding of small amounts of virus has been reported (Gerber and Kirschstein, 1962; Sabin and Koch, 1963; Black and Rowe, 1963), but this cannot be regarded as active virus production from the transformed cells themselves since in these studies the assay of SV40 was done by plating of infected cells on susceptible monkey cells (see below). It is now generally recognized that most transformed cells induced by SV40, polyoma, and adenoviruses are entirely free from infectious virus.

In clones of polyoma-transformed cells, neither infectious polyoma DNA nor virus capsid protein was detectable, and early attempts to rescue the virus by superinfection with mutant viruses or to induce infectious virus from cells by the agents effective in induction of lysogenized bacteriophages were unsuccessful (Vogt and Dulbecco, 1962). However, the presence of at least a portion of the viral genome in these polyoma-transformed cells has been suggested by three lines of experimentation. The first evidence is based on the demonstration of a new antigen in transformed cells which relates to neither normal cell nor viral capsid antigens. This antigen is responsible for the rejection of transformed cells by immunologically competent host animals (Sjögren et al., 1961; Habel, 1962). Second, using two strains of polyoma virus differing in their antigenicity, Ting (1964) demonstrated the rescue of the antigen marker from transformed cells. Third, the presence of virus-specific DNA-like RNA (mRNA) in the transformed cells was demonstrated by the technique of hybridization (Benjamin, 1966).

Both virus-specific RNA and transplantation-rejecting antigens were found also in SV40- and adenovirus-induced tumor cells (Benjamin, 1966; Reich et al., 1966b; Fujinaga and Green, 1966; Aloni et al., 1968; Defendi, 1963; Trentin and Bryan, 1966). In addition, these transformed cells contain tumor-specific antigens which react with antibodies from tumor-bearing animals. These antigens, which are detectable by complement fixation or fluorescent antibody staining methods, are different from those in virus particles and, therefore, are called "tumor antigens" or "T-antigens" (Huebner, 1967a).

The presence of the viral genome of SV40 in transformed cells was also demonstrated by another method. Gerber and Kirchstein (1962) and Sabin and Koch (1963) reported that when SV40-induced tumors, from which no virus was detectable, were placed on a layer of normal living monkey cells, infectious virus was found in the latter cultures by plaque formation. The contact of the two types of cells seems to be essential for the activation of virus (Gerber, 1963). Later, it was shown that fusion of these cell types induced by UV-inactivated Sendai virus greatly enhances the formation of active SV40 (Gerber, 1966; Koprowski et al., 1967; Watkins and Dulbecco, 1967). These results strongly suggest that SV40 is produced by hetero-karyons formed by fusion between transformed cells and susceptible monkey cells. Of great interest is the finding that fusion of the cytoplasm is enough to induce the virus-specific change in the nuclei of transformed cells (Watkins and Dulbecco, 1967). This suggests that some cytoplasmic factor coming from monkey cells either negates some suppressive state existing in transformed cells or supplies missing functions in these tumor cells. It should be pointed out that there are some clones of transformed cells from which infectious virus could not be recovered by this technique (Koprowski et al., 1967; Watkins and Dulbecco, 1967). Infectious polyoma virus could not be recovered from transformed cells by the same technique (Watkins and Dulbecco, 1967). It is not known whether the failure to rescue results from difference in the size of integrated virus genome or from a different type of integration.

Among 31 human adenoviruses, some (types 12, 18 and 31) are classified as highly oncogenic and some others (types 3, 7, 14, 16 and 21) as weakly oncogenic, based on efficiency and the length of the latent period in tumor production. [Recently Freeman et al. (1967) demonstrated transformation of rat cells by type 2 adenovirus.] Green and co-workers demonstrated that adenoviruses of the same oncogenic class are closely related in viral DNA, as revealed by base ratios, homology between DNA–DNA, and homology between DNA and the virus-specific RNA formed in tumor cells (Pina and Green, 1965; Lacy and Green, 1964; Fujinaga and Green, 1966). From the data obtained in these homology experiments, they assumed that about one-half of the viral genome, at maximum, is either integrated into the tumor cells or transcribed to virus-specific RNA (Fujinaga and Green, 1966). Similarly, Aloni et al. (1968) estimated, from results of competition experiments between virus-specific RNA from transformed cells and the late RNA from virus-yielding cells, that only a third of the SV40 genome is transcribed in the transformed cells.

The requirement of only a part of the genome for transformation of cells was also suggested by the fact that the capacity of virus to transform cells is more radioresistant than the capacity to produce plaque (complete virus formation) (Benjamin, 1965; Basilico and DiMayorca, 1965; Latarjet et al., 1967). Much effort has already been devoted to the analysis of the functions of virus genomes in transformed cells, and this work will undoubtedly provide the most important clue for understanding the role of virus in cancer induction.

V. Hybrid of Adenovirus and SV40

A. ISOLATION AND PROPERTIES

Mutual interaction of tumor viruses has been shown between sarcoma and leukemia viruses of both chickens and mice. A different type of interaction was demonstrated with two distantly related DNA viruses—adenovirus and SV40.

In 1964, Huebner et al. (1964b) found that a preparation of adenovirus type 7 (adeno 7), designated as E46, produced tumors in hamsters which contained T-antigen specific to both adeno 7 and SV40. This adeno 7 preparation had once been contaminated with SV40 during passage in monkey kidney cell cultures and was, therefore, treated with antiserum for SV40 to eliminate this virus from the preparation. Although they contained SV40-induced tumor antigen, the tumors produced neither SV40 virus antigen nor complete SV40. The synthesis of SV40–T-antigen was also observed in cultured cells of monkey, human, rabbit, and hamster infected with E46 (Rowe and Baum, 1964; Rapp et al., 1964). The formation of SV40–T-antigen in cells was abolished by neutralization of E46 with antiadeno 7 but not with anti-SV40 serum, and by heating the virus at 56°C. for 10 minutes which inactivates the standard adeno 7 but not SV40 (Rowe and Baum, 1964; Rapp et al., 1964). These results suggested that the E46 preparation contains SV40 genomes in adenovirus capsids. This virus particle will be referred to as adeno 7–SV40+ in this chapter. In addition to the adeno 7–SV40+, the E46 stock also contained normal adeno 7, since the capacity to induce SV40–T-antigen was lost from plaque isolates obtained from terminal dilution passages in human embryo cells (Rowe and Baum, 1964).

The relationship between particles of the normal adeno 7 and adeno 7–SV40+ was further clarified by plating efficiency and virus production on two different host cells. In human embryo kidney (HEK) cells, adeno 7 grows to make plaques but SV40 does so only very poorly; however, in African green monkey kidney (GMK) cells, adeno 7 cannot grow but SV40 can make plaques. The E46 stock produced plaques equally well in both HEK and GMK cultures. The lysates of either culture contained both adeno 7 and adeno 7–SV40+, but no SV40 virus (Rapp et al., 1965; Rowe and Baum, 1965). The plaque formation in HEK cells by the E46 stock followed a one-hit dose response, but the dose response of plaque formation on GMK cells was of the two-hit type (Boeyé et al., 1966; Rowe and Baum, 1965). The number of plaques formed by E46 on GMK cells was enhanced

20- to 300-fold by the addition of excess amounts of adeno 7, but not by excess of SV40, and all of these plaques formed under conditions of enhancement released both adeno 7–SV40+ and adeno 7 viruses (Rapp et al., 1965).

These results were interpreted in the following way. Plaque formation on GMK cells requires double infection by adeno 7 and adeno 7–SV40+, but in HEK cells plaques are formed by either double infection or single adeno 7 infection. Since adenovirus itself cannot grow in GMK cells the production of adeno 7 from GMK plaques must be a result of assistance by adeno 7–SV40+. Likewise the replication of adeno 7–SV40+ in GMK cells depends on superinfection with adenovirus. Although SV40 cannot produce plaques in HEK cells, adeno 7–SV40+ replicates in cells doubly infected with adeno 7 and adeno 7–SV40+.

Because adeno 7–SV40+ alone cannot produce plaque either in GMK or HEK cells, this virus was defined as a defective virus which cannot replicate without the assistance of adenovirus. The adeno 7–SV40+ was designated as E46+ by Rowe and Baum (1965) and as "PARA," an acronym for "particles aiding and aided by replication of adenovirus," by Rapp et al. (1965).

In studies of enhanced plaque formation by adeno 7–SV40+ in the presence of excess adenovirus, the effects of other types of adenovirus were examined (Rapp et al., 1965; Rowe, 1965). Enhanced plaque formation was also obtained with adenovirus types 2 and 12. The resultant plaques contained adeno 2 or adeno 12 and adeno 7–SV40+ in the capsids of either adenovirus. This phenomenon was called the transfer of SV40 determinant or *transcapsidation*. Double infection of GMK cells with SV40 and adeno 2 also produced SV40 coated with adenocapsids. But in this case the SV40 genome is not defective and is capable of reproducing infectious SV40 in infected cells (Lewis et al., 1966).

B. The Nature of the Hybrid Virus

The biological properties of adeno 7–SV40+ described above indicate that this particle consists of at least a defective genome of SV40 and adenovirus capsids which can be either of type 2, 7 or 12. The following biological and biophysical studies showed the presence of adeno 7 DNA in the virus particle. Rowe and Pugh (1966) demonstrated that T-antigen specific to adeno 7 is produced in the cells infected with adeno 7–SV40+ encapsidated by adeno 2. Since the virus preparation contained only adeno 2 as associated virus, the result indicates the presence of the adeno 7 genome in the virus particle together with the SV40 genome. The presence of SV40 DNA in the adeno 7–SV40+ particle was demonstrated by hybridization of viral DNA with RNA complementary to SV40 (Reich et al., 1966a; Baum et al.,

1966). Baum *et al.* (1966) also showed that DNA obtained from E46, which contains a comparable amount of both adeno 7–SV40+ and adeno 7, sedimented as a single peak at a position close to adeno DNA and separate from SV40 DNA. The RNA's complementary to both SV40 and adeno 7 were bound with this single peak DNA. Therefore it was concluded that adeno 7–SV40+ has a single hybrid DNA molecule having both a density and molecular weight similar to adenovirus DNA. In this molecule, SV40 DNA was estimated to be linked to adeno 7 DNA by a covalent bond, and the ratio of the DNA content of SV40 and adenovirus components was thought to be about 1:20 (Baum *et al.*, 1966).

The basis for the defectiveness of this virus is not known. Probably the information carried by the DNA of SV40 and adeno 7 in the hybrid virus is not sufficient to code for either component alone. However, alternatives, such as configurational hindrance or mutual suppression of gene functions, are equally conceivable.

C. Cell Transformation by the Hybrid Virus

The transforming ability of this hybrid virus was studied by many investigators (Black and Todaro, 1965; Rabson *et al.*, 1966; Black, 1966; Black and White, 1967; Black *et al.*, 1967). Three hybrids of adeno 7–SV40+ coated by capsids of adeno 2, 7 and 12, respectively, produced transformation in hamster cells. The transformed cells induced by the first two hybrid viruses were morphologically similar to cells transformed by SV40, and those induced by the adeno 12 encapsidated virus more closely resembled the transformed cells induced by adeno 12. The last result is naturally due to the presence of adenovirus 12 in the virus preparation. Such transformed cells contained T-antigen specific to SV40 but produced neither SV40 nor adenovirus. Tumors were produced by transplantation of these transformed cells into hamsters (Igel and Black, 1967) or direct infection of baby hamsters (Rapp *et al.*, 1968). In the latter study, adeno 7–SV40+ hybrids coated with types 1, 2, 5, and 6 adenovirus were shown to be active in tumor formation.

Dose–response experiments indicate that transformation events followed one-hit type kinetics. This suggests that the defective hybrid virus may be capable of transforming cells by itself (Black, 1966), and, although, the characteristics of transformed cells are those of SV40 the role of the adeno 7 genome of the hybrid virus in cell transformation remains to be determined. Recently the presence of T-antigen specific to adeno 1 or 2 was demonstrated in every tumor and transformed cell induced by type 1 or 2 adenovirus grown together with SV40, respectively. Since large amounts of adenovirus are present in these virus inocula, the T-antigen formation may be simply due to normal adenovirus. But it is also conceivable that hybrid virus similar to adeno 7–SV40+ is produced from these adenoviruses and SV40 (Black *et al.*, 1967).

D. Complementation of Adenovirus by SV40

One of the unique characteristics of the interaction between adenovirus and the adeno 7–SV40+ hybrid is their mutual dependency for replication in monkey cells. It appears, therefore, that the defective SV40 genome in the hybrid virus somehow complements a missing function of adenovirus in monkey cells. This complementation was observed also with infectious SV40. Adenoviruses 2, 7, and 12 grow in GMK cells when the cells are preinfected with SV40. Since input adenovirus persisted in GMK cultures, even without SV40, the phenomenon was first recognized as enhancement of adenovirus growth by SV40 (O'Conor *et al.*, 1963; Rabson *et al.*, 1964; Schell *et al.*, 1966). However, quantitative assays of adenovirus in cultures with and without SV40 revealed that the presence of SV40 is essential for the growth of the adenovirus (Feldman *et al.*, 1966; Butel and Rapp, 1966).

Despite their failure to mature into complete virus in GMK cells, adenoviruses induce a specific T-antigen in the cell nuclei (Feldman *et al.*, 1966). The step at which the adenovirus is blocked in GMK cells and the role of SV40 in this phenomenon are not known.

VI. Adenovirus-Associated Virus

Another type of complementation was found between adenovirus and a DNA virus newly isolated from adenovirus preparations. Although it may not relate directly to oncogenesis by adenovirus, the nature of this virus, which is widely distributed among simian and human adenoviruses, will be described briefly. Atchison *et al.* (1965), Melnick *et al.* (1965), and Hoggan (1965) found small virus particles of about 20 mμ in diameter in stocks of various simian and human adenoviruses. Surprisingly, this small virus appeared to replicate only in the presence of an adenovirus (Atchison *et al.*, 1965; Hoggan, 1965). The new defective virus was named adenovirus-associated virus (AAV). Four antigenically distinct AAV have been isolated (Hoggan *et al.*, 1966; Parks *et al.*, 1967a) which also differ serologically from any of the known adenoviruses. The AAV can be separated from adenovirus on the basis of particle size using filtration through membranes or gradient centrifugation (Atchison *et al.*, 1965). In addition to the simian and human adenoviruses, mouse adenovirus and infectious canine hepatitis virus are active as helper virus for AAV (Hoggan *et al.*, 1966; Casto *et al.*, 1967a).

In view of its association with adenovirus and its small size, the possibility of the AAV particle being a subunit of adenovirus was initially considered. However, it is dissimilar to adenovirus in its DNA as well as its serological properties. Rose *et al.* (1966) characterized the DNA of AAV type 1 (AAV-1), which was isolated from human adenovirus 7, as a double-stranded molecule having 54.2% GC (guanine + cytosine) content and a molecular weight of 3.1×10^6 daltons. Similar observations were made on the DNA of AAV-4 isolated from simian adenovirus SV15 (Parks *et al.*, 1967a).

Adenovirus-associated virus shows a certain resemblance to the defective satellite virus found in tobacco necrosis virus (Kassanis, 1962). The satellite virus is a small RNA virus which depends on tobacco necrosis virus for its replication because its RNA (mol. wt.: 4×10^5) carries only enough genetic information for its coat protein (Reichmann, 1964). However, the studies on AAV–DNA show that the resemblance to satellite virus may be only superficial since the size of AAV–DNA is equivalent to that of papovaviruses which are not defective at all.

The replication of AAV was studied by Parks *et al.* (1967b) and by Blacklow *et al.* (1967a). Growth kinetics of AAV closely followed that of the helper adenovirus, and preinfection with adenovirus shortened the eclipse period for AAV growth from 12 to 4 hours. These results suggest that AAV depends on adenovirus in some late step of the replication cycle. In these studies the amount of AAV was estimated by particle count under electron microscopy or by staining with a fluorescent antibody. More recently, AAV was found to induce interference in plaque formation of adenovirus (Casto *et al.*, 1967b). Since the establishment of the interference requires a complete (noninactivated) AAV and the degree of interference is proportional to the dose of input AAV, interference is also useful for measuring the amount of AAV present. The interference by AAV is not mediated by an interferon (Casto *et al.*, 1967b; Parks *et al.*, 1968). The origin of AAV is not known, although antibody to AAV was recently found in monkey and human cells (Blacklow *et al.*, 1968), and two types of AAV were isolated from children who had previously experienced adenovirus infection (Blacklow *et al.*, 1967b).

VII. Comments

As can be expected from their structural and functional diversity, various tumor viruses establish different interactions with their host cells. The typical interactions discussed in this chapter are summarized in Table II. The diversity is amplified by the variety of types and species of host cells and their physiological conditions. At the moment no unified scheme can be solidly drawn for these interactions. Yet, the recent progress described here reveals some fundamental similarities between several systems. It may not be surprising that close similarities exist between viruses having similar dimensions and structures, such as papovaviruses or avian and murine leukemia–sarcoma virus complexes. But even among DNA and RNA viruses, there seems to be some resemblance in virus production and behavior of virus genomes in transformed cells. Both of them induce specific antigens in transformed cells, and sometimes these transformed cells do not release infectious virus which, however, can subsequently appear following rescue by co-culture with sensitive cells or superinfection with a helper virus. Biological characteristics of cells transformed by all tumor viruses, of course, are similar in morphological and metabolic alterations and unrestricted growth. Therefore, despite their obvious differences in structure and biological functions, there is good reason to speculate that different oncogenic viruses may elicit a common key reaction for malignant transformation to occur.

In order to analyze this transformation process, knowledge on the functions of the virus genomes present in transformed cells is essential, and several functions have already been identified for integrated genes of papovaviruses (Sachs, 1965; Dulbecco, 1966, 1967). However, a question still remains as to whether or not these viral genomes in the transformed cells directly determine the malignant behavior of the cells. The persistence of the viral genome may merely be a consequence of virus–cell interaction and not responsible for continued maintenance of the malignant state. So far only one experiment presented suggestive evidence for the role of the virus genome in the malignant expression of cells. With RSV-infected hamster cells, Macpherson (1965) found the appearance of morphologically normal cells from clones of transformed cells. The revertant normal-appearing cells had lost their oncogenic potentials, and RSV could not be rescued from them by co-culture with chicken cells. The genome of RSV may be lost from these cells during their rapid growth, resulting in the reversion to apparently normal cells. It was not determined, however, whether the RSV genome is completely lost from the cells or whether it exists in a somewhat altered form unable to be rescued by the co-culture method. As pointed out by Dulbecco (1967), the isolation of conditionally lethal mutants may give a more definite answer to this question.

Interaction among tumor viruses involves different principles, such as phenotypic mixing, recombination, and complementation. In studies on some tumor viruses, one has to be cautious about possible combinations of these interactions. Frequent occurrence of such interactions may be one of the characteristics of the tumor viruses. Since in transformed cells oncogenic viruses do not have a short life-span like ordinary cytocidal viruses, there is ample opportunity for them to interact with a second virus either deliberately added or naturally present in the host cells. Many properties of avian and murine sarcoma viruses are subject to significant alteration by growing in host cells naturally infected with leukemia viruses.

TABLE II

Summary of Virus Reproduction and Interaction with Other Viruses in Cells Transformed by Some Oncogenic Viruses

Viruses	Virus production in infected cells		Recovery of infectious virus from nonproducing transformed cells by co-culture with	Possible interaction with
	Nontransformed	Transformed		
RNA viruses				
Rous sarcoma virus		+ Chicken − Mouse − Rat − Hamster − Monkey	+ Chicken cells	Avian leukosis viruses (phenotypic mixing)
Murine sarcoma virus		+ Mouse + Rat − Hamster	+ Mouse cells	Murine leukemia viruses (phenotypic mixing)
DNA viruses				
Polyoma virus	+ Mouse	− Hamster − Mouse − Rat	—	
SV40	+ Monkey	− Hamster − Mouse − Human, Monkey	± Monkey cells	Adenoviruses (complementation)
Adenoviruses	+ Human	− Hamster	NT[a]	SV40 and adeno 7–SV40+ (complementation)
Adeno 7–SV40+	± Monkey ± Human (in the presence of adenovirus)	− Hamster	—	Adenoviruses (complementation)

[a] NT = not tested.

The concept of virus defectiveness has been introduced to explain the nature of some tumor viruses which depend on other viruses in their replication. The term defectiveness is used here in either a broad or narrow sense. Operationally expressed, a virus may be defective in one cell and functionally normal in another. However, in its strict sense the term defectiveness should be applied only to a virus that lacks some function essential for its replication. Some transducing phages and the satellite virus of tobacco necrosis virus are defective in this sense, and adeno 7–SV40+ may also belong to this group of virus. But RSV is certainly not defective because it can replicate in some host cells without the aid of another virus.

This article has described several examples of relatively well-studied tumor virus–host cell interactions in transformed cells, but many other tumor viruses have not been included. A number of important findings are now being made in studies with other tumor viruses, such as the nature of "masked" papilloma virus, hormonal effect on mammary tumor virus infection, and interaction between leukemia virus and hematopoïetic cells. Unique virus–cell interactions other than those described here may be revealed by studies with these viruses. It should also be remembered that some of the foregoing statements may oversimplify complex and dynamic phenomena, and new developments may originate from these exceptional findings.

REFERENCES

Ahlström, C. G., and Forsby, N. 1962. *J. Exptl. Med.* **115**, 839–852.

Ahlström, C. G., and Jonsson, N. 1962. *Acta Pathol. Microbiol. Scand.* **54**, 136–144.

Aloni, Y., Winocour, E., and Sachs, L. 1968. *J. Mol. Biol.* **31**, 415–429.

Atchison, R. W., Casto, B. C., and Hammon, W. McD. 1965. *Science* **149**, 754–756.

Bader, J. P. 1964. *Virology* **22**, 462–468.

Baluda, M. A. 1966. *In* "Subviral Carcinogenesis" (Y. Ito, ed.), pp. 19–35. Editorial Comm. 1st Intern. Symp. Tumor Viruses, Nagoya.

Bases, R. E., and King, A. S. 1967. *Virology* **32**, 175–183.

Basilico, C., and DiMayorca, G. 1965. *Proc. Natl. Acad. Sci. U.S.* **54**, 125–128.

Bauer, H., and Schäfer, W. 1966. *Virology* **29**, 494–497.

Baum, S. G., Reich, P. R., Huebner, R. J., Rowe, W. P., and Weissman, S. M. 1966. *Proc. Natl. Acad. Sci. U.S.* **56**, 1509–1515.

Benjamin, T. L. 1965. *Proc. Natl. Acad. Sci. U.S.* **54**, 121–124.

Benjamin, T. L. 1966. *J. Mol. Biol.* **16**, 359–373.

Black, P. H. 1966. *In* "Subviral Carcinogenesis" (Y. Ito, ed.), pp. 220–234. Editorial Comm. 1st Intern. Symp. Tumor Viruses, Nagoya.

Black, P. H., and Rowe, W. P. 1963. *Proc. Natl. Acad. Sci. U.S.* **50**, 606–613.

Black, P. H., and Todaro, G. J. 1965. *Proc. Natl. Acad. Sci. U.S.* **54**, 374–381.

Black, P. H., and White, B. J. 1967. *J. Exptl. Med.* **125**, 629–646.

Black, P. H., Lewis, A. M., Jr., Blacklow, N. R., Austin, J. B., and Rowe, W. P. 1967. *Proc. Natl. Acad. Sci. U.S.* **57**, 1324–1330.

Blacklow, N. R., Hoggan, M. D., and Rowe, W. P. 1967a. *J. Exptl. Med.* **125**, 755–765.
Blacklow, N. R., Hoggan, M. D., and Rowe, W. P. 1967b. *Proc. Natl. Acad. Sci. U.S.* **58**, 1410–1415.
Blacklow, N. R., Hoggan, M. D., and Rowe, W. P. 1968. *J. Natl. Cancer Inst.* **40**, 319–327.
Boeyé, M., Melnick, J. L., and Rapp, F. 1966. *Virology* **28**, 56–70.
Butel, J. S., and Rapp, F. 1966. *J. Bacteriol.* **91**, 278–284.
Casto, B. C., Atchison, R. W., and Hammon, W. McD. 1967a. *Virology* **32**, 52–59.
Casto, B. C., Armstrong, J. A., Atchison, R. W., and Hammon, W. McD. 1967b. *Virology* **33**, 452–458.
Courington, D., and Vogt, P. K. 1967. *J. Virol.* **1**, 400–414.
Crittenden, L. B., and Okazaki, W. 1965. *J. Natl. Cancer Inst.* **35**, 857–863.
Crittenden, L. B., Okazaki, W., and Reamer, R. 1963. *Virology* **20**, 541–544.
Crittenden, L., Stone, H. A., Reamer, R. H., and Okazaki, W. 1967. *J. Virol.* **1**, 898–904.
Defendi, V. 1963. *Proc. Soc. Exptl. Biol. Med.* **113**, 12–16.
Dougherty, R. M., and Di Stefano, H. S. 1965. *Virology* **27**, 351–359.
Dougherty, R. M., and Rasmussen, R. 1964. *Natl. Cancer Inst. Monograph* **17**, 337–350.
Duesberg, P. H., and Robinson, W. S. 1966. *Proc. Natl. Acad. Sci. U.S.* **55**, 219–227.
Duesberg, P. H., and Robinson, W. S. 1967. *Virology* **31**, 742–746.
Dulbecco, R. 1963. *Science* **142**, 932–936.
Dulbecco, R. 1966. *Perspectives Biol. Med.* **9**, 298–305.
Dulbecco, R. 1967. *Sci. Am.* **216**, No. 4, 28–37.
Febvre, H., Rothschild, L., Arnoult, J., and Haguenau, F. 1964. *Natl. Cancer Inst. Monograph* **17**, 459–466.
Feldman, L. A., Butel, J. S., and Rapp, F. 1966. *J. Bacteriol.* **91**, 813–818.
Freeman, A. E., Black, P. H., Vanderpool, E. A., Henry, P. H., Austin, J. B., and Huebner, R. J. 1967. *Proc. Natl. Acad. Sci. U.S.* **58**, 1205–1212.
Fujinaga, K., and Green, M. 1966. *Proc. Natl. Acad. Sci. U.S.* **55**, 1567–1574.
Gerber, P. 1963. *Science* **140**, 889–890.
Gerber, P. 1966. *Virology* **28**, 501–509.
Gerber, P., and Kirschstein, R. L. 1962. *Virology* **18**, 582–588.
Goldé, A. 1966. *Compt. Rend.* **262D**, 329–331.
Goldé, A., and Latarjet, R. 1966. *Compt. Rend.* **262D**, 420–423.
Goldé, A., and Vigier, P. 1966. *Compt. Rend.* **262D**, 2793–2796.
Habel, K. 1962. *Cold Spring Harbor Symp. Quant. Biol.* **17**, 433–439.
Haguenau, F., and Hanafusa, H. 1968. *Virology* **34**, 275–281.
Hanafusa, H. 1964. *Natl. Cancer Inst. Monograph* **17**, 543–556.
Hanafusa, H. 1965. *Virology* **25**, 248–255.
Hanafusa, H. 1968. *In* "Methods in Virology" (K. Maramorosch and H. Koprowski, eds.), Vol. 4, pp. 321–350. Academic Press, New York.
Hanafusa, H., and Hanafusa, T. 1966a. *Proc. Natl. Acad. Sci. U.S.* **55**, 532–538.
Hanafusa, H., and Hanafusa, T. 1966b. *In* "Subviral Carcinogenesis" (Y. Ito, ed.), pp. 283–295. Editorial Comm. 1st Intern. Symp. Tumor Viruses, Nagoya.
Hanafusa, H., and Hanafusa, T. 1968. *Virology* **34**, 630–636.
Hanafusa, H., Hanafusa, T., and Rubin, H. 1963. *Proc. Natl. Acad. Sci. U.S.* **49**, 572–580.
Hanafusa, H., Hanafusa, T., and Rubin, H. 1964a. *Proc. Natl. Acad. Sci. U.S.* **51**, 41–48.
Hanafusa, H., Hanafusa, T., and Rubin, H. 1964b. *Virology* **22**, 591–601.
Hanafusa, T., and Hanafusa, H. 1967. *Proc. Natl. Acad. Sci. U.S.* **58**, 818–825.
Hanafusa, T., Hanafusa, H., and Rubin, H. 1964. *Virology* **22**, 643–645.
Harris, R. J. C., and Chesterman, F. C. 1963. *Proc. Roy. Soc. Med.* **56**, 307–308.

Hartley, J. W., and Rowe, W. P. 1966. *Proc. Natl. Acad. Sci. U.S.* **55**, 780–786.
Harvey, J. J. 1964. *Nature* **204**, 1104–1105.
Hirst, G. K., and Gotlieb, T. 1953. *J. Exptl. Med.* **98**, 41–51.
Hlavayova, E., Smida, J., Altaner, C., and Švec, F. 1964. *Folia Biol. (Prague)* **10** 301–306.
Hoggan, M. D. 1965. *Federation Proc.* **24**, 248.
Hoggan, M. D., Blacklow, N. R., and Rowe, W. P. 1966. *Proc. Natl. Acad. Sci. U.S.* **55**, 1467–1474.
Huebner, R. J. 1967a. *Perspectives Virol.* **5**, 147–166.
Huebner, R. J. 1967b. *Proc. Natl. Acad. Sci. U.S.* **58**, 835–842.
Huebner, R. J., Armstrong, D., Okuyan, M., Sarma, P. S., and Turner, H. C. 1964a. *Proc. Natl. Acad. Sci. U.S.* **51**, 742–749.
Huebner, R. J., Chanock, R. M., Rubin, B. A., and Casey, M. J. 1964b. *Proc. Natl. Acad. Sci. U.S.* **52**, 1333–1340.
Huebner, R. J., Hartley, J. W., Rowe, W. P., Lane, W. T., and Capps, W. I. 1966. *Proc. Natl. Acad. Sci. U.S.* **56**, 1164–1169.
Igel, H. J., and Black, P. H. 1967. *J. Exptl. Med.* **125**, 657–663.
Ishizaki, R., and Vogt, P. K. 1966. *Virology* **30**, 375–387.
Kassanis, B. 1962. *J. Gen. Microbiol.* **27**, 477–488.
Kelloff, G., and Vogt, P. K. 1966. *Virology* **29**, 377–384.
Klement, V., and Svoboda, J. 1963. *Folia Biol. (Prague)* **9**, 181–188.
Koprowski, H., Jensen, F. C., and Steplewski, Z. 1967. *Proc. Natl. Acad. Sci. U.S.* **58**, 127–133.
Lacy, S., and Green, M. 1964. *Proc. Natl. Acad. Sci. U.S.* **52**, 1053–1059.
Latarjet, R., Cramer, R., and Montanier, L. 1967. *Virology* **33**, 104–111.
Lewis, A. M., Jr., Prigge, K. O., and Rowe, W. P. 1966. *Proc. Natl. Acad. Sci. U.S.* **55**, 526–531.
Macpherson, I. 1965. *Science* **148**, 1731–1733.
Melnick, J. L., Mayor, H. D., Smith, K. O., and Rapp, F. 1965. *J. Bacteriol.* **90**, 271–274.
Moloney, J. B. 1966. *Natl. Cancer Inst. Monograph* **22**, 139–142.
Munroe, J. S., and Southam, C. M. 1964. *J. Natl. Cancer Inst.* **32**, 591–623.
Negroni, G. 1963. *Advan. Cancer Res.* **7**, 515–561.
Novick, A., and Szilard, L. 1951. *Science* **113**, 34–35.
O'Connor, T. E., and Fischinger, P. J. 1968. *Science* **159**, 325–329.
O'Conor, G. T., Rabson, A. S., Berezesky, I. K., and Paul, F. J. 1963. *J. Natl. Cancer Inst.* **31**, 903–917.
Parks, W. P., Green, M., Pina, M., and Melnick, J. L. 1967a. *J. Virol.* **1**, 980–987.
Parks, W. P., Melnick, J. L., Rongey, R., and Mayor, H. D. 1967b. *J. Virol.* **1**, 171–180.
Parks, W. P., Casazza, A. M., Alcott, J., and Melnick, J. L. 1968. *J. Exptl. Med.* **127**, 91–108.
Payne, F. E., Solomon, J. J., and Purchase, H. G. 1966. *Proc. Natl. Acad. Sci. U.S.* **55**, 341–348.
Payne, L. N., and Biggs, P. M. 1964. *Virology* **24**, 610–616.
Pina, M., and Green, M. 1965. *Proc. Natl. Acad. Sci. U.S.* **54**, 547–551.
Piraino, F. 1967. *Virology* **32**, 700–707.
Purchase, H. G. 1965. *Avian Diseases* **9**, 127–145.
Rabotti, G. F., Raine, W. A., and Sellers, R. L. 1965. *Science* **147**, 504–506.
Rabotti, G. F., Bucciarelli, E., and Dalton, A. J. 1966. *Virology* **29**, 684–686.
Rabson, A. S., O'Conor, G. T., Berezesky, I. K., and Paul, F. J. 1964. *Proc. Soc. Exptl. Biol. Med.* **116**, 187–190.

Rabson, A. S., Malmgren, R. A., and Kirschstein, R. L. 1966. *Proc. Soc. Exptl. Biol. Med.* **121**, 486–489.

Rapp, F., and Melnick, J. L. 1966. *Progr. Med. Virol.* **8**, 349–399.

Rapp, F., Melnick, J. L., Butel, J. S., and Kitahara, T. 1964. *Proc. Natl. Acad. Sci. U.S.* **52**, 1348–1352.

Rapp, F., Butel, J. S., and Melnick, J. L. 1965. *Proc. Natl. Acad. Sci. U.S.* **54**, 717–724.

Rapp, F., Jerkofsky, M., Melnick, J. L., and Levy, B. 1968. *J. Exptl. Med.* **127**, 77–90.

Reich, P. R., Baum, S. G., Rose, J. A., Rowe, W. P., and Weissman, S. M. 1966a. *Proc. Natl. Acad. Sci. U.S.* **55**, 336–341.

Reich, P. R., Black, P. H., and Weissman, S. M. 1966b. *Proc. Natl. Acad. Sci. U.S.* **56**, 78–85.

Reichmann, M. E. 1964. *Proc. Natl. Acad. Sci. U.S.* **52**, 1009–1017.

Rich, M. A., and Moloney, J. B., eds. 1966. *Natl. Cancer Inst. Monograph* **22**.

Rich, M. A., and Siegler, R. 1967. *Ann. Rev. Microbiol.* **21**, 529–572.

Robinson, H. L. 1967. *Proc. Natl. Acad. Sci. U.S.* **57**, 1655–1662.

Robinson, W. S., Pitkanen, A., and Rubin, H. 1965. *Proc. Natl. Acad. Sci. U.S.* **54**, 137–144.

Rose, J. A., Hoggan, M. D., and Shatkin, A. J. 1966. *Proc. Natl. Acad. Sci. U.S.* **56**, 86–92.

Rowe, W. P. 1965. *Proc. Natl. Acad. Sci. U.S.* **54**, 711–717.

Rowe, W. P., and Baum, S. G. 1964. *Proc. Natl. Acad. Sci. U.S.* **52**, 1340–1347.

Rowe, W. P., and Baum, S. G. 1965. *J. Exptl. Med.* **122**, 955–966.

Rowe, W. P., and Pugh, W. E. 1966. *Proc. Natl. Acad. Sci. U.S.* **55**, 1126–1132.

Rubin, H. 1960. *Proc. Natl. Acad. Sci. U.S.* **46**, 1105–1119.

Rubin, H. 1964. *Sci. Am.* **210**, No. 6, 46–52.

Rubin, H. 1965. *Virology* **26**, 270–276.

Sabin, A. B., and Koch, M. A. 1963. *Proc. Natl. Acad. Sci. U.S.* **50**, 407–417.

Sachs, L. 1965. *Nature* **207**, 1272–1274.

Sarma, P. S., Vass, W., and Huebner, R. J. 1966. *Proc. Natl. Acad. Sci. U.S.* **55**, 1435–1442.

Sarma, P. S., Cheong, M. P., Hartley, J. W., and Huebner, R. J. 1967. *Virology* **33**, 180–184.

Schell, K., Lane, W. T., Casey, M. J., and Huebner, R. J. 1966. *Proc. Natl. Acad. Sci. U.S.* **55**, 81–88.

Shope, R. E. 1950. *In* "Viruses" (M. Delbrück, ed.), pp. 79–92. California Inst. of Technol., Pasadena, California.

Šimkovič, D., Svoboda, J., and Valentova, N. 1963. *Folia Biol. (Prague)* **9**, 82–91.

Sjögren, H. D., Hellström, I., and Klein, G. 1961. *Cancer Res.* **21**, 329–337.

Steck, F. T., and Rubin, H. 1966a. *Virology* **29**, 628–641.

Steck, F. T., and Rubin, H. 1966b. *Virology* **29**, 642–653.

Svet-Moldavsky, G. J. 1957. *Nature* **180**, 1299–1300.

Svoboda, J. 1960. *Nature* **186**, 980–981.

Svoboda, J. 1961. *Folia Biol. (Prague)* **7**, 46–60.

Svoboda, J. 1962. *Folia Biol. (Prague)* **8**, 215–220.

Svoboda, J., and Klement, V. 1963. *Folia Biol. (Prague)* **9**, 403–411.

Temin, H. M. 1962. *Cold Spring Harbor Symp. Quant. Biol.* **27**, 407–414.

Temin, H. M. 1963. *Virology* **20**, 577–582.

Thurzo, V., Smida, J., Smidova-Kovarova, V., and Šimkovič, D. 1963. *Acta, Unio Intern. Contra Cancrum* **19**, 304–305.

Ting, R. C. 1964. *Virology* **24**, 227–228.

Ting, R. C. 1966. *Virology* **28**, 783–785.

Trentin, J. J., and Bryan, E. 1966. *Proc. Soc. Exptl. Biol. Med.* **121**, 1216–1219.

Vigier, P., and Montagnier, L. 1966. *In* "Subviral Carcinogenesis" (Y. Ito, ed.), pp. 156–175. Editorial Comm. 1st Intern. Symp. Tumor Viruses, Nagoya.

Vigier, P., and Svoboda, J. 1965. *Comp. Rend.* **261D**, 4278–4281.

Vogt, M., and Dulbecco, R. 1962. *Virology* **16**, 41–51.

Vogt, P. K. 1965a. *Virology* **25**, 237–247.

Vogt, P. K. 1965b. *Advan. Virus Res.* **11**, 293–385.

Vogt, P. K. 1967a. *Proc. Natl. Acad. Sci. U.S.* **58**, 801–808.

Vogt, P. K. 1967b. *Virology* **33**, 175–177.

Vogt, P. K., and Ishizaki, R. 1965. *Virology* **26**, 664–672.

Vogt, P. K., and Ishizaki, R. 1966. *Virology* **30**, 368–374.

Vogt, P. K., Sarma, P. S., and Huebner, R. J. 1965. *Virology* **27**, 233–235.

Vogt, P. K., Ishizaki, R., and Duff, R. 1966. *In* "Subviral Carcinogenesis" (Y. Ito, ed.), pp. 297–310. Editorial Comm. 1st Intern. Symp. Tumor Viruses, Nagoya.

Waters, N. F., and Fontes, A. K. 1960. *J. Natl. Cancer Inst.* **25**, 351–357.

Watkins, J. F., and Dulbecco, R. 1967. *Proc. Natl. Acad. Sci. U.S.* **58**, 1396–1403.

Weiss, R. 1967. *Virology* **32**, 719–723

Zilber, L. A., and Kryukova, I. N. 1957. *Acta Virol. (Prague)* **1**, 156–160.

CELLULAR IMMUNITY AGAINST TUMOR ANTIGENS

Karl Erik Hellström and Ingegerd Hellström

Departments of Pathology and Microbiology, University of Washington
Medical School, Seattle, Washington

I. Introduction

Virtually all animal neoplasms studied contain tumor-specific transplantation antigens (TSTA) which are so called because they were first

detected by transplantation techniques: animals which have been properly immunized are specifically resistant toward challenge with transplanted syngeneic tumor cells. Methods have been developed by which immune reactions against TSTA can be identified *in vitro*. Such methods have been used in recent studies which indicate that certain human neoplasms also contain TSTA.

Immune reactions against specific antigens of syngeneic tumors are similar to allograft reactions, by which transplanted normal and tumor cells are rejected if they contain isoantigens which are foreign to the recipients. They are to a large extent mediated by immunologically competent cells, i.e., lymphocytes and macrophages. The role of cytotoxic humoral antibodies is less certain.

This article will first summarize the evidence that tumors possess TSTA. Techniques will be described by which cellular immunity to transplantation antigens can be demonstrated and different systems will be reviewed in which such techniques were used to detect lymphocyte-mediated immune reactions to TSTA. The possible role of cellular immunity to TSTA *in vivo* will be discussed and speculations will be offered why neoplasms often grow progressively *in vivo* in spite of the fact that their cells can be killed by immune lymphocytes *in vitro*. There will be a discussion of what implications for tumor therapy the findings of cellular immunity to TSTA might have. Possible mechanisms of tumor cell destruction by immune cells will be considered. Finally, the phenomenon of allogeneic inhibition will be reviewed, since this phenomenon has been postulated to operate in parallel to the immunological mechanisms as part of the organism's defense against antigenic neoplastic cells.

No attempts have been made to cover completely the vast literature in the field or to review all possible aspects of cellular immunity to tumor antigens. We have, instead, chosen to discuss some recent work in detail.

II. Demonstration of Tumor-Specific Transplantation Antigens in Animal and Human Tumors

This section is included to provide a background to the studies on cellular immunity to TSTA, which are discussed in Sections III to VIII. For details, the reader is referred to several reviews on TSTA which have been published (Prehn, 1963a; Old and Boyse, 1964; Sjögren, 1965; Hellström and Möller, 1965; Haddow, 1965; Klein, 1966; Smith, 1968).

A. Definition of Tumor-Specific Transplantation Antigens

Tumor-specific transplantation antigens are macromolecules present in tumor cells and absent from normal cells of the same individual and against which immune reactions can be demonstrated with transplantation techniques.

The transplantation methods used to demonstrate TSTA can involve immunization of recipient animals with tumor cells which have been rendered incapable of multiplication [by heavy X-irradiation (Révész, 1960) or by other means] or which are inoculated in subthreshold doses (Klein et al., 1960). Immunization can be also achieved by inoculation of living tumor cells and excision of the subsequent tumor nodule (Foley, 1953). The immunized animals are then challenged with a small dose of living syngeneic tumor cells and the neoplastic growth is compared with that in control animals (Klein, 1959).

B. DEMONSTRATION THAT ANIMAL TUMORS POSSESS TUMOR-SPECIFIC TRANSPLANTATION ANTIGENS

Early in this century it was claimed that tumors have specific antigens. These claims were, however, based on experiments with noninbred animals so that no distinctions could be made between TSTA and isoantigens which were present on both tumor and normal cells and, therefore, specific to the individual animal rather than to the tumor.

When inbred mice became available, it was possible to make meaningful searches for truly tumor-specific antigens. This field of research was pioneered by Gross (1943), Foley (1953), and by Prehn and Main (1957), all of whom presented evidence that tumor-specific antigens, indeed, exist. In the experiments of Prehn and Main, tumors were induced by methylcholanthrene (MCA) and transplanted to syngeneic mice in which they were allowed to form palpable nodules which were then surgically removed. These mice were subsequently rechallenged with the immunizing tumor. They were found to be more resistant to growth of the inoculated tumor than were control mice which were either untreated or sensitized against another, syngeneic MCA sarcoma. Normal tissues did not immunize against sarcoma growth, even when derived from the same mouse in which the challenge tumor had originated, and mice which were resistant to tumor challenge did not reject a skin graft derived from the same mouse in which the tumor had originated. It was concluded that MCA sarcomas have TSTA and that these are individually distinct for each neoplasm.

Klein et al. (1960) showed that immune reactions can also be demonstrated against autochthonous MCA sarcomas, following removal of a primary tumor and repeated treatment of the operated mouse with heavily (15,000 r) X-irradiated cells of that tumor.

Tumor-specific transplantation antigens were later demonstrated in tumors induced with chemical carcinogens other than MCA, as well as in tumors induced by ionizing radiation or by implantation of plastic or cellophane films (see Sjögren, 1965, for references). In all these cases, most neoplasms have been found to possess individually distinct TSTA.

Tumors of a known viral etiology behave differently from those discussed so far in that they have TSTA which are common to all neoplasms induced by the same virus and different for those induced by different viruses. Polyoma virus-induced mouse tumors were the first viral neoplasms in which TSTA were detected. Sjögren *et al.* (1961a,b) and Habel (1961, 1962) independently found that polyoma tumors grew less well when transplanted to syngeneic mice infected with the polyoma virus as adults than in mice which had not been infected with the polyoma virus. Resistance was also demonstrated in mice that had been immunized with non-virus-releasing allogeneic polyoma tumors and which lacked detectable antibodies against polyoma virions (Sjögren, 1961, 1964c). It was, therefore, postulated that polyoma tumors possess a cellular antigen which is immunologically unrelated to the antigen of the intact virus particle (Sjögren, 1961, 1964b; Habel, 1962)— a postulate of which the correctness could be proved by a direct *in vitro* assay of serum from mice which were immune to polyoma TSTA and polyoma virions, respectively (Hellström, 1965).

Since the discovery of TSTA in polyoma tumor cells, specific TSTA have been detected in a variety of both deoxyribonucleic acid (DNA) and ribonucleic acid (RNA) virus-induced neoplasms. Tumors induced by DNA viruses have TSTA which are immunologically distinct from the antigens of the virus particles, whereas such distinction cannot generally be made for RNA virus-induced neoplasms. There are only few exceptions in which virus-induced animal tumors were studied by transplantation techniques and found to be nonantigenic (Hare, 1967), and it may be questioned in these cases whether the lack of TSTA was complete (Klein, 1966).

So-called spontaneous tumors were long considered nonantigenic since the transplantation methods used to detect antigens in experimentally induced neoplasms failed to reveal any immunity to spontaneous mouse tumors. For example, Foley (1953) did not detect any immunity against mammary carcinomas in the mammary tumor virus (MTV)-carrying C3H strain, although the experimental system was the same as that which worked with MCA tumors, and Prehn and Main (1957) were unable to demonstrate immunity in mice against spontaneous fibrosarcomas. Révész (1960) did not find resistance in mice immunized with X-irradiated mammary carcinomas, using a procedure successfully employed to show immunity to MCA tumors. It appeared from such experiments that immunological studies on experimentally induced tumors may have little relevance for human neoplasms, since these are "spontaneous." It was, therefore, of great importance when Morton (1962) and Weiss *et al.* (1964) were able to show that spontaneous mammary carcinomas in MTV-carrying C3H mice contain a common TSTA. A special procedure had to be employed to detect the antigen: MTV-bearing C3H mice could not be immunized against it, whereas immunization was easily achieved by using C3Hf mice, which lacked MTV. It was postulated that C3H mice are immunologically non-reactive against a virus-induced common antigen of spontaneous mammary tumors because of their contact with MTV early in life (Weiss *et al.*, 1964; Morton *et al.*, 1965; Attia *et al.*, 1965). Recent studies indicate that it is possible to detect immunity against individually distinct TSTA of spon-taneous mammary carcinomas if sensitive techniques are used (Vaage, 1968; Heppner and Pierce, 1969). These findings would imply that mam-mary carcinomas in MTV strains have TSTA of two types, namely, an individually specific antigen and a common one which may be either determined by the viral genome or just represent virions at the tumor cell surface. It remains to be studied whether also viral neoplasms other than those associated with MTV have both common and individually distinct TSTA. If so, the individually distinct antigens might represent genetic differences between different tumors induced by the same virus, which can be detected by, for example, chromosome cytological techniques (Hellström *et al.*, 1963). It is not unlikely that the individually distinct TSTA of chemically induced mouse neoplasms also reflect a random genetical variation between different tumors. If a virus were involved in the etiology of these tumors, too, such a virus would probably be one naturally occurring in mice, against which these are likely to be tolerant; consequently, cross-reading TSTA among chemically induced tumors would not be detectable by the transplantation procedures generally used. It is interesting in this context that Old *et al.* (1968a) have demonstrated an antigen determined by the Gross virus in several tumors of chemical origin.

C. *In Vitro* Demonstration of Humoral Antibodies to Specific Antigens of Animal Tumors

Several *in vitro* techniques have been employed for the demonstration of humoral antibodies to tumor-specific antigens. Such methods are neces-sary when searching for antigens in human neoplasms. One of the first assays introduced was an indirect fluorescent antibody test developed by Möller (1961) for the detection of isoantigens in living normal and neo-plastic cells. In this assay, serum antibodies are demonstrated by their ability to bind to such antigens localized at the cell surface causing the membrane to fluoresce. Fluorescent antibody tests on living cells have been used by several groups of investigators in studies on immune reactions against virus-induced neoplasms (Klein and Klein, 1964, 1965; Tevethia *et al.*, 1965; Klein *et al.*, 1966a).

Short-time cytotoxic tests were introduced by Gorer and O'Gorman (1956). Target cells are incubated with antiserum and complement, and a cytotoxic effect is demonstrated by the uptake of supravital stains such as eosin or trypan blue. Sanderson (1964) and Wigzell (1965) modified the technique so that cell death can be detected by the outleak of an isotope label, such as ^{51}Cr. The cytotoxic assay has been frequently employed to demonstrate antibodies against specific antigens in murine lymphomas (Old et al., 1963; Haughton, 1965) but has been less useful with carcinomas and sarcomas. Studies by Winn (1960, 1962) and by Möller and Möller (1962) have shown that the cell death measured demands a certain critical amount of antibody-bound complement at the cell surface and that cells are more easily killed when they have a high concentration of those surface antigens to which the antibodies added in a particular test are directed.

The colony inhibition (CI) assay of humoral antibodies was introduced (Hellström and Sjögren, 1965; Hellström, 1965) as a more sensitive tool to measure essentially the same reaction as that detected with the short-time cytotoxic test. The target cells are incubated with various antisera and control sera in the presence of complement, after which they are seeded onto petri dishes in dilute concentrations. The number of colonies growing out is determined 4–7 days later. Many sera which had given negative results with the cytotoxic assay were found to contain specific antibodies when CI experiments were made (Hellström et al., unpublished).

The cytotoxic and CI assays probably detect the same tumor antigens as those that induce transplantation resistance and rejection of tumor syngrafts in vivo, i.e., the TSTA, since the immune reactions studied both in vivo and in vitro lead to target cell death (growth inhibition) and are likely directed against surface antigens of the tumor cells. Indirect fluorescent antibody tests on living cells also demonstrate reactions with surface antigens. It is possible, therefore, that these tests also detect TSTA. However, cell destruction is implicit in reactions against TSTA. This aspect of the immune defense cannot be investigated with the fluorescent antibody test. Furthermore, the rejection of antigenic tumors in vivo appears to be primarily mediated by immune cells (see Section IV). If one wants to investigate the immune status of a host to TSTA, investigations of cellular immunity appear, therefore, to be particularly relevant.

In addition to surface antigens, neoplastic cells often have other types of specific antigens. Work by Huebner et al. (1963), in particular, has shown that virus-induced tumor cells contain antigens which are present in their nuclei and can be detected by complement fixation (CF) techniques and by immunofluorescence assays on fixed cells (Pope and Rowe, 1964). This antigen has been called the CF, tumor (T), or neoantigen. It is common to all tumors induced by the same virus and different for tumors induced by different viruses. There are generally no cross-reactions between the CF antigen and TSTA, and it is not believed that an immune reaction against the CF antigen is involved in the rejection of transplanted tumor cells (Habel, 1965).

D. Searches for Humoral Antibodies against Human Tumor-Specific Transplantation Antigens

Many early claims that human tumor antigens exist had to be rejected because the immune reactions observed were primarily directed against normal histocompatibility antigens. It was not until the experience gained from animal work was used as a model for human studies that data could be obtained which gave at least suggestive evidence that certain human tumors have specific antigens (Southam, 1967). Work will be summarized here which indicates that some human tumor cells have specific surface antigens, against which humoral antibodies can be detected. Studies on other antigenic components of human tumor cells (e.g., possibly occurring CF antigens) will not be included.

Klein et al. have used the indirect fluorescent antibody assay on living cells to search for immunity against specific antigens of Burkitt lymphomas (1966b, 1967a,b). The same experimental approach was employed as when investigating Moloney virus-induced lymphomas. It was found that Burkitt lymphoma cells from fresh biopsies and from lines propagated in culture possess antigens which could be detected by incubation of the tumor cells with serum from Burkitt patients. The strongest reactions were observed with serum from patients whose disease was in remission. Burkitt patients who responded well to chemotherapy were more prone to have antibodies against their tumors than those patients in whom therapy had little effect. This finding suggested that the antibodies detected were involved in a host defense against Burkitt lymphomas (Klein et al., 1967b). It was not possible, however, to demonstrate any cytotoxic effect of the antibodies in vitro.

Klein et al. (1966b) also found quite a few positive reactions against Burkitt lymphoma cells when they studied sera from African patients with diseases other than Burkitt lymphoma. It is not likely, however, that the antibodies detected in Burkitt patient sera were directed against normal isoantigens, since they could bind to autochthonous as well as to allogeneic Burkitt cells, and since the active sera did not give specific fluorescence with other cells, such as normal cells from bone marrow of Burkitt patients, leukemic cells, and tissue culture lines derived from leukemias of non-Burkitt origin (Klein et al., 1967b).

Morton et al. (1968) obtained results somewhat analogous to those described by Klein et al. (1966b) when studying living melanoma cells with the indirect fluorescent antibody test. They found that patients with malignant melanoma contained antibodies which gave a specific fluorescence with melanoma cells (60%). Less frequently (20%), positive reactions were obtained with various control sera. Morton and Malmgren (1968) also found that sera from patients with osteogenic sarcomas and from relatives of such patients gave fluorescence with osteogenic sarcoma cells; their data therefore suggested the involvement of a virus in the disease.

Gold and Freedman (1965a,b) reported that carcinoma cells from the gastrointestinal tract possess an antigen, which is absent from normal cells of adult origin but present in embryonal tissues from the gastrointestinal tract. The antigen was, therefore, denoted as carcinoembryonic, and it was postulated that its appearance in carcinomas was due to genetic derepression. It is yet unclear whether the carcinoembryonic antigen is a TSTA, against which an immunological reaction can be mounted in tumor patients (Gold et al., 1968).

Cellular immunity to TSTA is thought to have a more significant role than humoral immunity as a host defense mechanism against neoplasia (Section IV). Studies which have demonstrated cellular immunity to certain human tumors are reviewed in Section IV. In part of these studies (Hellström et al., 1968b,c) a search was made for humoral antibodies in the plasma of tumor patients whose lymphocytes were found to be immune. Cytotoxic (growth inhibitory) effects of humoral antibodies were detected against neuroblastoma cells with plasma from patients who were symptom-free after therapy of neuroblastoma, but not from patients with progressive disease. These studies will be further discussed in connection with the demonstration of cellular immunity against human tumors (Section IV).

III. Assays of Cellular Immunity against Tumor-Specific Transplantation Antigens

Several systems have been developed by which cellular immune reactions against tumor antigens can be detected and quantitated. They were originally introduced for purposes other than tumor immunological studies, such as demonstration of graft destruction by sensitized allogeneic immune cells and detection of delayed hypersensitivity. The similarities between the organism's rejection of cells carrying TSTA and the allograft reaction (see Section VII for discussion), and between the allograft reaction and delayed hypersensitivity (Chase, 1953; Lawrence, 1960), have facilitated the development of these test systems.

This section will present different techniques which can be used for the demonstration of cellular immunity to TSTA. Findings obtained with these techniques will be reviewed in Sections IV to VI.

A. Adoptive Transfer of Immunity

If allografts of normal or neoplastic origin are transplanted to recipient animals, they will be rejected by a so-called first set reaction (Snell, 1957;

Medawar, 1958). If the transplants contain "strong" antigens, which are foreign to the recipients, such as the H-2 antigens in mice, they will be rejected after a short time period (8–10 days), whereas grafts which only differ at "weak" loci survive longer (up to 20 days or more). If animals which have undergone a first set reaction receive a second graft of the same origin as the first one, a second set reaction follows and is detected as a rapid rejection of the grafted tissue. As a rule, second set reactions destroy a graft within 6 to 8 days (Medawar, 1958).

Mitchison (1954, 1955, Mitchison and Dube, 1955) showed that immunity against H-2 incompatible tumor grafts can be adoptively transferred with lymph node cells. Experiments were performed in which mice were grafted with tumors that contained foreign H-2 antigens. When a first set reaction had destroyed the transplants, lymph node cells were harvested from the regional nodes, and inoculated intraperitoneally in untreated syngeneic mice which were subsequently grafted with the same allogeneic tumor. It was found that the tumor grafts were rapidly destroyed in those animals that had received specifically immune lymph node cells. Immunity could not be transferred with serum or with killed lymph node cells. Neither was it transferred with spleen cells nor cells from nodes other than those draining the grafts.

Billingham *et al.* (1954, 1963) found that immunity to allogeneic skin grafts could be transferred with syngeneic lymph node cells, and coined the term "adoptive immunity" for immunity transferred in this way.

The finding that allograft immunity can be adoptively transferred with lymph node cells provides a method which has been used to search for cellular immunity to TSTA, as well as to a variety of other antigens: a graft is immunogenic if lymphoid cells which have been exposed to its antigens can transfer an increased resistance to the graft, when inoculated into untreated recipients.

B. Neutralization Tests

So-called neutralization tests were introduced by Winn (1959, 1962) and used by him and by Klein and Sjögren (1960), Koldovsky (1961), Old *et al.* (1962, 1963), and others to demonstrate cell-mediated immune reactions. They are based on the finding that lymph node cells (LNC) from mice which have been immunized against the H-2 antigens of another mouse strain can inhibit the growth *in vivo* of tumors carrying the respective H-2 antigens, if tumor cells and LNC are mixed *in vitro* and inoculated into syngeneic recipients. The recipients are usually X-irradiated with a sublethal dose (300–400 r) in order to decrease their immunological reactivity against the transplanted cells. Controls are made with nonimmune allogeneic and syngeneic instead of immune allogeneic LNC. These controls are essential since the addition of LNC to tumor cells may have either a nonspecific cytotoxic or, alternatively, a stimulatory effect on the tumor cells. In order to detect a neutralizing effect, the proportion of LNC per target cell must be relatively large (as a rule 10–200 LNC per tumor cell) and the immune LNC must be intact.

As a rule, LNC from nonimmune allogeneic donors have a slight inhibitory effect as compared to syngeneic control LNC, and a strong inhibition with allogeneic LNC is detected if phytohemagglutinin is added to the LNC–target cell mixtures (Bergheden and Hellström, 1966; see also Section VIII).

Neutralization techniques have been frequently used to study immune reactions against TSTA. Syngeneic lymphocytes are usually added in the experimental groups and are derived from donors which are immune to the TSTA of the target cells according to transplantation tests.

C. Tissue Culture Assays of Target Cell Destruction by Immune Lymphocytes and Macrophages

A series of investigations has been published during the last decade in which tissue culture assays were used to demonstrate target cell destruction by immune cells. Govaerts (1961) described the destruction of explanted kidney cells by allogeneic rat LNC derived from rats which were immune to the isoantigens of the explants. A synergistic effect between LNC and serum from the immune animals was detected. Koprowski and Fernandes (1962) reported that lymphocytes from animals with allergic encephalitis destroyed nerve cells *in vitro* and that the destruction was preceded by aggregation of the lymphocytes around the targets. Rose *et al.* (1963) found that lymphocytes from rats with thyroiditis were cytotoxic to cultivated thyroid cells.

Rosenau and Moon (1961) published a study of target cell destruction by immune allogeneic lymphoid cells. Mouse L cells (of C3H origin) were seeded into culture tubes. Twenty-four hours after the tubes had been seeded, the medium was removed and each tube received spleen cells from BALB/c mice which had been repeatedly immunized against C3H. The ratio of lymphoid to target cells was 200:1. The controls received nonimmune BALB/c spleen cells. Immune spleen cells were found to aggregate around the target cells within approximately 18 hours after they were added to the cultures, whereas no aggregation was observed in the controls. After 48 hours of cultivation, the number of living target cells was counted. These cells could be distinguished from the added lymphoid cells by their difference in size and morphology. Those tubes that had received immune BALB/c spleen cells had fewer living L cells than the controls. It was thus concluded that the immunocytes had destroyed most of the L cells.

Later studies (Rosenau, 1963; Rosenau and Morton, 1966; Rosenau and Moon, 1964, 1966b; Brondz, 1964, 1965; Wilson, 1963, 1965a) showed that cells other than L cells can also be used as targets and that the destruction mediated by immune allogeneic LNC is specific, so that LNC which are immune to antigens absent from the target cells are not cytolytic. The cytotoxic effect of immune LNC was found to be greater when no serum was present in the cultures during the addition of the LNC (Brondz, 1964). Consequently, the addition of guinea pig serum as a source of complement decreases cytotoxicity (Brondz, 1964).

Ginsburg (1968) cultivated mouse cells *in vitro* and found that LNC from rats which had been immunized against mice of different strains could destroy the mouse cultures. The degree of destruction was greater when the LNC were harvested from rats which had been immunized against the mouse strain of target cell origin than when they came from rats immunized against other H-2 genotypes.

Vainio *et al.* (1964) introduced isotope techniques to assess the cytotoxic effect of immunologically competent cells, and such techniques have been subsequently used by Holm and Perlmann (1965, 1967; Holm *et al.*, 1964), Ming *et al.* (1967), and others. In the experiments of Vainio *et al.* (1964), target cells were labeled with ^{14}C thymidine and the amount of ^{14}C label in their DNA was determined after exposure to immune cells. The outleak of ^{51}Cr from labeled target cells has been utilized as another assay of lymphocyte-mediated immune reactions. The reutilization of ^{51}Cr released from damaged cells was small enough to be discounted. The ^{51}Cr technique is rapid, objective, and well suited for experiments designed to detect immunity against a minor fraction of cells within a mixed population.

Granger and Weiser (1964) introduced the so-called "plaque assay" to detect cell destruction by immune macrophages. The target cells are grown in petri dishes to establish continuous cell layers. A drop of immune macrophages in tissue culture medium is then added carefully on top of the cell layer. Drops containing immune and nonimmune (control) macrophages are added at different places on the same layer, so that controls are built into each experiment. Between 24 and 96 hours after addition of the macrophages, plaques are detected at the sites of immune macrophage addition. The macrophages are also destroyed upon interaction with the target cells, and it is, therefore, possible to reverse the protocol by cultivating the macrophages in the petri dishes and adding drops of tumor cells on them.

Möller and Möller (1965) have used the plaque technique to study the phenomenon of allogeneic inhibition (Section VIII); in these experiments drops of LNC are added upon continuous cell layers of normal or neoplastic mouse cells. The plaque assay has also been used in studies of immune reactions against human tumors (see Section IV).

The CI technique was introduced to study humoral antibodies (Hellström and Sjögren, 1965; Hellström, 1965). It was later modified to detect also cellular immunity (Hellström, 1967). In this test, tumor cells are plated onto petri dishes in numbers sufficient to yield 50–80 colonies per dish in untreated controls. The following day, after their attachment to the petri dish surface, the culture medium is removed and the target cells are covered with a suspension containing immune lymphocytes, each petri dish receiving 1–5 × 10⁶ LNC or blood lymphocytes. Following 45 minutes of incubation, culture medium containing fetal calf serum is added and the dishes incubated for another 2 to 5 days, at which time the colonies are stained and counted. Controls include groups in which nonimmune allogeneic and syngeneic LNC are added, as well as groups with LNC which are immune to antigens absent from the target cells. In other controls, lymphocytes are plated alone; they rarely form colonies under the conditions of the CI tests. Complement is not added, and the sera supplied with the culture media are heat-inactivated (30 minutes at 56°C.).

The CI assay has been used in searches of cellular immunity against TSTA of a variety of tumors, including human neoplasms, and in studies on allogeneic inhibition (see Section IV and VIII). Its advantages are its sensitivity and reproducibility (even with tumors which have a low plating efficiency), the relatively small amounts of lymphocytes and target cells needed, and the fact that the results can be quantitated. Its sensitivity is probably due to the possibility that slight damage to the target cells may inhibit their multiplication even when it is not sufficient to cause cell death. The ratio of lymphocytes per target cell seems high, but, in fact, the majority of LNC added onto the petri dishes falls between target cells where no contact is established. It can be much decreased by incubating mixtures of target cells and LNC in test tubes, after which they are seeded onto petri dishes and target cell plating efficiency is measured. The degree of variation in colony counts on different petri dishes has, however, shown to be higher when mixtures of target cells and LNC are plated than when the target cells are plated first.

Brunner et al. (1966) have developed a technique which is similar to the CI assay and have used it for the demonstration of cellular immunity to H-2 isoantigens. Ascites tumor cells are mixed with immune LNC and plated in agar, where they form colonies unless destroyed by the LNC. Brunner's system seems to have an advantage over the CI technique when studying tumor cells that do not plate well in petri dishes, e.g., leukemic cells.

D. Lymphocyte Transformation *in Vitro*

If lymphocytes from peripheral blood, lymph nodes, or the thoracic duct are harvested from sensitized donors and exposed *in vitro* to the antigen used for sensitization, they undergo a "transformation," which means that they develop into lymphoblasts, synthesize DNA, and, finally, divide (Hirschhorn et al., 1963; Dutton, 1965; Bach and Hirschhorn, 1964; Bach et al., 1964; Bach, 1968). For example, lymphocytes from tuberculin-sensitive donors undergo transformation when exposed to the tuberculin antigen (PPD) in vitro (Pearmain et al., 1963). If the lymphocyte donors have not been sensitized, addition of the foreign antigen has little or no effect.

The transformation test has been used to study the interaction of lymphocytes derived from donors with different histocompatibility antigens (Bain et al., 1964; Dutton, 1965, 1966; Chapman and Dutton, 1965; Bach and Hirschhorn, 1964; Bach, 1968). If LNC from mice of two strains differing at the H-2 locus are mixed in vitro, some of the cells start to synthesize DNA, thus undergoing transformation (Dutton, 1965, 1966). The transformation occurs regardless of whether the LNC donors have been immunized against each other. It differs in this respect from the transformation detected after addition of PPD and similar antigens, where the lymphocyte donors must be immune.

Bach and Voynow (1966) showed that lymphocytes which have been treated with mitomycin C are still capable of inducing transformation but cannot undergo transformation themselves. One-way reactions can, therefore, be studied by mixing lymphocytes from two individuals after treatment of one of the cell populations with mitomycin C. By using such a one-way test for histocompatibility typing of patients, it was found that antigenic differences between two individuals at the strong HLA locus, but not minor incompatibilities, can be detected. Findings obtained on a large series of cases agreed well with studies by other techniques, such as typing with known cytotoxic antisera (Bach and Amos, 1967).

It is believed that only a small fraction (1–4%) of all lymphocytes in a population are capable of reacting with a given antigen and that exposure of that fraction to the antigen causes its selective transformation and proliferation (Dutton, 1965; Bach, 1968). If animals are immunologically tolerant to an antigen, the lymphoid cell clones capable of reacting with it may have been depleted, since it was shown that LNC from rats which were tolerant to the isoantigens of another rat strain were not transformed when exposed to cells from the latter strain (Wilson et al., 1967; Schwarz, 1968). There was no decrease in their ability to become transformed after exposure to other isoantigens. The lymphocyte transformation test may, therefore, be used as an in vitro assay for immunological tolerance, and may be employed, e.g., to determine whether or not immunological tolerance to TSTA exists.

It remains to be seen whether the lymphocyte transformation test is useful when studying immunity to TSTA. However, unless identical twins are involved, it may be difficult to prove whether a lymphocyte transformation detected is directed against TSTA or against normal isoantigens. These difficulties may be circumvented by studying autochthonous neoplasms. Preliminary findings by Stjernswärd *et al.* (1968) are promising in this respect: these workers studied patients with postnasal carcinoma and observed that cells from lymph nodes which were distal to the tumors underwent transformation when exposed to the tumor cells *in vitro* and that the frequency of transformation was higher when lymphocytes from the nodes regional to the tumors were studied, indicating that the latter lymphocytes were immune *in vivo*.

E. Demonstration of Delayed Hypersensitivity to Transplantation Antigens

The similarities between delayed hypersensitivity and the allograft reaction (Chase, 1953; Medawar, 1958; Lawrence, 1960), and between the allograft reaction and the mechanisms by which cells with TSTA are rejected (see Section VII), indicates that it is worth while to search for delayed hypersensitivity to TSTA.

Brent *et al.* (1962) found that guinea pigs previously sensitized by skin grafts have a delayed skin reaction to an extract of splenic cells from the donor of the skin graft. Churchill *et al.* (1968) have investigated the possibility that TSTA might also be detected by delayed skin reactions in sensitized guinea pigs. Hepatomas were induced in strain-2 guinea pigs by diethylnitrosamine, and syngeneic animals were immunized against the tumor, after which they were inoculated intradermally with hepatoma cells and found to develop a skin reaction of which the rate of development, onset, duration, histological features, and specificity were characteristics of delayed hypersensitivity in guinea pigs.

It is likely that attempts to demonstrate delayed hypersensitivity reactions to TSTA may be very profitable also in species other than guinea pigs, e.g., in man. We feel, however, that an *in vitro* test of delayed hypersensitivity can be easier controlled and quantitated than *in vivo* tests and may involve less complications when human tumors are studied.

One *in vitro* assay of delayed hypersensitivity, the so-called macrophage inhibition test, has proved to be very sensitive and specific (David and Paterson, 1965; Bloom and Chase, 1967; David, 1968). It is based on the finding that macrophages from immune donors are inhibited from migrating when exposed to the antigens toward which they are immune. Macrophages, obtained, e.g., from peritoneal washings, are drawn up into a capillary tube which is placed upon a glass or plastic surface and surrounded by tissue culture medium (George and Vaughan, 1962). They soon start migrating out of the tube onto the flat surface and the extension of their migration can be quantitied. If the macrophages are harvested from a sensitized donor and the specific antigen added to the culture medium, the migration of the macrophages will be inhibited (David *et al.*, 1964a; Al-Askari *et al.*, 1965; Bloom and Chase, 1967). This inhibition is highly specific, and control antigens, toward which the macrophage donor is not immune, will not inhibit. If the macrophage donors are sensitized against a series of closely related haptens, each of which is added individually to the culture medium, the degree of inhibition depends on the extent to which the haptens are related and shows a strong correlation with *in vivo* tests for delayed hypersensitivity (David *et al.*, 1964a; David, 1968).

The presence of 2.5% or more of lymphocytes in the macrophage population is needed for the migration inhibition to occur (David *et al.*, 1964b). If lymphocytes from an immune donor are admixed with pure macrophages from an untreated control, the macrophages will be inhibited, whereas pure macrophage populations are not inhibited. It has been shown that immune lymphocytes release a factor, MIF, upon contact with the specific antigen which is taken up by the macrophages and inhibits their migration in a nonspecific way (Bloom and Bennett, 1966; David, 1966). Its chemical nature is still not known, but it is probably distinct from any known antibodies (David, 1968).

The macrophage inhibition test has so far not been used for the demonstration of immune reactions toward tumor antigens. However, the great sensitivity of this technique in other types of delayed hypersensitivity reactions indicates that it might become a valuable tool for studies on tumor immunity.

IV. Demonstration of Cellular Immunity to Tumor-Specific Transplantation Antigens

There are good reasons to believe that the resistance of properly immunized mice against syngeneic tumor transplants has an immunological explanation (see Section VII for discussion). Experiments will be reviewed in which cellular immunity to tumor antigens has been detected. Studies carried out in inbred animals, primarily mice, will be dealt with first, after which investigations will be discussed which were performed to search for cellular immunity to tumors in outbred populations, including man. Since transplantation techniques cannot be satisfactorily employed in such work, *in vitro* tests, guided by the experience gained from studies of tumors in inbred animals, are necessary.

A. Neutralization Tests with Animal Tumors

A priori, it might be suggested that transplantation resistance to syngeneic and autochthonous tumors is mediated by (*a*) cellular immunity,

(b) humoral antibodies, or (c) both. This question was first approached with MCA-induced mouse sarcomas in experiments carried out with the neutralization technique (Klein et al., 1960; Old et al., 1962, 1963). Mice were immunized against syngeneic MCA-induced sarcomas which had TSTA according to transplantation tests, and their LNC were mixed with tumor cells in vitro. Then the mixtures were inoculated to sublethally irradiated syngeneic mice. Living LNC from specifically immunized animals gave a clear-cut neutralization, whereas disrupted LNC did not work. Serum taken from the same mice as the LNC had no effect when admixed with the tumor cells in the presence of guinea pig complement. It was concluded that the major part of the reaction by which an animal rejects MCA sarcoma cells is mediated by immune lymphocytes—a conclusion analogous to that reached for the rejection of cells with foreign H-2 antigens (Mitchison, 1954, 1955; Winn, 1959; Klein and Sjögren, 1960).

Neutralization tests have since been performed in several other systems. Sjögren et al. (1961b; Sjögren, 1964b) showed that LNC from mice which had been infected with the polyoma virus as adults or immunized by transplantation of allogeneic polyoma tumors neutralized the outgrowth of polyoma tumor cells in syngeneic recipients; killed LNC gave no neutralization. Lymph node cells from control mice which had been immunized with other kinds of tumors did not neutralize. Positive effects were occasionally obtained with serum from the same mice as the LNC and mixed with the tumor cells together with complement. Slettenmark and Klein (1962) found that LNC from mice which had been immunized against the TSTA of Gross lymphomas were also effective in neutralization tests. Klein et al. (1963) found that LNC from mice immunized against syngeneic plastic disc-induced sarcomas could specifically inhibit the outgrowth of tumor cells of the line to which they were immune. Mikulska et al. (1966) used the neutralization test in studies of immunity to autochthonous chemically induced sarcomas in the rat. These workers found that spleen cells taken 20 days or more after removal of the tumors neutralized the outgrowth of autochthonous sarcoma cells in syngeneic recipients. On the other hand, no clear-cut neutralization was obtained when spleen cells were harvested from rats with progressively growing tumors. Fefer et al. (1968) found that LNC from mice in which Moloney sarcomas had regressed spontaneously, inhibited the growth of Moloney sarcomas in vivo.

The findings mentioned indicate that immune cells have a greater importance than serum for the rejection of specifically antigenic tumors. The same conclusion has been drawn for the rejection of H-2 incompatible grafts. However, the role of cytotoxic antibodies for graft rejection in vivo should not be excluded for several reasons. Coggin and Ambrose (1969) have shown that SV40 virus-induced hamster tumor cells are destroyed (or inhibited from growing) when placed into cell-impermeable diffusion chambers which are inserted into hamsters specifically immune to SV40 tumors. Antibodies inhibitory to Moloney sarcoma cells both *in vitro* and *in vivo* have been detected in the serum of mice in which such sarcomas have regressed (Hellström *et al.*, 1969a). Cytotoxic (or growth inhibitory) effects of humoral antibodies against cells with TSTA have been demonstrated *in vitro* against certain human tumor cells when the antibodies are derived from patients who have not been artifically immunized and are tested against the autochthonous tumor cells (Hellström *et al.*, 1968b,c). Finally, cytophilic antibodies (Boyden, 1963) may arm nonimmune macrophages so that these become capable of target cell destruction (Tsoi and Weiser, 1968b).

B. Tissue Culture Experiments with Animal Tumors

Tissue culture assays were introduced as a more sensitive tool than the neutralization test for studies on lymphocyte-mediated reactions to TSTA.

Yoshida found (Yoshida and Southam, 1963; Yoshida, 1965) that spleen cells from mice from which autochthonous MCA sarcomas had been removed aggregated around and destroyed sarcoma cells *in vitro*. These data were presented, however, with considerable reservation, since "positive" reactions were inconsistently observed and were difficult to judge objectively (Southam, 1967).

Rosenau and Morton (1966) studied MCA-induced mouse sarcomas which had been kept in transplantation during 1 to 2 passages before explantation. The tumors were trypsinized and seeded into tubes, to which LNC were added from immunized and from nonimmune donors. In agreement with the findings from *in vivo* tests that different MCA sarcomas have individually distinct TSTA (Prehn and Main, 1957), it was observed that the LNC added in the experimental groups specifically decreased the target cell numbers. The effects observed were, however, generally small.

The colony inhibition (CI) technique has been used to investigate cellular immunity to a variety of mouse tumors and to tumors in rabbits and man, as discussed below. It was introduced by Hellström (1967) who studied polyoma tumors, against which a cellular immunity had already been demonstrated with neutralization tests (Sjögren *et al.*, 1961b). She found that LNC from polyoma-immune mice reduced target cell colony formation, but there was no reduction with control LNC. The polyoma-immune LNC were almost as inhibitory as allogeneic LNC from donors which were immune to the H-2 antigens of the target cells. The sensitivity of the CI assay as a tool for detection of immune reactions against TSTA was thereby established.

Cellular immunity against adenovirus 12-induced mouse sarcomas was detected by Hellström and Sjögren (1967) in experiments in which the tumor cells were exposed to syngeneic LNC from mice which had been immunized against the adeno 12-induced transplantation antigen by repeated inoculation of allogeneic adeno 12 tumor cells. The immunity was specific so that control LNC did not inhibit, regardless of whether they were derived from donors immune to TSTA other than those induced by adeno 12 or from donors immune to H-2 antigens which were absent from the target cells. Humoral antibodies were commonly found in sera from mice immunized in the same way as the donors of the reactive LNC and gave a complement-dependent inhibition of colony formation by adeno 12-induced tumors.

The CI assay has been used for investigations of immune reactions against mouse sarcomas which were induced by MCA or by implantation of plastic discs (I. Hellström and Hellström, 1967; Hellström et al., 1968a). These studies will be discussed in detail since it is felt that they may be valid as models for a similar approach to human neoplasms and since they seem to give some insight into the interaction between an organism and its antigenic tumor.

The first step in these investigations was an attempt to detect cellular immunity against autochthonous MCA-induced tumors. Sarcomas were induced in the legs of mice, which were amputated, after which the tumors were trypsinized and explanted in vitro. Between 3 and 8 days later, the operated mice were killed and their LNC tested by CI assays for inhibition of the respective tumors which had been removed; regional as well as distal nodes were used as the source of LNC. Controls were made with LNC from mice which were either untreated or had been immunized against unrelated MCA sarcomas or from which an unrelated primary MCA sarcoma had been removed. It was found that autochthonous LNC constantly decreased colony formation of the target tumor cells as compared to control LNC. No differences were seen between LNC from control mice which were untreated or from which an unrelated primary MCA tumor had been removed.

The finding of a cellular immunity to MCA sarcomas, mediated by autochthonous LNC, implied that either the primary tumors grew in vivo in spite of the fact that their cells could be inhibited by LNC in vitro or that the LNC reaction was established during the time interval between tumor removal and the tests. The latter alternative was tested in experiments with LNC from mice which carried progressively growing transplanted MCA sarcomas. Since a LNC-mediated colony inhibition was detected also in these cases, it followed that the MCA tumors probably existed in vivo in spite of the fact that the host LNC could inhibit (kill) their cells in vitro.

The time interval necessary for the appearance of CI-detectable immunity after transplantation of living MCA sarcoma cells was then studied. Experiments showed that LNC harvested only 3 days after the transplantation of approximately 10^7 tumor cells were inhibitory to the tumor line transplanted. These data agree with the demonstration by Rosenau and Moon (1966a) of lymphoblasts in regional lymph nodes of mice within 2 to 3 days after they had been transplanted with syngeneic MCA sarcomas. A corollary of the findings is that transplanted MCA tumor cells apparently have to overcome an immune response in their host but, nevertheless, are generally able to grow progressively *in vivo*.

The surgical removal of an autochthonous or transplanted tumor was found to be the most efficient way of immunization against MCA tumor cells, as far as this could be detected with the CI assay. The effect of immunization with multiple doses of X-irradiated (15,000 r) cells was less clear. It was found that mice given 2–7 doses of irradiated tumor cells, as a rule, had less inhibitory LNC than mice which had been given only 1 dose.

In order to determine whether or not the MCA tumor system is a useful model for investigations on neoplasms originating in outbred populations, such as man, experiments were made with allogeneic instead of syngeneic LNC in the control groups, since syngeneic LNC donors are, obviously, not available in outbred populations. It was found that such LNC could, indeed, be used as controls and that the specific effects with immune syngeneic LNC were still detected. However, the allogeneic controls were unsatisfactory if they were immune to any isoantigens present on the target cells or if phytohemagglutinin (PHA) was included in the culture medium. In the presence of PHA, allogeneic inhibition (see Section VIII) was generally detected as a decrease in colony numbers in groups treated with allogeneic as compared to syngeneic LNC.

Plastic disc-induced sarcomas are generally less antigenic than MCA sarcomas, according to transplantation experiments (Prehn, 1963b; Klein *et al.*, 1963). These findings were parallelled by CI tests: only a weak inhibition was seen with LNC from mice which had been immunized by transplantation of living or X-irradiated plastic disc-induced sarcomas (Hellström *et al.*, 1968a).

Comparisons were made between cellular and humoral immunity against TSTA, using MCA and plastic disc tumors as targets. The sera were commonly harvested from the same donors as the LNC. Guinea pig and rabbit sera were used as sources of complement. Only occasionally could humoral antibodies be detected by the CI technique in sera from mice of which the autochthonous MCA tumors had been removed or mice which had been transplanted with living tumor cells or which carried progressively growing sarcomas. On the other hand, inhibition of colony formation was almost regularly obtained with serum from mice which had received multiple doses of X-irradiated MCA or plastic disc-induced tumors. The serum findings are thereby in contrast to the findings on cellular immunity. It cannot, of course, be excluded that the mice had humoral antibodies to their tumors which could not be detected under the conditions of the experiments.

For several reasons, Moloney virus-induced sarcomas offer a good material for tumor immunological studies (Fefer et al., 1967a,b, 1968). They appear within 5 to 10 days at the site of virus inoculation. The tumors can be induced in adult mice, but sarcomas which appear in mice inoculated with the virus as adult as a rule regress spontaneously, unless the immunological reactivity of the mice has been diminished by whole-body X-irradiation. Colony inhibition tests were made with LNC from mice in which Moloney sarcomas had regressed, from mice with progressively growing tumors, and from mice transplanted with sarcoma cells which had not yet formed a palpable tumor (Hellström et al., 1968b, 1969a). The controls were either untreated or had been immunized against other tumors. Lymph node cells from mice in which the tumors had regressed and from mice with progressively growing neoplasms were both active, and the degree of reactivity was approximately the same.

Mammary carcinomas in MTV-carrying mice were long considered to be nonantigenic (Foley, 1953; Révész, 1960), until it was shown by Morton (1962) and by Weiss et al. (1964) that such tumors have a common antigen against which transplantation immunity can be built up in mice which are MTV-free. Neither Morton nor Weiss succeeded in immunizing mice which possessed MTV from birth against any antigen common to transplanted syngeneic mammary tumors; failure to do so suggested that these animals might be tolerant to the common tumor antigen. The fact that mammary tumors are "spontaneous" makes them particularly relevant models for human neoplasms. Heppner and Pierce (1969), therefore, applied the CI assay to mammary carcinomas which had appeared in BALB/c f C3H mice which contained MTV by foster nursing on C3H. The following findings were obtained. (1) Lymph node cells from mice the primary carcinomas of which had been removed approximately 20 days before they were added to the target cells consistently inhibited cells from autochthonous tumors but inhibited only 10% of mammary carcinomas from other BALB/c f C3H mice. (2) An equally good inhibition of autochthonous carcinomas was seen when LNC from tumor-bearing mice were removed from the mice at the same time as the tumors and plated together in vitro. (3) Inhibition was seen in 90% of the experiments in which BALB/c mice were immunized by transplantation of cells of the target tumor line but only in about half of the experiments in which BALB/c mice were immunized by a mammary tumor other than the target tumor. (4) Lymph node cells derived from BALB/c f C3H mice, which did not have mammary carcinoma or from normal BALB/c mice, were not inhibitory. It was concluded that cellular immunity can, indeed, be demonstrated against TSTA of spontaneous tumors and that spontaneous mammary carcinomas appear to have individually distinct TSTA in addition to the common antigens previously detected by transplantation tests.

The Shope virus induces papillomas in rabbits, which commonly regress after a few weeks. They may progress to carcinomas, however, and the probability of regression varies between different strains of rabbits. Evans and Ito have found (1966) that DNA prepared from the Shope virus can induce papillomas in previously untreated rabbits and in rabbits which have a persistent Shope papilloma. On the other hand, it will not induce papillomas in rabbits in which tumors previously regressed. This finding suggests that the "regressor" rabbits are immune to TSTA induced by the Shope virus (Evans and Ito, 1966). It cannot be attributed to antiviral antibodies which are found both in regressor rabbits and in animals with persistent tumor.

The Shope system was chosen for CI studies because spontaneous tumor regressions occur, the mechanisms of which deserve thorough investigation, and because it provided a tumor material in an outbred population which appeared to be useful when trying to bridge the gap between tumors in inbred mice and in man (Hellström et al., 1969b, and unpublished findings).

Shope papillomas and carcinomas were used as targets in the experimental groups, and normal skin fibroblasts from the same rabbits were studied in parallel controls. Papillomas were induced on the back of the rabbits, and regional axillary lymph nodes were harvested for the experiments. Colony inhibition of papilloma cells was regularly found after exposure to autochthonous LNC from rabbits in which either a papilloma had regressed or which had a persistent tumor. Such LNC also inhibited papilloma cells from other rabbits, which indicated that these cells contained a cross-reacting TSTA. No inhibition was detected with LNC from rabbits which had not been exposed to the Shope virus or tumors induced by it. Normal skin fibroblasts from the same rabbits as the tumor cells were not inhibited. The fact that allogeneic LNC could serve as valid controls suggested that investigations of cellular immune reactions against human tumor antigens might be feasible.

The finding that lymphocytes from both regressor and persistor rabbits gave colony inhibition agrees with studies on mouse MCA and Moloney sarcomas, in which lymphocytes from animals with progressively growing neoplasms were active.

C. NEUTRALIZATION TESTS WITH HUMAN TUMORS

The neutralization technique has been applied when searching for cellular immunity to autochthonous human neoplasms (Brunschwig et al.,

1965; Southam *et al.*, 1964, 1966; Southam, 1967). This technique had been previously used to detect cellular immune reactions to mouse tumors induced by MCA and by different viruses. Experiments were made in which tumor cells were mixed with blood leukocytes (lymphocytes and granulocytes) from the autochthonous patient and subsequently inoculated subcutaneously to the patient; leukocytes from healthy donors were used in the controls. The patients were followed for the development of a palpable tumor nodule at the site of inoculation.

In the few cases in which there was sufficient growth of the transplanted tumors to produce a measurable nodule, it appeared that the patient's own leukocytes often had some inhibitory effect upon the growth of the transplanted tumor cells, whereas leukocytes from a healthy donor showed no consistent effect (Southam *et al.*, 1966). These results might suggest a specific cell-mediated reaction against the individual's own cancer; however, the data were too few to be conclusive (Southam, 1967).

D. TISSUE CULTURE STUDIES OF HUMAN TUMORS

It seems, *a priori*, to be likely that at least some human tumors possess TSTA against which cellular immune reactions occur, since such reactions have been demonstrated against virtually all animal tumors studied with sensitive techniques. Furthermore, specific surface antigens have been demonstrated in certain human tumors by the indirect fluorescent antibody assay (Klein *et al.*, 1966b, 1967a,b; Morton *et al.*, 1968; Morton and Malmgren, 1968).

Chu *et al.* (1967) used the plaque assay of Granger and Weiser (1964) to search for immunity against postnasal carcinomas from African patients, tumors which may be chemically induced. Confluent layers of tumor cells were established in petri dishes; droplet suspensions of blood lymphocytes were then added on top of these layers. Autochthonous lymphocytes were tested in the experimental groups and compared to lymphocytes from patients with nonneoplastic disease. Controls were made in which the same lymphocyte suspensions were added to layers of normal skin fibroblasts established from the patients whose tumor cells were studied. Each test included parallel groups in which lymphocytes of the same origin were added to the target cells with and without PHA. When PHA was added, plaques were observed both in carcinoma and in fibroblast cultures at the sites of both allogeneic and autochthonous lymphocyte addition. When skin fibroblasts were used as target cells, the plaques were more frequent at the sites of allogeneic lymphocyte drops than at the points where autochthonous lymphocyte drops had been placed. If PHA was excluded from the system, plaques were more common where the tumor cultures had been exposed to autochthonous lymphocytes than where control lymphocytes had been added. No such differences were seen in the fibroblast cultures. The data suggested that the postnasal carcinomas studied possessed TSTA. Additional data were reported by Stjernswärd et al. (1968), who found that subcutaneous inoculation of X-irradiated postnasal carcinoma cells into a site drained by the inguinal nodes, conferred an increased ability of the inguinal node lymphocytes to form plaques on tumor layers *in vitro*, as compared to control inguinal LNC. Although the data by Chu et al. and by Stjernswärd et al. tend to suggest that cellular immunity exists against autochthonous postnasal carcinomas, the published material is rather small and a nonquantitative technique has been used so that no statistical evaluation has been possible. It is difficult, therefore, to draw any firm conclusions.

The demonstration of immune reactions against a variety of animal tumors with the CI assay suggested that this technique might be useful in the search for immune reactions against human TSTA. Neuroblastomas were selected for the initial phase of such a study (Hellström et al., 1968b,c) because occasional spontaneous regressions occur and because patients with these tumors are not infrequently cured even if they have widespread metastases (Everson and Cole, 1966). Tumors removed at operation were explanted *in vitro* and exposed to blood lymphocytes from the autochthonous patients, from other patients with neuroblastomas, from patients with other kinds of tumors, from control patients with nonneoplastic disease, and from healthy subjects. In addition, neuroblastoma cells were exposed to lymphocytes from the autochthonous patients' mothers, from mothers of other children with neuroblastomas, and from mothers of children who did not have neuroblastomas. In order to rule out false positive findings due to nonspecific toxicity or reactions against normal histocompatibility antigens, control tests were made against skin fibroblasts from the tumor donors.

Lymphocytes from neuroblastoma patients inhibited colony formation by neuroblastoma cells as compared to control lymphocytes. The controls included patients with Wilms' tumor, who had received the same treatment as the neuroblastoma patients. Their lymphocytes did not inhibit colony formation any more than did lymphocytes from healthy children. Autochthonous lymphocytes from neuroblastoma patients were tested and found to be as inhibitory as allogeneic lymphocytes from such patients. Lymphocytes both from neuroblastoma patients who were symptom-free and from those with progressive disease were inhibitory to the tumor cells.

Colony formation by skin fibroblasts was not reduced after exposure to lymphocytes from neuroblastoma patients as compared to lymphocytes from controls; the same lymphocyte suspensions as those used in the tumor experiments were tested on the fibroblasts.

Lymphocytes from the mothers of 4 patients in whom the diagnosis of neuroblastoma was made within 1 to 2 years after birth, inhibited colony formation of neuroblastoma cells from their own and other children in comparison with control lymphocytes which had been derived either from mothers who had healthy children of approximately the same age or from mothers of children with Wilms' tumor. It is important to note that the mothers of children with neuroblastomas inhibited the tumors from their own children and from other children equally well, and that they did not inhibit skin fibroblasts from their own or other children with neuroblastomas.

The present findings can be explained by postulating that neuroblastomas possess TSTA, toward which lymphocyte-mediated immune reactions can be detected with the CI assay. There are several strong arguments against the possibility that inhibition was due to nonspecific toxicity of certain samples of lymphocytes or to immune reactions against normal histocompatibility antigens.

First, lymphocytes from children with neuroblastomas inhibited the growth of neuroblastoma cells in culture but did not affect the growth of skin fibroblasts from the same donors. Autochthonous and allogeneic tumor cells were inhibited to the same extent. Occasionally, lymphocytes inhibited both neuroblastoma cells and fibroblasts, but this happened with only 2 of 50 control lymphocyte suspensions tested and the skin fibroblasts were at least as sensitive as the tumor cells to this inhibition. In no case did lymphocytes from healthy controls, from patients with nonneoplastic disease, nor from patients with other kinds of tumor selectively inhibit the growth of neuroblastoma cells.

Second, lymphocytes from mothers who had given birth to children with neuroblastomas reduced colony formation of neuroblastoma cells, but they did not inhibit skin fibroblasts from the same patients whose tumors were used as targets. Their lymphocytes were not more effective against their own children's tumor than they were against neuroblastomas from other children. These findings are in sharp contrast to those with lymphocytes from control mothers, who were matched with the mothers of neuroblastoma patients for age, number of pregnancies, and time interval between their last pregnancy and the test.

The finding of cross-reacting TSTA in neuroblastoma cells can be explained by postulating that such tumors have been induced by a virus, a postulate supported by the finding that lymphocytes from the patients' mothers inhibited colony formation by neuroblastoma cells. It is plausible that the common antigenicity is caused by derepression of some gene(s) normally expressed in less differentiated cells, as has been suggested to occur in mouse hepatomas (Abelev, 1965) and in human carcinomas of the gastrointestinal tract (Gold and Freedman, 1965a,b); of course, such carcinoembryonic antigens may still be virus induced. It cannot be definitely excluded that the inhibitory effects of the patients' lymphocytes were due to autoimmunity to organ-specific antigens of nerve cells. However, such an explanation appears unlikely since active lymphocytes could be derived from cured patients, in whom no signs of autoimmune disease could be detected. Furthermore, the effects obtained with maternal lymphocytes cannot be explained by autoimmunity.

The experiments performed with neuroblastoma suggest that the CI assay may be a useful tool to demonstrate immune reactions against other types of human neoplasms. Preliminary experiments of this nature have been performed to search for cellular immune reactions against a variety of autochthonous human neoplasms, including colon carcinoma, malignant melanoma, thyroid carcinoma, squamous cell carcinoma, and mammary carcinoma. In all of a total of 19 cases tested, cultivated neoplastic cells were inhibited by the patients' own autochthonous lymphocytes, while normal skin fibroblasts (or colon epithelial cells in tests with colon carcinomas) were not inhibited (Hellström et al., 1968d). The data indicated that adenocarcinomas of the colon possess common TSTA(s), in agreement with findings of Gold and Freedman (1965a,b) and of Gold et al. (1968), which were obtained by other techniques and which did not permit distinctions between TSTA and antigens of other types. On the basis of animal experiments performed with the CI assay (Heppner and Pierce, 1969) and transplantation tests (Vaage, 1968), it appears likely that those human tumors that have common antigens will, in addition, have individually distinct ones. Such antigens may be difficult to detect, however, because of the influence of allogeneic inhibition, by which allogeneic lymphocytes, immune to one antigen, may be as inhibitory as autochthonous lymphocytes that are immune to two antigens (Hellström and Hellström, 1967). Colony inhibition was detected independently of whether the lymphocytes tested were harvested from patients whose tumors had been completely removed or whether they were taken from patients with progressive neoplastic disease (Hellström et al., 1968d).

V. Discussion of the Possible Role of Cellular Immunity to Tumor Antigens in Vivo

Data reviewed in Section IV have shown that lymphoid cells from tumor-bearing animals and from some tumor patients can destroy neoplastic cells in vitro. Some implications of these findings will be commented on in this section.

We shall first discuss whether it is likely that there is an ongoing immunological destruction of tumor cells in some or possibly most cases of neoplasia. We shall then review work pertaining to the seemingly paradoxical situation that tumors develop in vivo in spite of the fact that their cells contain TSTA against which an immunity can be detected with *in vitro* techniques. The next section (Section VI) is a discussion of experiments performed to establish new ways for tumor prophylaxis and therapy on the basis of cellular immunity to tumor antigens.

Burnet has postulated (1961, 1964) that the survival value of cellular immune reactions is the protection offered the organism against antigenic neoplastic cells, which appear spontaneously or as a result of contact with tumor viruses and chemical carcinogens. According to this postulate, tumors develop when the immunological surveillance does not function properly, for one reason or another.

There are many experimental data which support Burnet's view that immunological mechanisms protect the organism against neoplasia. Neonatal thymectomy, which decreases cellular immunity (Miller *et al.*, 1962), makes experimental animals so much more sensitive to viral oncogenesis that even room infection with the polyoma virus can induce neoplasms (Ting and Law, 1967). Certain virus-induced tumors regress spontaneously, and this regression can be abrogated by whole body X-irradiation or treatment of the animals with immunosuppressants (Allison, 1966; Fefer *et al.*, 1967b). Patients with immunological deficiencies are prone to develop neoplasms, particularly in the lymphoreticular system (Good, 1967; Penn *et al.*, 1969).

Some samples of spontaneous regression of human tumors have been reported (Everson and Cole, 1966). Such regressions have been most common among chorioepitheliomas, which are known to contain isoantigens, foreign to the patients. Regression of such tumors can be relatively easily induced by drugs, which destroy the majority of the neoplastic cells. Childhood neuroblastomas represent other tumors in which complete remissions of metastases have been detected when only the primary tumors could be removed. Burkitt lymphomas make up a third category, in which the disappearance of large tumor masses has been repeatedly seen in spite of the fact that the therapy given was not possibly capable of destroying every tumor cell (Clifford *et al.*, 1967). The evidence cited indicates that immunological reactions against TSTA occur *in vivo* and that progressive neoplastic growth may be counteracted by an immunological defense mounted by the patients. It is, therefore, not surprising that accumulation of lymphocytes around a tumor and the appearance of lymphoblasts in the nodes draining it offer good prognostic signs, at least in certain cases of neoplasia (Black and Speer, 1958; Berg, 1959; Southam, 1960).

If we assume that certain human neoplasms grow in spite of an immunological response directed against their antigens (which can be detected, e.g., with the CI test), the elimination of most tumor cells from a patient (by surgery, X-irradiation, hormones, drugs, etc.) may be sufficient to allow the immune response to destroy the remaining ones. However, this is, obviously, possible only when therapy offered has not destroyed the immunologically competent cells. The best therapeutic goal might, therefore, be not to treat the patients so extensively that there are substantial risks that the doses of chemotherapy or radiation given will strongly depress the immune response. It is likely that *in vitro* techniques will become helpful for monitoring the patients' immune status toward their tumors during therapy.

The immunological mechanisms are, obviously, not capable of coping with all antigenic tumors and it, therefore, has to be explained why tumors grow in spite of the fact that they are antigenic. In 1957, Prehn and Main explained the observation that primary MCA tumors develop by postulating that chemical carcinogens such as MCA depress the immune response of the organism so that antigenic tumor cells can grow. They derived some support for this postulate from studies by Malmgren *et al.* (1952) and by Davidsohn *et al.* (1956) which indicated that chemical carcinogens, including MCA, depress antibody formation. Subsequent works by Linder (1962), Prehn (1963b), Berenbaum (1964), Stjernswärd (1965, 1966, 1967), and others have proven that doses of chemical carcinogens sufficient for tumor induction decrease the immunological reactivity of mice toward transplants which contain either weak isoantigens or foreign TSTA and also inhibit the sensitization of lymphocytes against sheep erythrocytes, as detectable by the assay of Jerne *et al.* (1963). Certain viruses, including some tumor viruses, also depress immune responses, cellular and humoral as well (Parfentjev and Duran-Reynals, 1951; Rubin, 1964; Dent *et al.*, 1965; Salaman and Wedderburn, 1966).

The demonstration of cellular immunity to TSTA (see Section IV) implies that autochthonous neoplasms appear in the presence of immune LNC which can destroy their cells at least *in vitro*. Therefore, the well-documented depressive effect of carcinogens and viruses on cellular immunity cannot, alone, suffice to explain why antigenic tumors grow progressively *in vivo*. Furthermore, it gives no leads why transplanted tumors with TSTA are not eliminated by the immune response.

Another hypothesis introduced to explain the progressive growth of antigenic tumors *in vivo* is that the organism is immunologically tolerant to the specific antigens of its own tumor. Evidence for this hypothesis has been derived from Weiss' *et al.* (1964) and Morton's *et al.* (1965) studies on immune reactions to MTV-associated mammary carcinomas: mice with MTV from birth do not become immune to the common antigen of these "spontaneous" tumors. The fact that most viruses must be inoculated within the neonatal period in order to induce tumors has been interpreted as additional evidence for immunological tolerance to TSTA. Data by

Rubin (1962), Klein and Klein (1964), and others also indicate that animals which have been exposed to a tumor virus early in life have a much diminished immunological reactivity to the antigens of tumors, induced by the respective viruses. However, Sjögren et al. found (1961a) that mice which had been injected with the polyoma virus when newborn were more resistant than untreated controls to challenge with polyoma tumor transplants, indicating that the virus infection did not make them tolerant. On the other hand, Stjernswärd (1968) demonstrated that mice from which primary MCA sarcomas had been removed were more sensitive than controls to challenge with cells of the same but not of other MCA sarcomas. He speculated that the increased susceptibility to autochthonous tumor grafts was probably caused by immunological tolerance to TSTA. Other possible interpretations, such as immunological enhancement, could not be critically excluded, however.

The finding of tumor cell destruction in vitro by LNC from animals with autochthonous tumors, induced by MCA, Moloney sarcoma virus, or Shope virus, indicates that immunological tolerance does not play any major role against TSTA, if tolerance is defined as a phenomenon in which an organism is depleted of clones of immunologically competent cells capable of reacting in vivo or in vitro against a given antigen (Burnet, 1959, 1961; Wilson et al., 1967; Schwarz, 1968).

Since some of the most convincing data in favor of immunological tolerance to TSTA were obtained in studies of mammary tumors in MTV-carrying strains of mice (Weiss et al., 1964; Morton et al., 1965), recent findings by Heppner and Pierce (1969) are of particular interest. They reported that colony formation of mammary carcinoma cells in vitro was inhibited after exposure of the target cells to autochthonous LNC, even when the LNC were derived from a tumor-bearing host, which implies that even if immunological tolerance plays a role against the common antigen of MTV-induced mammary carcinomas, it does not operate against their individually specific antigens.

The fact that primary tumors generally develop from small cell numbers led Old et al. to postulate (1962; Old and Boyse, 1964) that small numbers of neoplastic cells may be able to "sneak through" an immunological defense, because they may not provide sufficient antigenic stimulation to immunize their host until the number of tumor cells is so great that the immune reaction cannot overcome the neoplastic growth. The "sneaking through" mechanism appears to offer the simplest explanation why tumors grow progressively in vivo in spite of the fact that their cells are inhibited by immune LNC in vitro. The immune response detected in vitro may, indeed, be capable of inhibiting neoplastic cells in vivo but it is not sufficient for coping with a rapidly growing tumor mass. If the sneaking through explanation is correct, the introduction or recruitment of more immune cells into a tumor bearing animal should have a therapeutic effect, regardless of whether the immune cells are supplied by the adoptive transfer of lymphocytes or develop within the animal in response to vaccination or to a nonspecific stimulation. Experiments on adoptive transfer of immune cells are discussed in Section VI.

It may be argued that the failure of immune LNC to destroy tumors *in vivo* is owing to the fact that the TSTA which are recognized by LNC *in vitro* are not expressed in the majority of neoplastic cells growing *in vivo*. Lack of expression of the antigens can have several causes. Tumors undergo continuous genetic changes and may, therefore, be prone to lose (or change) their antigens just as they can lose normal isoantigens and thereby gain the possibility of growing in mice in which they would be otherwise rejected (Klein and Klein, 1958; Klein and Möller, 1963). Losses and changes of the TSTA of MCA may occur upon serial transplantation *in vivo* but they appear to be infrequent (Prehn and Main, 1957; Klein and Klein, 1962; Old *et al.*, 1962). It is even less likely that antigenic losses occur amongst virus tumors, which have common TSTA even after they have been propagated during many serial passages *in vivo* (Sjögren, 1965). Quantitative decreases in tumor antigenicity have been detected in Moloney virus-induced leukemias (Fenyö *et al.*, 1968) but not absolute losses. Where MCA-induced sarcomas and other neoplasms with individually distinct antigens are concerned, the possibility may be considered that those cells that at a given moment grow progressively *in vivo* do not contain the TSTA against which the LNC react *in vitro;* their predecessors may have possessed the antigen and become replaced by cells against the TSTA of which no immunity has yet developed. Such an explanation is unlikely, however, since the same TSTA have been detected when studying cellular immunity against MCA tumors which have been propagated over several passages *in vivo* (Hellström *et al.*, unpublished observations).

We shall now consider the phenomenon of antigenic modulation which may offer an explanation why certain tumors can grow *in vivo*, although they possess TSTA which are recognized by immune lymphocytes *in vitro*. Old *et al.* found (1968a,b) that mouse lymphoma cells which contain a surface antigen, TL, detectable by cytotoxic tests, will lose this antigen when propagated in syngeneic mice which have been immunized against TL, but that the antigen will reappear after transfer of the tumor cells to nonimmune mice; the term "antigenic modulation" was introduced to denote the shift in antigenicity. The TL-positive cells became negative when exposed *in vitro* to antibodies directed against the TL antigen (in the absence of complement) (Old *et al.*, 1968a,b). The TL antigen is not a strict TSTA, since positive cells which were transplanted to immune TL-negative recipients grew as well in these animals as in untreated mice. Studies on TSTA of animal neoplasms have not demonstrated any antigenic losses subsequent to transplantation of tumor cells to immune animals—the antigenic cells are generally killed in such recipients and when tumors have been harvested after passage in immune animals they still contain their original TSTA (Sjögren, 1965). It may, therefore, be argued that antigenic modulation does not explain why the majority of antigenic animal tumors can grow *in vivo*. However, it cannot be excluded that the ease by which antigenic modulation occurs varies for different tumors, leaving the possibility that most solid tumors do not modulate rapidly enough so as not to be rejected when transplanted to immune recipients. It is not known to what extent antigenic modulation of certain human tumor antigens may occur. The finding by Klein *et al.* (1966b) of specific immunity against freshly biopsied material from Burkitt lymphomas indicates, however, that TSTA in these tumors were probably present also on neoplastic cells growing *in vivo*.

Arguments have been presented that the progressive growth of most tumors *in vivo* is not due to any loss of their TSTA and that it may be due, at least in part, to lack of sufficient numbers of specifically immune cells. Factors that will facilitate the growth of antigenic tumors in the presence of immune cells will now be discussed. The following remarks are based on the assumption that tumors and immune cells may co-exist *in vivo* because the tumors are to some extent protected from being destroyed by immune cells.

Since tumor cell death or inhibition depends upon close contact with immunocytes (Section VII), interference with this contact may protect the neoplastic cells. There are several ways by which a contact might be prevented. For example, immune cells may not leave the blood circulation in sufficient amounts to penetrate into a growing tumor. Alternatively, the neoplastic cells may be surrounded by some protective coating (Currie and Bagshawe, 1967). Findings by Sanford (1967) are of interest in this connection. She observed that cells of the ascites carcinoma TA3 grew nonspecifically in foreign mouse strains and were only slightly sensitive to cytotoxic H-2 antibodies and complement. However, the tumor cells became sensitive in cytotoxic tests and lost their ability to grow in H-2 incompatible mice if they were incubated with neuraminidase. It was likely that the enzymic treatment of TA3 cells removed a protective coating of sialomucin and thereby made them vulnerable to an immunological attack.

Immunological enhancement offers another mechanism by which tumors can be protected *in vivo* from the cytolytic effect of immune cells. The term enhancement was introduced to denote a phenomenon in which humoral antibodies were found to facilitate the growth of transplanted H-2 incompatible mouse tumors (Kaliss, 1958, 1962; Snell *et al.*, 1960; Möller,

1963a,b,c). The antibodies could be injected into the recipient mice or admixed with the tumor cells. Billingham *et al.* (1956) have distinguished between afferent, central, and efferent forms of enhancement. Afferent enhancement occurs if serum antibodies bind to antigens released from the grafted cells and thereby weaken the antigenic stimulus. In the central type of enhancement, antibodies directly repress the immunocytes. Efferent enhancement is defined as the protective coating of tumor cells by humoral antibodies which bind to the TSTA and protect these cells from a lytic immune response. The antibodies mediating efferent enchancement must, obviously, be nontoxic or less toxic than the cytolytic immune response which they counteract, and are, therefore, likely to be immunochemically different from the cytotoxic antibodies (Bloch, 1965; Bubenik and Koldovsky, 1966; Chard, 1968). It is possible that a noncytotoxic antibody may also protect a cell from destruction by a cytotoxic, complement-fixing antibody by competition for the same antigenic receptors (Chutna and Rychlikova, 1964).

Enhancement of the afferent type cannot explain the findings that immune LNC are found by *in vitro* assays when a tumor grows progressively *in vivo*. A central type of enhancement might offer an explanation if it is postulated that antibodies can block the function of lymphocytes which are already immune rather than inhibiting them from becoming immune. An efferent type of enhancement may well protect tumors from being killed by immune lymphocytes *in vivo*. *In vitro* models of such protection have been established by experiments demonstrating that cultures of tumor cells are not killed by immune H-2 incompatible LNC if they have been previously incubated with serum directed against those of their H-2 antigens that are foreign to the LNC (Möller and Möller, 1965; Brunner *et al.*, 1968; Hellström and Hellström, unpublished observations). The protective effect of target cell exposure to humoral antibodies is probably due to coverage of those antigens that may otherwise be recognized as foreign by immune LNC.

Only little is known about the extent to which immunological enhancement exists against TSTA. Möller (1964) and Bubenik *et al.* (1965; Bubenik and Koldovsky, 1965, 1966) have reported that MCA-induced mouse sarcomas grow better in mice which had been inoculated with serum from syngeneic donors immunized with MCA tumors. Attia and Weiss (1966) found that mice which were immunized with a mixture of living and X-irradiated mammary carcinoma cells developed serum antibodies which facilitated the growth of transplanted mammary tumors into untreated syngeneic mice. It has to be pointed out that an efferent type of immunological enhancement would offer an explanation of the paradox that LNC may be destructive *in vitro* but not *in vivo*.

The CI assay has been recently employed to study the combined effect of lymphocytes and serum from tumor-bearing animals. Four different types of experimental material were used as a source of target cells: Moloney virus-induced sarcomas in mice, Shope papillomas in rabbits, spontaneous mammary carcinomas in mice, and, finally, two adenocarcinomas of the colon and two adenocarcinomas of the lung in humans. The neoplasms studied had been shown previously to possess tumor-specific antigens, against which cellular immunity could be detected *in vitro*. In all four systems, it was found that sera from hosts with progressively growing neoplasms could abrogate the inhibitory effect of lymphocytes which were immune to TSTA of the corresponding tumor type (Hellström *et al.*, 1969b). The serum effect was found to have a relatively high degree of specificity: Sera from mice with Moloney sarcomas protected target cells of that type from destruction by specifically immune lymphocytes but did not protect mammary tumor cells or cells from MCA induced sarcomas (Hellström *et al.*, unpublished findings). Sera from mice with mammary carcinomas or MCA induced sarcomas did not protect Moloney sarcoma cells. The protective effect could be specifically removed from the sera by absorption with the respective types of tumor cells (Hellström *et al.*, 1969b). Sera from rabbits, in which Shope papillomas had regressed, or from mice, in which Moloney sarcomas had regressed, did not protect the corresponding types of target cells from destruction by immune lymphocytes, indicating that the molecules mediating protection are different from the cytotoxic antibodies present in these sera. The finding that antisera to mouse gammaglobulin could remove the protective effect from sera harvested from mice with Moloney sarcomas (Hellström *et al.*, unpublished findings) suggests that the protection is mediated by some immunoglobulin, a suggestion also supported by its specificity. Although the serum effect detected may be easiest ascribed to efferent immunological enhancement, it might, alternatively, be attributed to antigenic modulation. Independently of which of the two explanations is correct, the experiments described have shown that the inhibitory effect of specifically immune lymphocytes from tumor-bearing animals (or patients) can be abrogated by factor(s) present in the serum of the tumor hosts.

Finally, tumor patients and animals with progressively growing neoplasms may contain some "factor(s)" which in a nonspecific way depresses the effect of immune cells or, alternatively, lack some factor(s) needed for the immune cells to function (Copperband *et al.*, 1968). The low immunological reactivity of tumor patients to a variety of antigens (Southam *et al.*, 1957; Southam, 1960) may thereby be explained. Sera from patients with Hodgkin's disease contain a factor, possibly an α-globulin, which inhibits lymphocytes from healthy persons to transform after contact with phytohemagglutinin or foreign isoantigens (Chase, 1966). It is of interest that delayed hypersensitivity reactions, as well as allograft reactions, are strongly decreased in patients with certain neoplasms, particularly those with Hodgkin's disease (Miller, 1967).

Mowbray (1963, 1967) has described another serum factor, which interferes with the immune response. His factor is an RNase which decreases the organism's ability to become immune after immunization. On the other hand, it does not effect an immunity once established. It cannot, therefore, explain the paradox of lymphocyte reactivity *in vitro* and tumor growth *in vivo*.

In conclusion, it is not possible to give one definite answer to the question why tumors grow *in vivo* in spite of the fact that they have TSTA and can be killed by autochthonous lymphocytes *in vitro*. It is likely that several of the mechanisms discussed (such as sneaking through, efferent immunological enhancement, and antigenic modulation) operate together in protecting the growth of antigenic neoplasms *in vivo*. Other, yet unknown, mechanisms may also be involved.

VI. Possible Therapeutic Implications of the Findings on Cellular Immunity to Tumor-Specific Transplantation Antigens

The experimental demonstration of cellular immunity to TSTA offers some hopes for immunotherapy of tumors although phenomena such as immunological enhancement (Section V) may complicate clinical attempts to prevent and cure tumors by immunological means. Relatively little work has been done to establish animal model systems for immunotherapy, and the results obtained with human neoplasms are not impressive. A review on immunotherapy of tumors has been published recently (Alexander, 1968).

It has been relatively easier to prevent the development of some primary tumors by immunological means than to cure animals with established neoplasms, which may be owing in part to the fact that a less vigorous immunological attack is needed to destroy a small amount of scattered neoplastic cells than to eliminate a large progressively growing tumor mass.

Eddy *et al.* (1964), Deichman and Kluchareva (1964), and Goldner *et al.* (1964) pioneered the field of immunological prevention of antigenic tumors. These workers studied SV40 tumorigenesis in hamsters and compared the frequency of primary SV40 sarcomas in animals which had been inoculated with the virus when newborn and which were subsequently either left untreated or given several additional doses of SV40 virus within a 3-month period. A significantly lower number of tumors was seen in those hamsters that had repeated virus doses. Goldner *et al.* (1964) also demonstrated that repeated doses of heavily X-irradiated SV40 tumor cells could be given instead of infectious virus partly to prevent SV40 tumorigenesis; vaccine prepared from homogenized SV40 sarcomas gave no protection but, instead, shortened the latency period before tumor appearance in treated animals. Girardi found (1965) that human fibroblasts which had been transformed to tumorlike cells by SV40 virus infection *in vitro* to some extent protected hamsters against primary SV40 sarcomas, when inoculated repeatedly within the first few months after a tumor-inducing neonatal dose of SV40 virus. The fact that the human cells did not release infectious SV40 virus particles *in vitro* suggested that the immunity was evoked by TSTA present on the transformed cells.

It is not yet known by what mechanisms the prevention experiments performed succeeded in decreasing the numbers of primary virus-induced tumors. The most likely explanation appears to be that the immunization procedures employed established a good systemic immunity and, hence, counteracted primary tumors from appearing by a sneaking through process (Section V).

Neonatal thymectomy renders normally resistant C57BL mice susceptible to polyoma virus oncogenesis; the susceptibility is probably due to the depressive effect of thymectomy on cellular immune responses (Ting and Law, 1967). Law *et al.* investigated (1967) what prophylactic effects could be achieved by an adoptive transfer of specifically immune cells to C57BL mice which had been thymectomized at birth and afterward inoculated with the polyoma virus. In part of the experiments, syngeneic LNC were inoculated intravenously from C57BL mice which had been immunized against the polyoma TSTA. It was found that such treatment when given up to 30 days after the virus gave a good protection against the development of primary polyoma tumors. Furthermore, it was demonstrated that the immune LNC actually destroyed scattered foci of virus-induced tumor cells which could be detected in the parotid glands of mice at a time point when the adoptive transfer of LNC still prevented tumorigenesis. Nonimmune C57BL LNC did not protect against tumors, and neither did allogeneic LNC from immune donors nor serum from mice of which the LNC were effective.

Immunotherapy of established tumors has been far less successful than tumor prevention. It has been approached following different lines, some of which appear to involve cellular immunity and, therefore, will be discussed here. Studies will be first reviewed in which nonimmune syngeneic and allogeneic lymphocytes were inoculated into tumor-bearing animals in an attempt to restore a defective cellular immune response. Experiments will then be summarized in which, instead, specifically immune lymphoid cells (or "messenger" derived from such cells) were inoculated. Finally, possibilities will be discussed for increasing the cellular immunity *in vivo* without the addition of extraneous lymphoid cells.

Woodruff and Symes (1962) reported that transplanted mouse tumors underwent partial regressions after the mice had been inoculated with large doses of allogeneic or xenogeneic spleen cells from nonimmune donors. A similar approach was tried with patients with far advanced cancer by inoculating large doses of allogeneic spleen cells (Woodruff and Nolan, 1963). The therapeutic effect of such treatment was slight and did not encourage its continuation.

Nadler and Moore (1966) have applied a somewhat similar approach. They immunized patients with far advanced neoplasia by allografting tumor cells from another patient, after which, 10–14 days later, they harvested blood leukocytes and inoculated large doses (10^9 cells approximately) to the patients whose tumors had been used as antigens for the immunization. A few remissions were obtained in this way. The facts that the transfused leukocytes may be immune not only to TSTA but to normal isoantigens as well and that they will be recognized as antigenically foreign and rejected, complicates the experiments and makes it difficult to conclude whether the tumor remissions observed occurred "spontaneously," were the results of previous (nonimmunological) treatment, or were due to a nonspecific stimulation of the immune response.

Mathé et al. (1967) treated leukemia patients by a lethal dose of whole-body X-irradiation followed by inoculation of bone marrow from healthy donors and observed some retardation of the neoplastic disease but no cures. The rationale behind these experiments was that the transfused cells might become sensitized to the leukemic cells and thereby destroy them. Great risks for secondary disease are involved, however.

A priori, it appears to be more feasible to cure an experimentally induced tumor by transfusion of specifically immune syngeneic cells than by transfusion of nonimmune cells or cells which are immune to normal isoantigens as well (or may become so). Experimental approaches to tumor therapy with cells immune to TSTA have been made with sarcomas induced by benzpyrene in rats and by the Moloney virus in mice. Related experiments by Law et al. (1967) with polyoma tumors have been already mentioned.

Haddow and Alexander (1964) studied primary sarcomas in the rat, which had been induced by benzpyrene. Tumors were partially removed, X-irradiated, and inoculated subcutaneously on repeated occasions. It was found that the growth of the remaining tumor mass was retarded in treated animals, as compared to rats which had not received any irradiated tumor cells or which were inoculated with irradiated cells from another sarcoma with noncross-reacting TSTA. As a second step, tumor-bearing rats were inoculated with lymphoid cells from syngeneic animals which had been sensitized to the respective tumors (Alexander, 1965; Delorme and Alexander, 1964). Retardation of tumor growth was observed, but there were very few, if any, cures. Experiments were subsequently made in which xenogeneic sheep LNC were used instead of rat lymphoid cells (Alexander *et al.*, 1966). Sheep were inoculated with rat sarcoma cells into a region drained by a prefemoral lymph node and LNC were harvested 3 days later by cannulation of the efferent lymphatic vessel from the node. The LNC were inoculated in large doses (10^9 cells approximately) to rats carrying the tumors used for immunization. Retardation of tumor growth was observed, whereas no such effect was detected with LNC from sheep which were untreated or which had been sensitized by inoculation of rat tumors with noncross-reacting TSTA. No harmful complications, such as graft-versus-host reactions, were observed in spite of the fact that the sheep LNC were immune not only to TSTA but to many of the antigens which distinguish rat from sheep.

It was postulated that the therapeutic effects observed in Alexander's experiments were not due to tumor cell destruction by inoculated LNC but were mediated by host cells which had become immune to TSTA by the uptake of some "messenger" factor (Fishman and Adler, 1963) released from the transfused lymphocytes (Alexander and Hamilton-Fairley, 1967; Alexander, 1967). This postulate was based, largely, on mouse experiments with labeled immune lymphocytes. When lymphocytes are inoculated to syngeneic mice which carry an allograft to which the lymphocytes are immune, they do not localize preferentially at the site of the allograft but are evenly distributed over the recipient which indicates that rejection of the antigenic graft is largely mediated by host cells (Najarian and Feldman, 1962). The following step in Alexander's experiments (Alexander *et al.*, 1966) was, therefore, to inoculate RNA-containing extracts from immune sheep lymphocytes into tumor-bearing rats. A therapeutic effect was detected in this case, too. It cannot be excluded that the RNA-containing extracts functioned as "superantigens" (Campbell, 1963), i.e., as strongly immunogenic complexes of antigen bound to RNA.

The Moloney virus sarcoma system offers certain advantages over most other systems when studying cellular immunity to TSTA. The virus induces tumors at the site of injection, appearing within approximately 7 days. When the virus is injected into BALB/c mice which are less than 30 days old, tumors appear which grow progressively and kill their hosts. Mice inoculated at the age of 30 days or more also get tumors, but these almost always regress spontaneously (Fefer *et al.*, 1967a,b). Lymph node cells from such regressors inhibit colony formation by Moloney sarcoma cells *in vitro* (Hellström *et al.*, 1968b, 1969a), which indicates that the regression is at least partly mediated by cells which are immune to TSTA of the sarcoma cells. To test whether LNC from regressor mice had any therapeutic effect on Moloney sarcomas *in vivo*, experiments were performed in which 1–2 × 10⁸ LNC from regressors were inoculated every third day into syngeneic (BALB/c) mice in which primary Moloney sarcomas had been induced before the age of 7–14 days and were growing progressively. A therapeutic effect (growth retardation) was detected in many of the tumors and approximately 30% of the tumors were erradicated (Hellström *et al.*, 1968b, 1969a). No such effects were seen in controls which were untreated and less than 5% regression was detected in controls given syngeneic nonimmune LNC. Small Moloney sarcomas proved to be much easier to treat than larger ones (Hellström *et al.*, 1969a).

Fefer *et al.* (to be published) combined chemotherapy and immunotherapy of transplanted BALB/c Moloney virus-induced lymphomas. Some (BALB/c × DBA)F₁ mice were specifically immunized against the TSTA of Moloney leukemias and their lymphoid cells inoculated into mice in which grafted syngeneic Moloney lymphoma cells were growing progressively. The immune lymphocytes had a strong therapeutic effect on the transplanted lymphomas if the mice were pretreated with cytoxan, whereas cytoxan or immunocytes alone had a moderate effect, only. These experiments have two important aspects—they show that immunotherapy may be more effective when applied in combination with other therapy than when given alone and they indicate that drugs such as cytoxan can depress the host's immunological response sufficiently for acceptance of allogeneic immune cells.

Another approach to immunotherapy was recently introduced and involved human skin tumors (basal and squamous cell carcinomas) (Helm and Klein, 1965; Klein, 1967, 1968). Tumors were treated by focal application of chemical agents which are prone to elicit delayed hypersensitivity reactions. Several patients were cured, which indicates that the procedure applied may be the most successful one so far for immunotherapy of human neoplasms. It may be speculated that the cures obtained were the outcome of lymphocyte–carcinoma cell interaction and that the lymphocytes had become more able to attack the tumor cells *in vivo* for several reasons: the chemical agents applied caused inflammation with accumulation of lymphocytes, they may have changed the vascular permeability making it easier for the lymphocytes to penetrate into the tumors, and they might have modified TSTA so they became more immunogenic.

The limited attempts which have been made to prevent and cure animal neoplasms by immunological means and the recent studies of skin carcinomas by Klein's group offer some hope for immunotherapy of certain human tumors to be applied together with already existing forms of therapy. As discussed in Section V, it is likely that many neoplasms grow in spite of ongoing immunological defense reactions and that treatment which can weigh the balance in favor of the host (chemotherapy of Burkitt lymphomas, for example) sometimes makes it possible for the immune system to eliminate surviving tumor cells (Clifford *et al.*, 1967). Procedures aimed at increasing the number of immune cells *in vivo* are likely to have a therapeutic value, at least in certain tumor systems, irrespective of whether the increase is established by the adoptive transfer of immune cells (or "messenger" prepared from them), by recruitment of more such cells following some vaccination procedure, or by a nonspecific stimulation of the immune system, such as can be achieved by inoculating mice with Bacillus Calmette Guérin (BCG) (Old *et al.*, 1961; Weiss *et al.*, 1961; Sjögren and Ankerst, 1969) or with a methanol insoluble residue prepared from tubercle bacilli (Weiss *et al.*, 1966). The findings of Evans *et al.* (1962a,b) are of interest in this respect; regression of Shope papillomas was demonstrated in rabbits after vaccination with a preparation of Shope papillomas and could have been caused by either an induced immunity against TSTA present in the vaccine or by nonspecific stimulation of the immune response.

We want to conclude this section by warning against premature enthusiasm which may lead to an uncritical immunization of cancer patients with tumor antigens in ways which might induce enhancement, instead of cellular immunity. Immunological treatment of tumors is faced with a dilemma. On the one hand, those patients who have advanced neoplasia will probably not respond to immunotherapy, as animals with advanced cancer will not, so that trials of immunological treatment of such patients may lead only to discouragement. On the other hand, immunotherapy is not ready to be tried on patients who have a relatively hopeful prognosis with already existing procedures for treatment. The best candidates for immunotherapy seem to be patients whose prognosis is pessimistic, according to experience but whose tumors are not yet in an advanced state. It is hoped that *in vitro* methods such as the CI assay can be employed to monitor the possible occurrence of immunological enhancement to human TSTA (Hellström *et al.*, 1969b) and that further guidelines for immunotherapy will be reached from animal studies.

VII. Mechanisms of Cellular Immune Reactions to Tumor-Specific Transplantation Antigens

The rejection of specifically antigenic tumor cells is mediated by an immunological reaction which is essentially identical to the allograft reaction (see below). Since many reviews have been published on the mechanisms of the allograft reaction (Gorer, 1956, 1962; Snell, 1957; Brent, 1958; Amos, 1962; Gowans and McGregor, 1965; Hellström and Möller, 1965; Wilson and Billingham, 1967; Rosenau, 1968), several of which appeared recently, the present discussion will be limited to only certain aspects.

A. Similarities between the Allograft Reaction and the Rejection of Tumor Syngrafts

Host resistance to transplants which contain TSTA (Section IV) is, primarily, of an immunological nature, although nonimmunological mechanisms such as allogeneic inhibition (Section VIII) may also be involved. Some characteristics will be listed which are valid both for the rejection of allografts and for syngrafts containing TSTA. First, the rejection is specific in that mice sensitized against unrelated tumors are as sensitive as untreated controls (Prehn and Main, 1957). Second, animals can be immunized against both allografts and tumor syngrafts and will subsequently reject tissues containing the respective antigens by second set reactions (Sjögren, 1965). Third, whole-body X-irradiation with 350 to 500 r suppresses primary allograft reactions (Stoner and Hale, 1962) and host resistance to tumor syngrafts as well (Rosenau and Moon, 1967) but has little effect on second set reactions to both kinds of grafts (Stoner and Hale, 1962; Klein et al., 1960; Sjögren, 1964a). Fourth, thymectomy at birth decreases both the allograft reaction (Miller et al., 1962) and host resistance against TSTA (Ting and Law, 1967). Fifth, both types of reactions can be suppressed by treatment of the animals with antilymphocyte sera (Woodruff, 1967; Bremberg et al., 1967). Sixth, allograft reactions and immune reactions against tumor syngrafts can be passively transferred with lymphocytes but generally not with sera (see Section IV for discussion). Seventh, histological preparations from the sites of rejection of either allografts (Scothorne, 1957) or tumor syngrafts (Allison, 1966; Rosenau and Moon, 1966a; Krüger, 1967; Fefer et al., 1968) show a heavy infiltration of lymphocytes and, to a lesser extent, of plasma cells and macrophages. Lymphocytes from the immune animals destroy appropriate target cells in vitro (Rosenau and Moon, 1961; I. Hellström and Hellström, 1967).

B. Cell Types Involved

The role of the lymphocyte as a mediator of both the allograft reaction and the rejection of tumor syngrafts has been demonstrated beyond reasonable doubt by tissue culture experiments (Rosenau and Moon, 1961; Wilson, 1965a: Gowans and McGregor, 1965; Wilson and Billingham, 1967) and by neutralization tests in vivo (Winn, 1959; Klein and Sjögren, 1960; Klein et al., 1960).

Data have been presented which indicate that macrophages can also function as effector cells in the allograft reaction. Granger and Weiser (1964) utilized the plaque technique introduced by them and could demonstrate that macrophages from animals which are immune to certain isoantigens destroy target cells which carry these antigens. These findings suggested that macrophages may be involved in graft destruction *in vivo*. Tsoi and Weiser (1968a) performed neutralization tests and demonstrated that the outgrowth of Sarcoma I in syngeneic mice could be suppressed if the sarcoma cells were inoculated after a suspension of immune macrophages had been admixed with them and that a ratio as low as 1 macrophage per target cell was sufficient. It could be excluded that the findings were due to contamination with small numbers of lymphocytes. Pearsall and Weiser (1968) observed accelerated rejection of A/Jax skin grafts transplanted in allogeneic C57BL mice onto graft beds which had been seeded with C57BL macrophages from donors immune to the grafts. The macrophage population which had been seeded was contaminated with approximately 3% lymphocytes. The immune activity of the macrophages could be destroyed by mild trypsinization, suggesting that it was due to cytophilic antibodies. Immune lymphocytes were also capable of transferring immunity but only in numbers exceeding those contaminating the macrophage preparations by 2- to 4-fold. It is so far not known what roles, if any, macrophages have in the rejection of tumor syngrafts.

C. Mechanisms of Target Cell Destruction by Immune Cells

Immune cells destroy their targets in a specific way, at least *in vivo*. This can be exemplified by data (Klein and Klein, 1956) showing that 20 (compatible) A sarcoma cells admixed with 5×10^7 [incompatible $(A \times A.SW)F_1$] sarcoma cells and inoculated into A recipients grew out and formed tumors, implying that the allograft reaction against the incompatible cells did not concomitantly destroy the compatible cells. The immune cells have generally to be alive and their action can be inhibited by the addition of antimetabolites that interfere with protein synthesis (Wilson, 1965b). A close contact between immune cells and their targets is a prerequisite for cytotoxicity (Rosenau and Moon, 1961; Möller, 1965b; Wilson, 1965a; Ginsburg, 1968). One specifically immune lymphocyte can kill one target cell, and only a minor fraction (below 10%) of all lymphocytes from a sensitized animal are immune to the respective antigen (Wilson, 1965a).

According to Rosenau and Moon (1961), Wilson (1965a), and Rosenau (1968), two steps are involved in a reaction between immunocytes and their targets: adherence of the immune cells and destruction of the targets. There are data indicating that the immune cells die during the reaction (Granger and Weiser, 1964) but this problem has not yet been solved.

Adherence of immune cells takes place within a few hours and precedes any detectable cytopathic changes. If close contact between immune and target cells is prevented, the cytotoxic effect of the immunocytes will be abrogated. Incubation of either the target cells or the lymphocytes with specific humoral antibodies will protect against destruction (Möller, 1965b, 1967).

The adherence of immunocytes to their targets can be studied by so-called rosette tests, in which animals are immunized with sheep red blood cells (SRBC) and the adherence between SRBC and lymphocytes or macrophages observed (Nota et al., 1964; Storb and Weiser, 1968). The attachment of the immunocytes is probably mediated by antibodies which are bound to their surface in minute concentrations and the action of which can be abolished by incubation of the immune cells with antiallotype antisera or with antilymphocyte sera (Pearsall and Weiser, 1969).

If animals are immunized to SRBC and rosette tests performed, only a small fraction of lymphocytes from their spleen and lymph nodes will attach to SRBC (usually below 10%) (Storb and Weiser, 1968). Macrophages, on the other hand, adhere readily. The discrepancy between the behavior of lymphocytes and macrophages is probably due to cytophilic antibodies (Boyden, 1963) which are present on the macrophages and bind to the antigens of SRBC (Storb and Weiser, 1968). Even macrophages from nonimmune animals will attach to SRBC after they have been incubated with sera containing cytophilic antibodies, whereas lymphocytes will not become more adherent after such treatment. The cytophilic antibodies are probably produced by plasma cells and lymphocytes and taken up by macrophages that are situated near the producer cells; if sufficient amounts of the antibodies are formed to get into the blood circulation, the macrophages will take up cytophilic antibodies also from the serum (Storb and Weiser, 1968). Therefore, the role of serum antibodies must not be neglected as an important component which may facilitate macrophage-mediated immune reactions (Tsoi and Weiser, 1968b).

The second step in the interaction between immunocytes and target cells is destruction of the latter. Its mechanisms are still unknown. Three hypotheses will be discussed. One important finding which any hypothesis must take into account is the great specificity of the allograft reaction in vivo, as previously mentioned. Another finding which may be relevant for understanding target cell destruction by immune cells is that nonimmune LNC are cytotoxic to cultivated homozygous cells, if they are either allogeneic or of F_1 hybrid origin and added together with PHA (see Section VIII for discussion). Holm et al. demonstrated (1964; Holm and Perlmann, 1965, 1967) that allogeneic and xenogeneic LNC from untreated animals were cytotoxic if PHA was added but not in its absence. Similar findings were made when cultures of mouse cells were exposed to nonimmune allogeneic and semisyngeneic LNC and lymphoma cells, whereas syngeneic lymphoid cells had a much smaller cytotoxic effect (Möller, 1965b;

Hellström *et al.*, 1965, 1967). The addition of PHA was required for the demonstration of cytotoxicity. It is unknown to what extent these studies provide a model for cellular immunity. Nevertheless, the fact that lymphoid cells from nonimmune animals are cytotoxic under certain conditions is relevant when interpreting lymphocyte-mediated cell destruction in other systems.

Probably the simplest hypothesis for the cytotoxic effect of immune cells is that they contain minute quantities of antibodies, by which they both adhere to and destroy their targets (Gorer, 1956; Karush and Eisen, 1962). If the amount of antibody per cell is very small, a sufficient concentration for cytotoxicity may be reached only at that part of the cell surface where an immunocyte adheres to a target cell. Humoral antibodies require complement for being cytotoxic, while the addition of complement does not potentiate cellular immune reactions; on the contrary, Brondz found (1964) that guinea pig complement decreased the cytolytic effect of immune allogeneic mouse lymphocytes. It may be, therefore, that classic antibodies are not involved as mediators of target cell destruction by immunocytes. However, it cannot be excluded that lymphocytes and macrophages contain sufficient amounts of complement to make further need superfluous or that target cell destruction by antibodies released from immunocytes does not have the same complement requirements as cell destruction by humoral antibodies.

The hypothesis that target cell death is caused by release of cytotoxic antibodies from immune cells is compatible with the great specificity of the reaction. It is particularly interesting in view of the fact that cytophilic antibodies eluted from immune macrophages are cytotoxic *in vitro* (Granger and Weiser, 1964), in the presence of complement. However, there is no proof that cytotoxic antibodies are released into the culture medium, when immune lymphocytes are brought into contact with and destroy appropriate target cells. The cytotoxic effect of PHA-treated nonimmune allogeneic and semisyngeneic lymphocytes on homozygous targets (Hellström and Möller, 1965) is not explained by this hypothesis.

The second hypothesis implies that the mechanism postulated for allogeneic inhibition (Hellström *et al.*, 1964) (see Section VIII for discussion) is also involved in the destruction of target cells by attached immune cells, i.e., destruction is caused by contact with foreign surface structures on the immunocytes, such as foreign isoantigens (Hellström and Möller, 1965). This hypothesis attempts to give a unified interpretation of target cell destruction by immune cells and by nonimmune lymphoid cells to which PHA has been added. It may be argued that the hypothesis does not explain how syngeneic lymphocytes can kill tumor cells which possess TSTA. This argument may not be valid since lymphocytes possess specific antigens which are absent from other cell types (Boyse *et al.*, 1968; Potworowski and Nairn, 1968) and since large doses of syngeneic LNC have been found to be cytotoxic, although less so than allogeneic LNC (Hellström *et al.*, 1967; Chu *et al.*, 1967). Some additional mechanism, however, must be postulated to explain why F_1 hybrid target cells are destroyed by parental strain lymphocytes (Möller and Möller, 1965) if they are intact but not if they are disintegrated (K. E. Hellström *et al.*, 1968). Such destruction could, for example, be caused by the release of cytotoxic substances from parental strain lymphocytes upon contact with foreign H-2 antigens of F_1 hybrid targets. If so, a similar release of cytotoxic substances would be possible also under other conditions when allogeneic or syngeneic lymphocytes come in contact with target cell antigens, which are foreign to them (cf. third hypothesis below).

According to the third hypothesis, cell destruction by immune lymphocytes and macrophages is caused by the release of a toxic factor from the immune cells upon their contact with specific antigens in the targets. *A priori*, such a factor might (*a*) be toxic to all kinds of cells, including syngeneic cells, (*b*) be toxic to those cells toward which the immunocytes have been specifically sensitized (and other cells with the same antigenicity), (*c*) to be toxic to all cells that are not syngeneic to the immunocytes from which the factor is released. It can be visualized that a factor may be nonspecifically toxic *in vitro* but not *in vivo* if the organism contains inhibitors by which its own cells are protected from destruction.

Experimental evidence in favor of the third hypothesis has been presented recently. Rudlde and Waksman (1967, 1969a,b), Granger and Kolb (1968) and Kolb and Granger (1968) found that rat and mouse lymphocytes released a toxic factor into the culture medium after they had been in contact with target cells which carried the isoantigens to which they were immune and that this factor in an apparently nonspecific way destroyed syngeneic, allogeneic, and xenogeneic cells. The same factor was also detected in the supernatant harvested from lymphocytes which were stimulated by PHA. The data tend to suggest that target cell destruction by immune cells is nonspecific after contact has been established between the immunocytes and the antigens to which they are immune. In order to reconcile these findings with the great specificity by which cellular immune mechanisms destroy antigenic cells *in vivo*, it must be postulated that (*a*) only a small amount of the factor is released upon contact between lymphocytes and target cells which is immediately taken up by the cells which are later destroyed or (*b*) that some inhibitor exists *in vivo* by which syngeneic cells are protected from destruction or (*c*) that the factor will prove to have some specificity when purified and carefully titrated. It appears to be important to find out what relationship exists, if any, between the cytotoxic factor and the factor that is detected in allogeneic and F_1 hybrid lymphocytes by its destruction of tumor and normal cells *in vitro* (Hellström *et al.*, 1964; Hellström and Möller, 1965; Fialkow, 1967; see Section VIII).

McIvor, Heise, and Weiser (1969) have identified another factor, which is different from that described by Ruddle and Waksman (1967) and by Granger and Kolb (1968). It is released from immune macrophages when they are confronted with the isoantigens of allogeneic cells toward which they are immune. It appears to destroy cultivated cells in a specific way. What possible role this (or the lymphocyte) factor may have *in vivo* is yet unknown.

VIII. Allogeneic Inhibition

In 1958, Snell discovered that mouse lymphomas of C57BL origin grew better when transplanted to syngeneic C57BL mice than they did in semi-syngeneic F_1 hybrids between C57BL and other strains (Snell, 1958; Snell and Stevens, 1961). This finding formed an exception to the so-called rules of transplantation, according to which F_1 hybrids are universal recipients of grafts from the parental strains (Snell, 1953).

Hellström (1963, 1966a; Hellström and Hellström, 1965) extended Snell's observation to a large spectrum of lymphomas, originating in different mouse strains and found, in addition, that carcinomas and sarcomas also grow less well in F_1 hybrids than in syngeneic animals. The preferential growth of homozygous tumor cells in syngeneic mice was called syngeneic preference and the inhibition seen in the hybrids was referred to as allogeneic inhibition. Huemer (1965), Oth *et al.* (1964), Klein and Möller (1963), and others have confirmed the observation of deficient growth of transplanted homozygous tumors in F_1 hybrid recipients, and Möller *et al.* (1969) have reported that allogeneic inhibition can be demonstrated in thymectomized X-irradiated F_1 hybrids and in tolerant mice as well.

It is possible that allogeneic inhibition, as detected with tumors, and the poor growth of homozygous bone marrow cells in F_1 hybrid recipients, which has been described by several investigators (Boyse, 1959; Cudkowicz and Stimpfling, 1964a; Goodman and Bosma, 1967), have a similar explanation; evidence both favoring (Goodman and Bosma, 1967) and disfavoring (Cudkowicz and Stimpfling, 1964b) such a view can be cited.

A review on allogeneic inhibition has been published recently (Hellström and Hellström, 1967b). This presentation can, therefore, be confined to aspects which illustrate two points relevant to the preceding sections of this article: (*a*) whether or not data exist which support the hypothesis that allogeneic inhibition plays a role in lymphocyte–target cell interaction as studied *in vitro* and (*b*) whether or not there are data indicating that allogeneic inhibition can act as a surveillance mechanism by which small numbers of antigenically foreign cell variants are eliminated without need for an immunity to develop.

Hellström *et al.* reported (1964) that mouse tumor cells cultivated *in vitro* were destroyed when exposed to homogenates or antigenic extracts which had been prepared from allogeneic spleen or tumor cells and which contained H-2 isoantigens foreign to the explants. It was postulated that the target cells were killed upon contact with such H-2 antigens in the added extracts which were foreign to them. It could not be excluded, however, that the cytotoxic effect was due to some cellular material which was associated with the H-2 antigens, rather than the antigens per se. Nevertheless, the findings suggested that allogeneic inhibition, as detected *in vivo*, may be due to contact between transplanted homozygous tumor cells with foreign surface structures of surrounding cells in the F_1 hybrid hosts.

Möller found (1965a) that allogeneic LNC from untreated mice were cytotoxic to mouse tumor cultures, as compared with syngeneic LNC. The cytotoxic effect was weak, however, unless PHA was added. With PHA it reached the same magnitude as that obtained with immune allogeneic LNC. Heteroimmune (rabbit antimouse) serum had a similar effect as PHA, whereas complement did not potentiate the cytotoxicity of allogeneic LNC. Semisyngeneic F_1 hybrid LNC were approximately as destructive to the target cells as allogeneic LNC. In a later investigation, Möller and Möller (1965) studied normal mouse embryonic cells and found that both allogeneic and F_1 hybrid LNC destroyed homozygous target cells, as compared to controls with syngeneic LNC.

Concomitant studies by Hellström *et al.* (1965; Hellström and Hellström, 1965) and by Bergheden and Hellström (1966), using the neutralization assay, gave results similar to those reported by the Möllers. Homozygous lymphoma cells were mixed with allogeneic or F_1 hybrid LNC (syngeneic LNC being used in the controls) in the presence of PHA, and the mixtures were inoculated to mice which were syngeneic to the target cells. Allogeneic and F_1 hybrid LNC inhibited tumor formation *in vivo*. X-irradiation of the LNC with up to 10,000 r did not abolish their effect. Inhibition was also seen when lymphoma cells of allogeneic and F_1 hybrid origin (instead of normal LNC) were admixed with the target cells (Bergheden and Hellström, 1966).

The CI technique was introduced as a more sensitive assay of the interaction between mouse tumor cells and LNC (Hellström and Hellström, 1966; K. E. Hellström *et al.*, 1967, 1968; Hellström and Hellström, 1967a,b,

1968). Experiments were done with tumor lines of A/Sn and A.SW origin, which were exposed to intact and disintegrated cells from allogeneic mouse strains, in the presence of PHA. The cells added to the targets were most commonly derived from four congeneic resistant mouse lines, which differed from each other only at locus H-2, namely, A,A.SW, A.CA, and A.BY (Snell, 1955) and from their semisyngeneic F_1 hybrids with the strain of target cell origin.

The following findings were obtained: (a) allogeneic and semisyngeneic F_1 hybrid LNC were equally inhibitory to homozygous target cells—since the F_1 hybrid LNC tested were derived from male and female hybrids of reciprocal crosses, the inhibition detected with such LNC could not have been due to immunological reactions against sex chromosome-determined histocompatibility antigens (Bailey, 1963; Rosenau and Horwitz, 1968); (b) allogeneic and F_1 hybrid lymphoma cells inhibited homozygous target cells to approximately the same extent as normal LNC in experiments with three lymphoma lines added to the targets, namely, a lymphoma of (A × A.SW)F_1 origin and isoantigenic variant lines (Klein and Klein, 1958) selected from it for compatibility with the A and A.SW parental strains; (c) syngeneic LNC and lymphoma cells were inhibitory when added in large doses, although their effect was slight as compared to that of allogeneic and F_1 hybrid cells; (d) ultrasound disintegration of lymphoid cells did not abrogate their inhibitory effect; (e) PHA was needed to detect any clear-cut inhibition with intact cells; (f) ultrasonicated parental strain LNC were not inhibitory to F_1 hybrid target cells; (g) target cell inhibition was greatest after exposure to LNC that contained foreign H-2 antigens. However, a significant reduction of colony formation was also detected with LNC which contained multiple foreign non-H-2 antigens.

Intact and disintegrated sarcoma cells were found also to inhibit tumor cells to which they had been added, if they contained foreign H-2 antigens (Hellström and Hellström, 1968; K. E. Hellström et al., 1968; Möller and Möller, 1967). The sarcomas to which the target tumors were exposed in these experiments had been passed during one transfer in F_1 hybrids so that they contained the same type of normal stroma cells irrespectively of whether they were allogeneic or syngeneic to the targets.

The finding that F_1 hybrid and allogeneic lymphoid cells inhibited homozygous tumors to the same extent cannot be explained by a classic immunological reaction, mediated by immunologically competent cells (or humoral antibodies) and specifically directed against target cell antigens. First, it is unclear whether parental strain-specific antigens exist, against which F_1 hybrids can react immunologically. Thus, it has not been possible to immunize F_1 hybrid mice against parental strain skin grafts (Martinez et al., 1959; Wigzell and Linder, 1961), except when the transplanted tissue contains sex chromosome-determined antigens which are absent from the hybrids (Bailey, 1963; Rosenau and Horwitz, 1968). Findings by Cudkowicz and Stimpfling (1964a,b) suggest that hematopoietic cells which are homozygous for the H-2b allele contain an antigen which is not expressed in F_1 hybrids, but these findings could not be confirmed by Goodman and Bosma (1967). Second, even if it is supposed that homozygous tumor and normal cells possess an antigen which is not expressed in F_1 hybrids, it is still difficult to explain why an immunological reaction occurring against this antigen and mediated by F_1 hybrid LNC should be as strong as a reaction mediated by allogeneic LNC, to which *both* the H-2 antigens of the target cells and the parental strain-specific antigens should be foreign. Third, the fact that target cell exposure to allogeneic sarcoma cells was inhibitory in CI tests and in neutralization experiments indicates that the inhibition studied was of a nonimmunological nature. The data, therefore, support the hypothesis of Hellström *et al.* (1964) that target cell contact with foreign surface structures (such as H-2 antigens) can lead to their destruction. This hypothesis was also supported by experiments in which the cytotoxic effect of intact or disrupted allogeneic lymphoid cells could be blocked by a heat-inactivated antiserum, with which the lymphoid cells were incubated before they were added to tumor cultures (Hellström and Hellström, 1966; Möller, 1967.

Findings which appear analogous to those reported by the Hellströms and Möllers have been obtained by other groups of investigators as well. Fialkow found that allogeneic but not autogeneic human lymphocyte extracts produced polyploidization, chromosomal breaks, and cytopathic changes, when added to human fibroblast cultures (Fialkow and Gartler, 1966; Fialkow, 1967). Chromosomal breaks and cytotoxicity were also detected in mouse embryo cell cultures, to which allogeneic or F_1 hybrid spleen and lymph node homogenates had been added, as compared to controls given syngeneic homogenates (Fialkow *et al.*, 1968). Ming *et al.* (1967) found that the addition of nonimmune allogeneic LNC inhibited DNA synthesis in mouse tumor cultures, as compared to controls with syngeneic LNC. Chu *et al.* (1967) observed that allogeneic blood lymphocytes were more cytotoxic to cultivated human fibroblasts than autogenic lymphocytes, both in the presence and in the absence of PHA. Holmgren and Merchant (1968) reported destruction of a tissue culture line of human epithelial cells, when it was co-cultivated with another human cell line. Treatment of the "aggressor" cells with a specific antiserum gave a partial protection from target cell damage.

It has been speculated that allogeneic inhibition may be involved in target cell destruction by immune lymphocytes (Möller, 1965b; Hellström and Möller, 1965). Such destruction is generally preceded by aggregation of the immunocytes around the cells to be destroyed (Rosenau and Moon, 1961) and would according to the speculation by Möller be caused by the close contact between the target cells and the foreign surface structures (antigens) of the lymphocytes. Arguments both for and against such a hypothesis were discussed in the preceding section. It suffices to state that data have been presented according to which target cell exposure to foreign surface structures in LNC can lead to their specific destruction.

Hellström et al. (1964; Hellström and Hellström, 1965, 1967b) and Klein (1966) have postulated that allogeneic inhibition is capable of eliminating cell variants the surface structure (antigenicity) of which differs from that of surrounding cells within a tissue without need for immunological reactions of the classic type. According to this postulate, allogeneic inhibition may be capable of eliminating single (possibly neoplastic) cell variants. By the same token, allogeneic inhibition can be looked upon as a more primitive mechanism for growth surveillance than that provided by the immunological system. It cannot handle large numbers of cells and it has no anamnestic response.

It may be speculated that allogeneic inhibition has an early phylogenetic origin and that its role for surveillance is most important in animals which lack classic immunological mechanisms (K. E. Hellström et al., 1968). In the lack of experimental proof for this hypothesis, it may be worth while to consider whether any examples are known from other than mammalian systems, where contact between cells with different surface structure leads to destruction of one or both of the partners. Two examples in which the "targets" are bacteria appear particularly interesting, since immunological reactions cannot possibly play a role there. First, it has been observed that large amounts of "male" bacteria which have the F factor can kill "female" bacteria of the same strain which only differ from the males by being F negative (Gross, 1963) and that disintegrated male bacteria can kill female bacteria probably because of a direct action of the F substance (Nomura, 1967). Second, there are certain (perhaps superficial) similarities in the interaction between colicins and bacteria, on the one hand, and the cellular "factors" responsible for allogeneic inhibition and their targets, on the other, which suggest that the colicin system might be considered as a tentative model for cellular interaction.

Colicins are bacterial toxins which may either destroy bacteria or inhibit their growth, different colicins having different actions (Nomura, 1967). Some colicins are so closely associated with the bacterial cell membrane that they were first considered to be bacterial surface antigens. Bacteria which are colicinogenic, i.e., which have the genetic potential to produce a colicin, are resistant to the colicin which they can produce but fully sensitive to other colicins. Bacterial cells can be made colicinogenic for different colicins and thereby acquire resistance to the action of the respective colicins. The resistance can be overcome by large colicin doses and is probably mediated by a specific "immunity substance" (Nomura, 1967). Cells can be selected which are relatively resistant to a colicin foreign to them and a state of tolerance has been described in which bacteria absorb a colicin but are not affected by it.

The postulate that a nonimmunological mechanism exists by which antigenically aberrant cells can be eliminated *in vivo* appears to be contradictory to the findings that chimeras can be established between isoantigenically foreign cells and that allophenic mice can be created in which cells of different antigenicity exist happily together (Mintz and Silvers, 1967). This conflict will not be solved unless some mechanism is detected, by which allogeneic inhibition between antigenically different cells can be abrogated in a specific way. Although such a mechanism has not been conclusively demonstrated, two sets of findings indicate possible means by which antigenically different cells can exist together *in vivo*. First, homozygous mouse lymphoma lines which were serially propagated in semisyngeneic F_1 hybrids became more transplantable to hybrids of the type in which they had been propagated than lines which had been kept in transplantation in homozygous mice, which suggests either that cells can become tolerant to allogeneic inhibition or that less sensitive variants can be selected (Hellström, 1966b). These findings may be related to the Barrett-Deringer effect (Barrett and Deringer, 1950; Barrett *et al.*, 1953) by which homozygous (A) tumors which have been transplanted during at least one passage in $(A \times B)F_1$ hybrids become more capable of growing in $(A \times B)F_2$ hybrids and in backcrosses to the resistant (B) strain. Second, allogeneic inhibition can be detected *in vivo* only after inoculation of relatively small cell doses, but large inocula grow as well in F_1 hybrids as in syngeneic mice. A tentative explanation of this finding is that cells within a large inoculum mutually protect each other against allogeneic inhibition. This explanation is supported (but not proved) by the demonstration (Hellström, unpublished observations) that small doses of homozygous tumor cells become less sensitive to allogeneic inhibition in F_1 hybrid mice when noiculated together with a large dose of X-irradiated cells of the same tumor, whereas added F_1 hybrid tumor cells do not work. Recent findings by Goodman and Wheeler (1968) can be interpreted similarly. She found that transplanted C57BL bone marrow cells which normally grow less well in F_1 hybrids could grow as well there as in syngeneic mice, if the hybrids were pretreated with large doses of C57BL spleen or thymus cells shortly before the bone marrow was transplanted into them; allogeneic or F' hybrid cells had no such effect. Since previous studies by Goodman and Bosma (1967) had made an immunological explanation of these findings unlikely, it was suggested that the stimulation of the transplants by spleen and thymus cells was due either to a specific interaction between cells with the same surface antigens or to a specific humoral factor which was released from the spleen and thymus cells. The problem is open to experimental analysis, which can be modelled on the studies performed with tumor target cells, lymphocytes immune to their T.STA and serum from the tumor-bearing animals, described in Section VII (Hellström et al., 1969b).

Acknowledgments

The work of the authors described in this article was supported by grants CA 10188 and CA 10189 from National Institutes of Health, U.S. Public Health Service and by grant T 453 from the American Cancer Society. The skillful technical assistance of Mrs. Ingalill Mosonov, Mrs. Kerstin Ragde, and Mrs. Sherrie Wilkie is gratefully acknowledged.

References

Abelev, G. I. 1965. *Progr. Exptl. Tumor Res.* **7**, 104–157.

Al-Askari, S., David, J. R., Lawrence, H. S., and Thomas, L. 1965. *Nat. Acad. Sci.— Natl. Res. Council, Publ.* **1229**, 17.

Alexander, P. 1965. *In* "Scientific Basis of Surgery" (W. T. Irvine, ed.), pp. 487–495. Churchill, London.

Alexander, P. 1967. *Cancer Res.* **27**, 2521–2526.

Alexander, P., 1968. *Prog. Exptl. Tumor Res.* **10**, 23–72.

Alexander, P., and Hamilton-Fairley, G. 1967. *Brit. Med. Bull.* **23**, 86–92.

Alexander, P., Delorme, E. J., and Hall, J. G. 1966. *Lancet* **i**, 1186–1189.

Allison, A. C. 1966. *J. Natl. Cancer Inst.* **36**, 869–876.

Amos, D. B. 1962. *Progr. Allergy* **6**, 468–538.

Attia, M. A. M., and Weiss, D. W. 1966. *Cancer Res.* **26**, 1787–1800.

Attia, M. A. M., DeOme, K. B., and Weiss, D. W. 1965. *Cancer Res.* **25**, 451–457.

Bach, F., and Hirschhorn, K. 1964. *Science* **143**, 813–814.

Bach, F., Hirschhorn, K., Schreibman, R. R., and Ripps, C. 1964. *Ann. N.Y. Acad. Sci.* **120**, 299–302.

Bach, F. H. 1968. *In* "Biological Recognition Processes," 4th Developmental Immunol. Workshop (R. A. Good and R. T. Smith, eds.), in press.

Bach, F. H., and Amos, D. B. 1967. *Science* **156**, 1506–1507.

Bach, F. H., and Voynow, N. K. 1966. *Science* **153**, 545–547.

Bailey, D. W. 1963. *Transplantation* **1**, 70–74.

Bain, B., Vos, M., and Loewenstein, L. 1964. *Blood* **23**, 108–116.

Barrett, M. K., and Deringer, M. K. 1950. *J. Natl. Cancer Inst.* **11**, 51–59.

Barrett, M. K., Deringer, M. K., and Hansen, W. H. 1953. *J. Natl. Cancer Inst.* **14**, 381–394.

Berenbaum, M. C. 1964. *Brit. Med. Bull.* **20**, 159–164.

Berg, J. W. 1959. *Cancer Res.* **12**, 714–720.

Bergheden, C., and Hellström, K. E. 1966. *Intern. J. Cancer* **1**, 361–369.

Berman, L. D. 1967. *J. Exptl. Med.* **125**, 983–999.

Billingham, R. E., Brent, L., and Medawar, P. B. 1954. *Proc. Roy. Soc. (London)* **B143**, 58–80.

Billingham, R. E., Brent, L., and Medawar, P. B. 1956. *Transplant. Bull.* **3**, 84–91.

Billingham, R. E., Silvers, W. K., and Wilson, D. B. 1963. *J. Exptl. Med.* **118,** 397–420.
Black, M. M., and Speer, F. D. 1958. *Surg. Gynecol. Obstet.* **106,** 163–175.
Bloch, K. J. 1965. *Federation Proc.* **24,** 1030–1032.
Bloom, B. B., and Chase, M. W. 1967. *Progr. Allergy* **10,** 151–255.
Bloom, B. R., and Bennett, B. 1966. *Science* **153,** 80–82.
Boyden, S. V. 1963. In "Cell-bound Antibodies" (B. Amos and H. Koprowski, eds.), pp. 7–14. Wistar Inst. Press, Philadelphia, Pennsylvania.
Boyse, E. A. 1959. *Immunology* **2,** 170–181.
Boyse, E. A., Old, L. J., Stockert, E., and Shigeno, N. 1968. *Cancer Res.* **28,** 1280–1287.
Bremberg, S., Klein, E., and Stjernswärd, J. 1967. *Cancer Res.* **27,** 2113.
Brent, L. 1958. *Progr. Allergy* **5,** 271–348.
Brent, L., Brown, J. B., and Medawar, P. B. 1962. *Proc. Roy. Soc. (London)* **B156,** 187–209.
Brondz, B. D. 1964. *Folia Biol. (Prague)* **10,** 164.
Brondz, B. D. 1965. *Transplantation* **3,** 356–367.
Brunner, K. T., Mauel, J., and Schindler, R. 1966. *Immunology* **11,** 499–506.
Brunner, K. T., Mauel, J., Cerottini, J. C., and Chapuis, B. 1968. *Immunology* **14,** 181–196.
Brunschwig, A., Southam, C. M., and Levin, A. G. 1965. *Ann. Surg.* **162,** 416–423.
Bubenik, J., and Koldovsky, P. 1965. *Folia Biol. (Prague)* **11,** 258–265.
Bubenik, J., and Koldovsky, P. 1966. *Folia Biol. (Prague)* **12,** 11–16.
Bubenik, J., Ivany, J., and Koldovsky, P. 1965. *Folia Biol. (Prague)* **11,** 426–433.
Burnet, F. M. 1959. "The Clonal Selection Theory of Acquired Immunity," 208 pp. Vanderbilt Univ. Press, Nashville, Tennessee.
Burnet, F. M. 1961. *Science* **133,** 307–311.
Burnet, F. M. 1964. *Brit. Med. Bull.* **20,** 154–158.
Campbell, D. H. 1963. *Advan. Immunol.* **3,** 261–313.
Chapman, N. D., and Dutton, R. W. 1965. *J. Exptl. Med.* **21,** 85–100.
Chard, J. 1968. *Immunology,* **14,** 583–589.
Chase, M. W. 1953. *In* "The Nature and Significance of the Antibody Response" (A. M. Pappenheimer, Jr., ed.), pp. 156–169. Columbia Univ. Press, New York.
Chase, M. W. 1966. *Cancer Res.* **26,** 1097–1120.
Chu, E., Stjernswärd, J., Clifford, P., and Klein, G. 1967. *J. Natl. Cancer Inst.* **39,** 595–618.
Churchill, W. H., Rapp, H. J., Kronman, B. S., and Borsos, T. 1968. *J. Natl. Cancer Inst.* **41,** 13–29.
Chutna, J., and Rychlikova, M. 1964. *Folia Biol. (Prague)* **10,** 197.
Clifford, P., Stjernswärd, J., Singh, S., and Klein, G. 1967. *Cancer Res.* **27,** 2578–2615.
Coggin, J. H., Jr., and Ambrose, K. R. 1969. *Proc. Soc. Exptl. Biol. Med.* **130** 246–247.
Cooperband, S. R., Bondevik, H., Schmid, K., and Mannick, J. A. 1968. *Science* **159,** 1243–1244.
Cudkowicz, G., and Stimpfling, J. H. 1964a. *Immunology* **7,** 291–306.
Cudkowicz, G., and Stimpfling, J. H. 1964b. *Nature* **204,** 450–453.
Currie, G. A., and Bagshawe, K. D. 1967. *Lancet* **ii,** 708–710.
David, J. R. 1966. *Proc. Natl. Acad. Sci. U.S.* **56,** 72–77.
David, J. R. 1968. *Federation Proc.* **27,** 6–12.
David, J. R., and Paterson, P. Y. 1965. *J. Exptl. Med.* **122,** 1161–1171.
David, J. R., Al-Askari, S., Lawrence, H. S., and Thomas, L. 1964a. *J. Immunol.* **93,** 264–273.
David, J. R., Lawrence, H. S., and Thomas, L. 1964b. *J. Immunol.* **93,** 274–282.

Davidsohn, I., Stern, K., and Sabat, L. 1956. *Proc. Am. Assoc. Cancer Res.* **2**, 102.

Deichman, G. J., and Kluchareva, T. E. 1964. *Virology* **24**, 131–137.

Delorme, E. J., and Alexander, P. 1964. *Lancet* **i**, 117.

Dent, P. B., Peterson, R. D. A., and Good, R. A. 1965. *Proc. Soc. Exptl. Biol. Med.* **119**, 869–871.

Dutton, R. W. 1965. *J. Exptl. Med.* **122**, 759–770.

Dutton, R. W. 1966. *J. Exptl. Med.* **123**, 655–671.

Eddy, B. E., Grubbs, G. E., and Young, R. D. 1964. *Proc. Soc. Exptl. Biol. Med.* **117**, 575–579.

Evans, C. A., and Ito, Y. 1966. *J. Natl. Cancer Inst.* **36**, 1161–1166.

Evans, C. A., Gorman, L. R., Ito, Y., and Weiser, R. S. 1962a. *J. Natl. Cancer Inst.* **29**, 277–285.

Evans, C. A., Weiser, R. S., and Ito, Y. 1962b. *Cold Spring Harbor Symp. Quant. Biol.* **27**, 453–462.

Everson, T. C., and Cole, W. H. 1966. "Spontaneous Regression of Cancer," 560 pp. Saunders, Philadelphia, Pennsylvania.

Fefer, A., McCoy, J. L., and Glynn, J. P. 1967a. *Cancer Res.* **27**, 962–967.

Fefer, A., McCoy, J. L., and Glynn, J. P. 1967b. *Cancer Res.* **27**, 1626–1631.

Fefer, A., McCoy, J. L., Perk, K., and Glynn, J. P. 1968. *Cancer Res.* **28**, 1577.

Fenyö, E. M., Klein, E., Klein, G., and Swiech, K. 1968. *J. Natl. Cancer Inst.* **40**, 69–90.

Fialkow, P. J. 1967. *Science* **155**, 1676–1677.

Fialkow, P. J., and Gartler, S. M. 1966. *Nature* **211**, 713.

Fialkow, P. J., Hellström, I., and Hellström, K. E. 1968. *Exptl. Cell Res.* **49**, 223–225.

Fishman, M., and Adler, F. L. 1963. *J. Exptl. Med.* **117**, 595–602.

Foley, E. J. 1953. *Cancer Res.* **13**, 835–837.

George, M., and Vaughan, J. H. 1962. *Proc. Soc. Exptl. Biol. Med.* **111**, 514–521.

Ginsburg, H. 1968. *Immunology* **14**, 621–636.

Girardi, A. J. 1965. *Proc. Natl. Acad. Sci. U.S.* **54**, 445–451.

Gold, P., and Freedman, S. O. 1965a. *J. Exptl. Med.* **121**, 439–462.

Gold, P., and Freedman, S. O. 1965b. *J. Exptl. Med.* **122**, 467–481.

Gold, P., Gold, M., and Freedman, S. O. 1968. *Cancer Res.* **28**, 1331–1334.

Goldner, H., Girardi, A. J., Larson, V. M., and Hilleman, M. R. 1964. *Proc. Soc. Exptl. Biol. Med.* **117**, 851–857.

Good, R. A. 1967. *In* "Immunopathology Fifth International Symposium" (P. A. Miescher and P. Grabar, eds.), 416–417.

Goodman, J. W., and Wheeler, H. B. 1968. *Transplantation* **6**, 173–186.

Goodman, J. W., and Bosma, G. C. 1967. *Immunology* **13**, 125–140.

Gorer, P. A. 1956. *Advan. Cancer Res.* **4**, 149–186.

Gorer, P. A. 1962. *Advan. Immunol.* **1**, 345.

Gorer, P. A., and O'Gorman, P. 1956. *Transplant. Bull.* **3**, 142–143.

Govaerts, A. 1961. *J. Immunol.* **85**, 516–522.

Gowans, J. L., and McGregor, D. D. 1965. *Progr. Allergy* **9**, 1–78.

Granger, G. A., and Kolb, W. P. 1968. *J. Immunol.* **101**, 111–120.

Granger, G. A., and Weiser, R. S. 1964. *Science* **145**, 1427–1429.

Gross, J. D. 1963. *Genet. Res.* **4**, 463–469.

Gross, L. 1943. *Cancer Res.* **3**, 326–333.

Habel, K. 1961. *Proc. Soc. Exptl. Biol. Med.* **106**, 722–725.

Habel, K. 1962. *J. Exptl. Med.* **115**, 181–193.

Habel, K. 1965. *Virology* **25**, 55–61.

Haddow, A. 1965. *Brit. Med. Bull.* **21**, 133–139.

Haddow, A., and Alexander, P. 1964. *Lancet* **i**, 452–455.

Hare, J. D. 1967. *Virology* **31**, 625–632.

Haughton, G. 1965. *Science* **147**, 506–507.

Hellström, I. 1965. *Nature* **208**, 652–653.

Hellström, I. 1967. *Intern. J. Cancer* **2**, 65–69.

Hellström, I., and Hellström, K. E. 1966. *Ann. N.Y. Acad. Sci.* **129**, 724–734.

Hellström, I., and Hellström, K. E. 1967. *Science* **156**, 981–983.

Hellström, I., and Sjögren, H. O. 1965. *Exptl. Cell Res.* **40**, 212–215.

Hellström, I., and Sjögren, H. O. 1967. *J. Exptl. Med.* **125**, 1105–1118.

Hellström, I., Hellström, K. E., and Pierce, G. 1968a. *Intern. J. Cancer* **3**, 467–483.

Hellström, I., Hellström, K. E., and Pierce, G. E. 1968b. *Proc. 8th Can. Cancer Conf.* in press.

Hellström, I., Hellström, K. E., Pierce, G. E., and Bill, A. H. 1968c. *Proc. Natl. Acad. Sci. U.S.* **60**, 1231–1238.

Hellström, I., Hellström, K. E., Pierce, G. E., and Yang, J. P. S. 1968d. *Nature* **220**, 1352–1354.

Hellström, I., Hellström, K. E., Pierce, G. E., and Fefer, A. 1969a. *Proc. Transpl. Soc.*, **1**, 90–94.

Hellström, I., Hellström, K. E., Evans, C. A., Heppner, G. H., Pierce, G. E., and Yang, J. P. S. 1969b. *Proc. Acad. Sci. U.S.* **62**, 362.

Hellström, K. E. 1963. *Nature* **199**, 614–615.

Hellström, K. E. 1966a. *Intern. J. Cancer* **1**, 349–359.

Hellström, K. E. 1966b. *Exptl. Cell Res.* **42**, 189–192.

Hellström, K. E., and Hellström, I. 1965. *In* "Isoantigens and Cell Interactions" (J. Palm, ed.), pp. 79–90. Wistar Inst. Press, Philadelphia, Pennsylvania.

Hellström, K. E., and Hellström, I. 1967a. *In* "Endogeneous Factors Influencing Host-tumor Balance" (R. W. Wissler, T. L. Dao, and S. Wood, Jr., eds.), pp. 177–183. Univ. of Chicago Press, Chicago, Illinois.

Hellström, K. E., and Hellström, I. 1967b. *Progr. Exptl. Tumor Res.* **9**, 40–76.

Hellström, K. E., and Hellström, I. 1968. *Federation Proc.* **27**, 39–41.

Hellström, K. E., and Möller, G. 1965. *Progr. Allergy* **9**, 158–245.

Hellström, K. E., Hellström, I., and Sjögren, H. O. 1963. *J. Natl. Cancer Inst.* **31**, 1239–1253.

Hellström, K. E., Hellström, I., and Haughton, G. 1964. *Nature* **204**, 661–664.

Hellström, K. E., Hellström, I., and Bergheden, C. 1965. *Nature* **208**, 458–460.

Hellström, K. E., Hellström, I., and Bergheden, C. 1967. *Intern. J. Cancer* **2**, 286–296.

Hellström, K. E., Hellström, I., and Motet, D. 1968. *In* "Biological Recognition Processes," 4th Developmental Immunol. Workshop (R. A. Good and R. T. Smith, eds.), in press.

Helm, F., and Klein, E. 1965. *Arch. Dermatol.* **91**, 142–144.

Heppner, G. H., and Pierce, G. E. 1969. *Intern. J. Cancer* **4**, 212–218.

Hirschhorn, K., Bach, F., Kolodny, R. L., Firschein, I. L., and Hasham, N. 1963. *Science* **142**, 1185–1187.

Holm, G., and Perlmann, P. 1965. *Nature* **207**, 818–821.

Holm, G., and Perlmann, P. 1967. *J. Exptl. Med.* **125**, 721–736.

Holm, G., Werner, B., and Perlmann, P. 1964. *Nature* **203**, 841–843.

Holmgren, N. B., and Merchant, D. J. 1968. *J. Natl. Cancer Inst.* **40**, 561–568.

Huebner, R. J., Rowe, W. P., Turner, H. C., and Lane, W. T. 1963. *Proc. Natl. Acad. Sci. U.S.* **50**, 379–389.

Huemer, R. F. 1965. *Nature* **205**, 48–50.

Jerne, K., Nuroin, A. A., and Henry, C. 1963. *In* "Cell-bound Antibodies" (B. Amos and H. Koprowski, eds.), pp. 109–116. Wistar Inst. Press, Philadelphia, Pennsylvania.

Kaliss, N. 1958. *Cancer Res.* **18**, 992–1003.

Kaliss, N. 1962. *Ann. N.Y. Acad. Sci.* **101**, 64–79.

Karush, F., and Eisen, H. N. 1962. *Science* **136**, 1032–1039.

Klein, E. 1967. *Federation Proc.* **26**, 430.

Klein, E. 1968. *Geriatrics* **23**, 154–175.

Klein, E., and Klein, G. 1964. *J. Natl. Cancer Inst.* **32**, 547–568.

Klein, E., and Klein, G. 1965. *Cancer Res.* **25**, 851–854.

Klein, E., and Möller, E. 1963. *J. Natl. Cancer Inst.* **31**, 347–364.

Klein, E., and Sjögren, H. O. 1960. *Cancer Res.* **20**, 452–461.

Klein, G. 1959. *Cancer Res.* **19**, 343–358.

Klein, G. 1966. *Ann. Rev. Microbiol.* **20**, 223–252.

Klein, G., and Klein, E. 1956. *Nature* **178**, 1389.

Klein, G., and Klein, E. 1958. *J. Cellular Comp. Physiol.* **52**, Suppl. 1, 125–168.

Klein, G., and Klein, E. 1962. *Cold Spring Harbor Symp. Quant. Biol.* **27**, 463–470.

Klein, G., Sjögren, H. O., Klein, E., and Hellström, K. E. 1960. *Cancer Res.* **20**, 1561–1572.

Klein, G., Sjögren, H. O., and Klein, E. 1963. *Cancer Res.* **23**, 84–92.

Klein, G., Klein, E., and Haughton, G. 1966a. *J. Natl. Cancer Inst.* **36**, 607–621.

Klein, G., Clifford, P., Klein, E., and Stjernswärd, J. 1966b. *Proc. Natl. Acad. Sci. U.S.* **55**, 1628–1635.

Klein, G., Klein, E., and Clifford, P. 1967a. *Cancer Res.* **27**, 2510–2520.

Klein, G., Clifford, P., Klein, E., Smith, R. T., Minowada, J., Kourilsky, F. M., and Burchenal, J. H. 1967b. *J. Natl. Cancer Inst.* **39**, 1027–1044.

Kolb, W. P., and Granger, G. A. 1968. *Proc. Natl. Acad. Sci.* **61**, 1250–1255.

Koldovsky, P. 1961. *Folia Biol. (Prague)* **7**, 115–121.

Koprowski, H., and Fernandes, M. V. 1962. *J. Exptl. Med.* **116**, 467–476.

Krüger, G. 1967. *J. Natl. Cancer Inst.* **39**, 1–15.

Law, L. W., Ting, R. C., and Leckband, E. 1967. *Proc. Natl. Acad. Sci. U.S.* **57**, 1068–1075.

Lawrence, H. S. 1960. *Ann. Rev. Med.* **11**, 207–230.

Linder, O. E. A. 1962. *Cancer Res.* **22**, 380–383.

McIvor, K. L., Heise, E. R., and Weiser, R. S. 1969. *In* "Biological Recognition Processes" (R. A. Good and R. T. Smith, eds.). 4th Developmental Immunology Workshop, (in press).

Malmgren, R. A., Bennison, B. E., and McKinley, J. W. 1952. *Proc. Soc. Exptl. Biol. Med.* **79**, 484–488.

Martinez, C., Shapiro, F., and Good, R. A. (1959). *Proc. Soc. Exptl. Biol. Med.* **101**, 658–660.

Mathé, G., Schwarzenberg, L., Amiel, J. L., Schneider, M., Cattan, A., and Schlumberger, J. R. 1967. *Cancer Res.* **27**, 2542–2553.

Medawar, P. B. 1958. *Harvey Lectures Ser.* **52**, 144–176.

Mikulska, Z. B., Smith, C., and Alexander, P. 1966. *J. Natl. Cancer Inst.* **36**, 29–35.

Miller, D. G. 1967. *Cancer* **20**, 579–588.

Miller, J. F. A. P., Marshall, A. H. E., and White, R. G. 1962. *Advan. Immunol.* **2**, 111–162.

Ming, S. C., Klein, E., and Klein, G. 1967. *Nature* **215**, 1390–1392.

Mintz, B., and Silvers, W. K. 1967. *Science* **158**, 1484–1486.

Mitchison, N. A. 1954. *Proc. Roy. Soc. (London)* **B142**, 72–87.

Mitchison, N. A. 1955. *J. Exptl. Med.* **102**, 157–177.
Mitchison, N. A., and Dube, O. L. 1955. *J. Exptl. Med.* **102**, 179–197.
Möller, E. 1965a. *Science* **147**, 873–879.
Möller, E. 1965b. *J. Exptl. Med.* **122**, 11–23.
Möller, E. 1967. *J. Exptl. Med.* **126**, 395–405.
Möller, E., and Möller, G. 1962. *J. Exptl. Med.* **115**, 527–553.
Möller, E., and Möller, G. 1967. *Cancer* **20**, 871–879.
Möller, E., Lapp, W., and Lindholm, L. 1969. *Proc. Transplant Soc.* **1**, 543–547.
Möller, G. 1961. *J. Exptl. Med.* **114**, 415–434.
Möller, G. 1963a. *J. Natl. Cancer Inst.* **30**, 1153–1175.
Möller, G. 1963b. *J. Natl. Cancer Inst.* **30**, 1177–1203.
Möller, G. 1963c. *J. Natl. Cancer Inst.* **30**, 1205–1226.
Möller, G. 1964. *Nature* **204**, 846–847.
Möller, G., and Möller, E. 1965. *Nature* **208**, 260–263.
Morton, D. L. 1962. *Proc. Am. Assoc. Cancer Res.* **3**, 346.
Morton, D. L., and Malmgren, R. A. 1968. *Science* **162**, 1279–1281.
Morton, D. L., Goldman, L., and Wood, D. A. 1965. *Proc. Am. Assoc. Cancer Res.* **6**, 47.
Morton, D. L., Malmgren, R. A., Holmes, E. C., and Ketcham, A. S. 1968. *Surgery* **64**, 233–240.
Mowbray, J. F. 1963. *Federation Proc.* **22**, 441.
Mowbray, J. F. 1967. *J. Clin. Pathol.* **20**, Suppl., 499–503.
Nadler, S. H., and Moore, G. E. 1966. *Ann. Surg.* **164**, 482–490.
Najarian, J. S., and Feldman, J. D. 1962. *J. Exptl. Med.* **115**, 1083–1093.
Nomura, M. 1967. *Ann. Rev. Microbiol.* **21**, 257–284.
Nota, N. R., Liacopoulos-Briot, M., Stiffel, C., and Biozzi, G. 1964. *Compt. Rend.* **259**, 1277–1280.
Old, L. J., and Boyse, E. A. 1964. *Ann. Rev. Med.* **15**, 167–186.
Old, L. J., Benacerraf, H., Clarke, D. A., Carswell, E. A., and Stockert, E. 1961. *Cancer Res.* **21**, 1281–1301.
Old, L. J., Boyse, E. A., Clarke, D. A., and Carswell, E. A. 1962. *Ann. N.Y. Acad. Sci.* **101**, 80–106.
Old, L. J., Boyse, E. A., Bennett, B., and Lilly, F. 1963. *In* "Cell-bound Antibodies" (B. Amos and H. Koprowski, eds.), pp. 89–99. Wistar Inst. Press, Philadelphia, Pennsylvania.
Old, L. J., Boyse, E. A., Geering, G., and Oettgen, H. F. 1968a. *Cancer Res.* **28**, 1288–1299.
Old, L. J., Stockert, E., Boyse, E. A., and Kim, J. H. 1968b. *J. Exptl. Med.* **127**, 523–539.
Oth, D., Robert, J., Michaud, C., and Crestin, M. 1964. *Compt. Rend. Soc. Biol.* **158**, 841.
Parfentjev, I. A., and Duran-Reynals, F. 1951. *Science* **113**, 690–691.
Pearmain, G., Lycette, R. R., and Fitzgerald, P. H. 1963. *Lancet* **i**, 637–638.
Pearsall, N., and Weiser, R. S. 1968. *RES, J. Reticuloendothelial Soc.* **5**, 121–133.
Pearsall, N., and Weiser, R. S. 1969. To be published.
Penn, I., Hammond, W., Brettschneider, L., and Starzl, T. E. 1969. *Proc. Transplant Soc.* **1**, 106–112.
Pope, J. H., and Rowe, W. P. 1964. *J. Exptl. Med.* **120**, 121–128.
Potworowski, E. F., and Nairn, R. C. 1968. *Immunology* **14**, 591–597.
Prehn, R. T. 1962. *M. D. Anderson Hosp. Symp. Fundamental Cancer Res.* 475–486.
Prehn, R. T. 1963a. *Can. Cancer Conf.* **5**, 387–395.
Prehn, R. T. 1963b. *J. Natl. Cancer Inst.* **31**, 791–805.
Prehn, R. T., and Main, J. M. 1957. *J. Natl. Cancer Inst.* **18**, 769–778.

Révész, L. 1960. *Cancer Res.* **20**, 443–451.
Rose, N. R., Kite, J. H., Doebbler, T. K., and Brown, R. G. 1963. *In* "Cell-bound Antibodies" (B. Amos and H. Koprowski, eds.), pp. 19–34. Wistar Inst. Press, Philadelphia, Pennsylvania.
Rosenau, W. 1963. *In* "Cell-bound Antibodies" (B. Amos and H. Koprowski, eds.), pp. 75–83. Wistar Inst. Press, Philadelphia, Pennsylvania.
Rosenau, W. 1968. *Federation Proc.* **27**, 33–38.
Rosenau, W., and Horwitz, C. 1968. *Lab. Invest.* **18**, 298–303.
Rosenau, W., and Moon, H. D. 1961. *J. Natl. Cancer Inst.* **27**, 471–478.
Rosenau, W., and Moon, H. D. 1964. *J. Immunol.* **93**, 910–914.
Rosenau, W., and Moon, H. D. 1966a. *Lab. Invest.* **15**, 1212–1224.
Rosenau, W., and Moon, H. D. 1966b. *J. Immunol.* **96**, 80.
Rosenau, W., and Moon, H. D. 1967. *Cancer Res.* **27**, 1973–1981.
Rosenau, W., and Morton, D. 1966. *J. Natl. Cancer Inst.* **36**, 825–835.
Rubin, B. A. 1964. *Progr. Exptl. Tumor Res.* **5**, 217–292.
Rubin, H. 1962. *Cold Spring Harbor Symp. Quant. Biol.* **27**, 441–452.
Ruddle, N. H., and Waksman, B. H. 1967. *Science* **157**, 1060–1063.
Ruddle, N. H., and Waksman, P. H. 1969a. *J. Exptl. Med.* **128**, 1237–1254.
Ruddle, N. H., and Waksman, B. H. 1969b. *J. Exptl. Med.* **128**, 1267–1280.
Salaman, M. H., and Wedderburn, N. 1966. *Immunology* **10**, 445–458.
Sanderson, A. F. 1964. *Nature* **204**, 250.
Sanford, B. H. 1967. *Transplantation* **5**, 1273–1279.
Schwarz, R. 1968. *J. Exptl. Med.* **128**, 879–889.
Scothorne, R. J. 1957. *Ann. N.Y. Acad. Sci.* **64**, 1028–1039.
Sjögren, H. O. 1961. *Virology* **15**, 214–219.
Sjögren, H. O. 1964a. *J. Natl. Cancer Inst.* **32**, 375–393.
Sjögren, H. O. 1964b. *J. Natl. Cancer Inst.* **32**, 645–659.
Sjögren, H. O. 1964c. *J. Natl. Cancer Inst.* **32**, 661–666.
Sjögren, H. O. 1965. *Progr. Exptl. Tumor Res.* **6**, 289–322.
Sjögren, H. O., and Ankerst, J. 1969. *Nature* **221**, 863–864.
Sjögren, H. O., Hellström, I., and Klein, G. 1961a. *Exptl. Cell Res.* **23**, 204–208.
Sjögren, H. O., Hellström, I., and Klein, G. 1961b. *Cancer Res.* **21**, 329–337.
Slettenmark, B., and Klein, E. 1962. *Cancer Res.* **22**, 947–954.
Smith, R. T. 1968. *New Engl. J. Med.* **278**, 1207–1214, 1268–1275, 1326–1331.
Snell, G. D. 1953. *J. Natl. Cancer Inst.* **14**, 691–700.
Snell, G. D. 1955. *Transplant. Bull.* **2**, 6–8.
Snell, G. D. 1957. *Ann. Rev. Microbiol.* **11**, 439–458.
Snell, G. D. 1958. *J. Natl. Cancer Inst.* **21**, 843–877.
Snell, G. D., and Stevens, L. C. 1961. *Immunology* **4**, 366–379.
Snell, G. D., Winn, H. J., Stimpfling, J. H., and Parker, S. J. 1960. *J. Exptl. Med.* **112**, 293–314.
Southam, C. M. 1960. *Cancer Res.* **20**, 271–291.
Southam, C. M. 1967. *Progr. Exptl. Tumor Res.* **9**, 1–39.
Southam, C. M., Moore, G. E., and Rhoads, C. P. 1957. *Science* **125**, 158–160.
Southam, C. M., Brunschwig, A., Levin, A. G., and Dizon, Q. 1964. *Proc. Am. Assoc. Cancer Res.* **5**, 60.
Southam, C. M., Brunschwig, A., Levin, A. G., and Dizon, Q. 1966. *Cancer* **19**, 1743–1753.
Stjernswärd, J. 1965. *J. Natl. Cancer Inst.* **35**, 885–892.
Stjernswärd, J. 1966. *J. Natl. Cancer Inst.* **37**, 505–512.
Stjernswärd, J. 1967. *J. Natl. Cancer Inst.* **38**, 515–526.

Stjernswärd, J. 1968. *J. Natl. Cancer Inst.* **40**, 13–22.
Stjernswärd, J., Clifford, P., Singh, S., and Svedmyr, E. 1968. *E. African Med. J.* **45**, 70–83.
Stoner, R. D., and Hale, W. M. 1962. *In* "The Effects of Ionizing Radiations of Immune Processes" (C. A. Gordon, ed.), pp. 183–219. Breach Sci. Publ. Co., New York.
Storb, U., and Weiser, R. S. 1968. *RES, J. Reticuloendothelial Soc.* **5**, 81–106.
Tevethia, S. S., Katz, M., and Rapp, F. 1965. *Proc. Soc. Exptl. Biol. Med.* **119**, 896–901.
Ting, R. C., and Law, L. W. 1967. *Progr. Exptl. Tumor Res.* **9**, 165–191.
Tsoi, M. S., and Weiser, R. S. 1968a. *J. Natl. Cancer Inst.* **40**, 23–30.
Tsoi, M. S., and Weiser, R. S. 1968b. *J. Natl. Cancer Inst.* **40**, 37–42.
Vaage, J. 1968. *Cancer Res.* **28**, 2477–2483.
Vaage, J. 1968. Ph.D. Thesis, Univ. of California, Berkeley, California.
Vainio, T., Koskinies, D., Perlmann, P., Perlmann, H., and Klein, G. 1964. *Nature* **204**, 453–455.
Weaver, J. M., Algire, G. H., and Prehn, R. T. 1955. *J. Natl. Cancer Inst.* **15**, 1737–1758.
Weiss, D. W., Bonhag, R. S., and DeOme, K. B. 1961. *Nature* **190**, 889–891.
Weiss, D. W., Faulkin, L. J., and DeOme, K. B. 1964. *Cancer Res.* **24**, 732–741.
Weiss, D. W., Bonhag, R. S., and Leslie, P. 1966. *J. Exptl. Med.* **124**, 1039–1065.
Wigzell, H. 1965. *Transplantation* **3**, 423–431.
Wigzell, H., and Linder, O. E. A. 1961. *Transplant. Bull.* **28**, 490–492.
Wilson, D. B. 1963. *J. Cellular Comp. Physiol.* **62**, 273–286.
Wilson, D. B. 1965a. *J. Exptl. Med.* **122**, 143–166.
Wilson, D. B. 1965b. *J. Exptl. Med.* **122**, 167–172.
Wilson, D. B., and Billingham, R. E. 1967. *Advan. Immunol.* **6**, 189–275.
Wilson, D. B., Silvers, W. K., and Nowell, P. C. 1967. *J. Exptl. Med.* **126**, 655.
Winn, H. J. 1959. *Natl. Cancer Inst. Monograph* **2**, 113–138.
Winn, H. J. 1960. *J. Immunol.* **84**, 530–538.
Winn, H. J. 1962. *Ann. N.Y. Acad. Sci.* **101**, 23–45.
Woodruff, M. F. A. 1967. *Ciba Found. Study Group* **29**, 108.
Woodruff, M. F. A., and Nolan, B. 1963. *Lancet* **ii**, 426–429.
Woodruff, M. F. A., and Symes, M. O. 1962. *Brit. J. Cancer* **6**, 707–715.
Yoshida, T. 1965. *Japan J. Exptl. Med.* **35**, 115–124.
Yoshida, T. O., and Southam, C. M. 1963. *Japan J. Exptl. Med.* **33**, 369–383.

PERSPECTIVES IN THE EPIDEMIOLOGY OF LEUKEMIA*

Irving I. Kessler and Abraham M. Lilienfeld

Department of Chronic Diseases, Johns Hopkins University School of Hygiene
and Public Health, Baltimore, Maryland

I. Introduction

During the past few years there has been increasing interest in the epidemiological aspects of leukemia. Encouraged by the possibility that leukemia may be a form of cancer that is etiologically related to viruses, efforts are being made to evaluate the consistency of epidemiological data with a viral hypothesis, in addition to the experimental quest for a leukemia virus. A chromosomal hypothesis has also been postulated as an outgrowth of the analysis of clinical and epidemiological data. These new concepts have been used to integrate a body of knowledge implicating several environmental agents in the etiology of leukemia. A general feeling

* Work done, as reported in this review, was aided in part by Training Grant No. CA-5165 from the National Cancer Institute and by Research Career Award No. K6-GM 13901 from the National Institute of General Medical Sciences.

also prevails that leukemia in man may very well be the next form of cancer for which the etiology will be elucidated. Consequently, it seems particularly appropriate at this point in time to review the epidemiological aspects of leukemia in the light of these current developments.

II. Mortality Statistics

The infrequency of leukemia makes it extremely difficult to obtain morbidity data for a sufficiently large population, and, therefore, it is necessary to rely upon the available routinely collected mortality statistics. In considering such data, one must bear in mind the variety of diagnostic methods used as well as the incomplete ascertainment of cases upon which these statistics are often based. For leukemia there was an additional limitation since data did not permit, until recently, adequately detailed distributions of leukemia mortality by histological type. Nevertheless, much has already been learned from the existing statistics on the frequency and distribution of leukemia.

A. INTERNATIONAL

Segi and Kurihara (1966) have tabulated the age-adjusted leukemia and aleukemia death rates for 24 countries in 1962–1963. These rates are

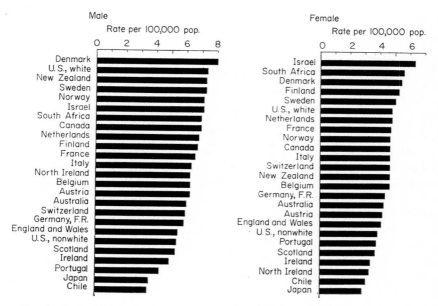

FIG. 1. Age-adjusted death rates from leukemia and aleukemia by country and sex, 1962–1963. (From Segi and Kurihara, 1966.)

highest in the Scandinavian countries, Israel, South Africa, and among U.S. whites and are lowest in Japan and Chile (Fig. 1). The highest death rates, for each sex, are about 2.3 × higher than the lowest rates (Table I). The range of variation in rates between the 24 different countries is narrower than for any other neoplasm examined by Segi and Kurihara (1966) (Table I), a fact which may be of some relevance in the quest for environmental leukemogens. In all of these countries the male death rates exceeded female rates. This is not surprising since sex ratios are high for most neoplasms, those of the thyroid, large intestine, and biliary tract being the major exceptions. However, leukemia sex ratios exhibit less variation in magnitude (between largest and smallest) than most other neoplasms (Table I). From this observation one might conclude that males irrespective of country are subject to a small but consistent enhancement in leukemia risk as compared to females. This conclusion gains support by the fact that, with the two exceptions, Northern Ireland and New Zealand, the countries with high male leukemia death rates also have high female rates and vice versa.

Variations in the reported mortality from the different countries for any given disease may reflect constitutional differences in susceptibility, environmental differences in carcinogenic exposure, or artifactual differences in reporting. One method for assessing the relative influence of each one of these factors on leukemia death rates is to compare the rates among natives of a particular country with the rates of those who have emigrated to another country. One thus attempts to estimate the effect of a change in environment while holding the genetic constitution constant.

Age-adjusted leukemia death rates were computed for a number of U.S. immigrant groups as well as for residents of the respective countries of origin in 1960 (Tables II and III). With only two exceptions (Swedish and Norwegian females), leukemia mortality in the countries of origin were below that of U.S. whites. The immigrant groups tended to approximate the mortality experience of the white population of the United States. For persons age 65 and over, the concordance of mortality rates between immigrants and total U.S. whites was especially remarkable. This suggests that for the elderly, at least, the environment plays a dominant role in leukemogenesis or, at least, in the reported mortality from leukemia. It should be noted, however, that the foreign born represented in these results comprise only about 73% of the total U.S. foreign born population. When the total foreign born group is considered, the age-adjusted leukemia death rates for male and female immigrants slightly exceed those for U.S. whites (Tables II and III), a finding that is consistent with other studies of the ethnic distribution of leukemia in the United States (Haenszel and Chiazze, 1965; Newill, 1961).

TABLE I

RANGE AND RATIO OF HIGHEST TO LOWEST AGE-ADJUSTED CANCER DEATH RATES AND SEX RATIOS, BY SEX AND PRIMARY SITE FOR SELECTED COUNTRIES,[a] 1962–1963

Primary sites	Males			Females			Sex ratio for selected countries		
	Highest (1)	Lowest (2)	Ratio (3) = (1/2)	Highest (4)	Lowest (5)	Ratio (6) = (4/5)	Highest (7)	Lowest (8)	Ratio (9) = (7/8)
All sites	199.4	108.2	1.84	140.3	82.8	1.69	177	94	1.88
Buccal cavity and pharynx	8.53	1.35	6.32	2.17	0.61	3.56	1160	131	8.85
Esophagus	13.04	2.54	5.13	5.01	0.63	7.95	1186	132	8.98
Stomach	67.96	9.78	6.95	41.04	5.10	8.05	231	149	1.55
Intestine except rectum	16.47	2.73	6.03	15.77	2.96	5.33	121	78	1.55
Rectum	11.48	2.05	5.60	6.10	2.43	2.51	201	84	2.39
Liver and biliary passages	14.88	2.36	6.31	13.49	2.66	5.07	161	39	4.13
Pancreas	8.78	3.33	2.64	5.76	2.11	2.73	210	128	1.64
Larynx	9.91	0.59	16.80	0.86	0.02	43.00	3376	196	17.22
Lung, bronchus, and trachea	71.57	9.70	7.38	9.38	2.44	3.84	1537	280	5.49
Breast (female)	—	—	—	24.38	3.76	6.48	—	—	—
Uterus (all parts)	—	—	—	23.96	6.55	3.66	—	—	—
Ovary, Fallopian tube, and broad ligament	—	—	—	11.02	1.69	6.52	—	—	—

Prostate	21.86	1.65	13.25	—	—	—	—	—	—
Bladder and other urinary organs	7.47	2.19	3.41	2.54	0.99	2.57	451	162	2.78
Skin	4.95	0.87	5.69	2.71	0.53	5.11	293	106	2.76
Thyroid gland	1.23	0.14	8.79	1.44	0.47	3.06	85	13	6.54
Leukemia and aleukemia	8.00	3.44	2.33	6.32	2.76	2.29	191	112	1.71
Leukemia and aleukemia (ages)									
<15	5.17	2.47	2.09	4.68	1.02	4.59	412	97	4.25
15–54	4.10	2.78	1.47	4.19	2.05	2.04	162	87	1.86
55 and over	29.62	4.96	5.97	22.53	3.33	6.77	211	122	1.73

a From data of Segi and Kurihara (1966).

TABLE II

AGE-ADJUSTED LEUKEMIA DEATH RATES PER 100,000 MALES, FOR
SELECTED COUNTRIES OF ORIGIN AND UNITED STATES, 1959–1961[a]

Country of origin	Age group	Residents of country	Immigrants to U.S.A.[d]	Total U.S. whites[d]
Sweden	All ages	6.9[b]	5.4	7.7
	65 and over	35.1[b]	49.4	43.8
Norway	All ages	6.7[b]	5.1	7.7
	65 and over	36.5[b]	41.3	43.8
Canada	All ages	6.3[b]	10.0	7.7
	65 and over	34.0[b]	44.6	43.8
Finland	All ages	6.2[b]	3.8	7.7
	65 and over	28.6[b]	43.2	43.8
Austria	All ages	6.2[b]	13.3	7.7
	65 and over	23.9[b]	60.0	43.8
Ireland	All ages	6.1[b]	6.8	7.7
	65 and over	14.6[b]	61.4	43.8
Germany	All ages	5.9[b]	8.0	7.7
	65 and over	26.2[b]	42.9	43.8
Czechoslovakia	All ages	5.8[c]	6.8	7.7
	65 and over	24.7[c]	42.6	43.8
Italy	All ages	5.8[b]	8.5	7.7
	65 and over	18.9[b]	46.7	43.8
United Kingdom	All ages	5.6[b]	6.7	7.7
	65 and over	25.7[b]	25.5	43.8
Hungary	All ages	5.5[c]	10.2	7.7
	65 and over	19.3[c]	48.7	43.8
Poland	All ages	4.0[c]	14.5	7.7
	65 and over	8.6[c]	46.2	43.8
Yugoslavia	All ages	3.7[c]	7.4	7.7
	65 and over	9.0[c]	42.3	43.8
Mexico	All ages	1.6[c]	5.9	7.7
	65 and over	5.8[c]	16.4	43.8
Total foreign born	All ages	—	8.7	7.7
	65 and over	—	44.3	43.8

[a] Rates adjusted to total U.S. population, 1940 (U.S. Bureau of Census, 1943).

[b] Segi and Kurihara (1966); data for 1960.

[c] World Health Organization (1963); data for 1960.

[d] Kessler (1968); data for 1959–1961.

The apparent effect of emigration was unusual in several of the nativity groups studied. Leukemia mortality in male migrants from the United Kingdom age 65 and over failed to show any rise in the direction of the higher U.S. white rate. Since a rate increase was experienced by the younger migrant groups from the United Kingdom, one in this instance may be dealing with a cohort effect of some kind. The older migrants may have

TABLE III

AGE-ADJUSTED LEUKEMIA DEATH RATES PER 100,000 FEMALES, FOR
SELECTED COUNTRIES OF ORIGIN AND UNITED STATES, 1959–1961[a]

Country of origin	Age group	Residents of country	Immigrants to U.S.A.[d]	Total U.S. whites[d]
Sweden	All ages	5.5[b]	10.0	5.0
	65 and over	26.0[b]	25.1	25.3
Norway	All ages	5.3[b]	3.5	5.0
	65 and over	24.7[b]	25.6	25.3
Canada	All ages	4.7[b]	5.9	5.0
	65 and over	22.1[b]	24.5	25.3
Finland	All ages	4.7[b]	2.6	5.0
	65 and over	15.9[b]	20.7	25.3
Germany	All ages	4.6[b]	4.1	5.0
	65 and over	19.3[b]	25.5	25.3
Hungary	All ages	4.1[c]	4.6	5.0
	65 and over	10.8[c]	22.2	25.3
Italy	All ages	4.1[b]	4.3	5.0
	65 and over	10.3[b]	27.1	25.3
Austria	All ages	4.0[b]	8.9	5.0
	65 and over	16.6[b]	36.0	25.3
Czechoslovakia	All ages	3.9[c]	4.3	5.0
	65 and over	13.8[c]	33.3	25.3
United Kingdom	All ages	3.8[b]	4.3	5.0
	65 and over	15.8[b]	18.7	25.3
Ireland	All ages	3.4[b]	4.7	5.0
	65 and over	12.9[b]	35.5	25.3
Poland	All ages	3.0[c]	5.3	5.0
	65 and over	5.6[c]	29.8	25.3
Yugoslavia	All ages	2.7[c]	4.9	5.0
	65 and over	4.5[c]	27.1	25.3
Mexico	All ages	1.4[c]	3.8	5.0
	65 and over	3.1[c]	11.1	25.3
Total foreign born	All ages	—	5.5	5.0
	65 and over	—	26.8	25.3

[a] Rates adjusted to total U.S. population, 1940 (U.S. Bureau of Census, 1943).
[b] Segi and Kurihara (1966); data for 1960.
[c] World Health Organization (1963); data for 1960.
[d] Kessler (1968); data for 1959–1961.

undergone less exposure to environmental leukemogens before their emigrating many years earlier, or, perhaps they emigrated at a relatively old age and were, therefore, less exposed to leukemogens in the U.S. or exposed at an age of reduced susceptibility to leukemia initiation. These explanations are not completely satisfying since the elderly female migrants from the United Kingdom did undergo an increase in leukemia mortality.

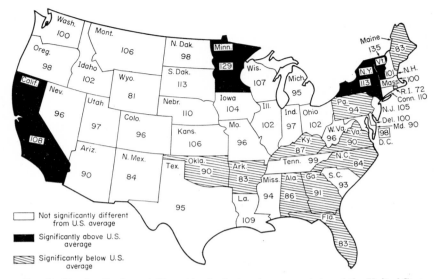

Fig. 2. Standardized mortality ratios for leukemia among states of the United States, 1949–1951 (significance where shown is at level of $p = 0.05$ or less). (From Walter and Gilliam, 1956.)

Immigrants of both sexes from Norway and Finland, Swedish males, and German females underwent reductions in leukemia mortality below the levels of their countries of origin. Without exception, however, mortality among those 65 and over rose to approximate that in the total U.S. white group. The selective emigration of young, disease-free persons from these countries would help to explain these findings, although it leaves unanswered the question of why such a phenomenon should be limited to migrants from these particular countries.

In several nativity groups, leukemia mortality among immigrants exceeded that of both the country of origin and the United States. This was especially noteworthy for the Austrians whose migrant leukemia rates among both the elderly as well as among persons of all ages were clearly elevated. Mortality among Canadian migrants of both sexes (excepting those 65 and over) was also maximal as was true for male Hungarians, Poles, and Italians and female Swedes. No immediate explanation for these findings is apparent. A selective migration of leukemia-prone individuals to the United States is one possibility although it is difficult to see how such a selective process would come about. It would no doubt be helpful to learn the mean duration of residence or the mean age at migration for each of the migrant groups. Wide variation in either of these factors could account for some of the observed differences. The noncompensating errors in the numerators or denominators entering into the calculated rates for these nativity groups might also contribute to the existing differences (Lilienfeld *et al.*, 1968).

B. REGIONAL DIFFERENCES

Additional clues to the etiology of leukemia are suggested by the study of regional differences in leukemia mortality within a particular country or geographic region. Such studies have been undertaken in the United States, England and Wales, Denmark, Scotland, Milan Province as well as three midwestern states, among others described below.

The geographic distribution of leukemia mortality within the United States has been studied over two time periods: 1949–1951 (or 1949–1953 in another study) and 1959–1961. Walter and Gilliam (1956) compare the observed number of leukemia deaths in each state from 1949 to 1951 with the expected number if age-, sex-, and race-specific rates for the United States as a whole applied. The results in standardized mortality ratios are shown in Fig. 2. Leukemia mortality is somewhat higher in the northern United States as compared with the South, especially the Southeast. This gradient was observed for both white and nonwhite males and females, but MacMahon (1957) finds that it was lower in 1949–1953 than it had been in 1938–1942. Analysis by geographic region showed that there was an excessive leukemia mortality in the West North Central, Middle Atlantic, and Pacific regions but it becomes clear from Fig. 2 that this is a reflection of the pattern of three individual states (New York, Minnesota, and California) rather than that of three geographic regions. The preliminary results of a study of leukemia mortality during 1959 to 1961 show essentially a similar distribution of deaths (Lilienfeld *et al.*, 1968). Consistent with international comparisons, the range in variation of leukemia mortality ratios between states is narrower than for other neoplasms. Even without adjusting for the effect of urban–rural differences there is only a 1.5-fold difference between states with the highest and the lowest leukemia death rates for females, and a 2.7-fold difference for males. This compares, for example, with the differences of 3.9-fold for female stomach cancer and 4.1-fold for male rectum cancer.

MacMahon (1957) found that the differences between the states correlated only slightly with urbanization, showed more correlation with median income, and showed the highest correlation with density of physicians. These differences also appear to increase with age at death (Fig. 3). Thus, distinctions in certain aspects of medical care or diagnosis may be responsible, at least in part, for the geographic variation in leukemia mortality. The generally acknowledged improvement in the standards of medical practice in the United States in recent years could account for the

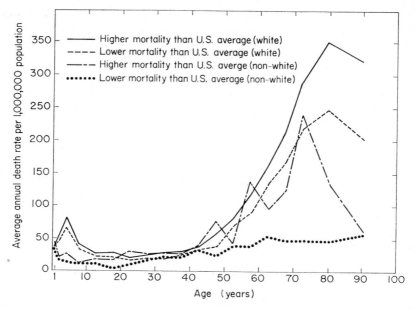

FIG. 3. Leukemia mortality rates by age and race: selected groups of states with significantly ($p = 0.05$ or less) high and significantly low mortality from leukemia, 1949–1951. (From Walter and Gilliam, 1956.)

secular decrease in these interstate leukemia mortality gradients discussed. However, certain states with low physician–population ratios have high leukemia rates, and it is clear that other factors must be operative as well. It is interesting to note that the 1959–1961 mortality data for the United States show essentially no urban–rural differences for leukemia (Lilienfeld *et al.*, 1968). Urban rates exceeded rural at all ages in 1944–1948 (Meadors, 1956) but by the following decade the differential was either absent or found only in children (Stark and Oleinick, 1966). This is in marked contrast to respiratory tract neoplasms, for instance, which show consistent urban–rural differences.

A geographic gradient in leukemia mortality has been apparent in England and Wales for a number of years, consisting of a region of relatively low rates in the north and west and a region of relatively high rates in the south and east (Hewitt, 1960). Consistent with the pattern in the United States, this gradient has been diminishing in magnitude over time as the leukemia rates have increased relatively more rapidly in the areas of lower reported leukemia mortality. Each cytologic type of leukemia has contributed to the observed geographic differences, the lymphatic type somewhat more than the myeloid. Apparently this is an age-related phenomenon, since the regional gradient increases with age, just as it does in the United States.

When the population of England and Wales was divided into more urban and less urban halves, no differences were noted in leukemia mortality during 1950–1956 below age 65, whereas among the elderly, the more urbanized were found to be at greater risk (Hewitt, 1960). Professional persons, as opposed to the unskilled, experienced increased leukemia mortality at all but especially at the older ages. Leukemia mortality in England and Wales was found to be negatively correlated with total mortality, infant mortality, and proportion of deaths certified as "senility," but it was positively correlated with physician density. As with the United States data, one is tempted to attribute the leukemia pattern to certain aspects of medical care and to some extent this must be valid. However, a significant correlation was also found between leukemia mortality and

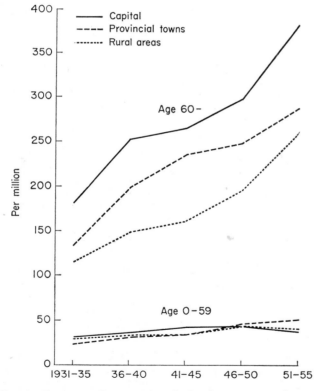

FIG. 4. Standardized mortality rates from leukemia among men by age groups and degree of urbanization for quinquennial periods 1931–1955, Denmark. (From Clemmesen, 1965.)

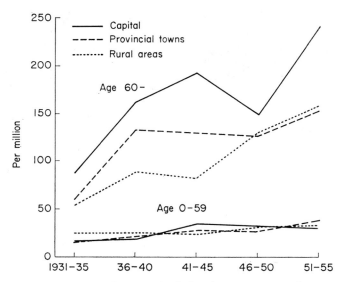

Fig. 5. Standardized mortality rates for leukemia among women by age groups and degree of urbanization for quinquennial periods 1931–1955, Denmark. (From Clemmesen, 1965.)

population density of architects. Thus, the pattern may reflect broader social factors than medical care alone.

The marked effect of age upon the geographic distribution of leukemia is also seen in Denmark. Clemmesen (1965) found little or no urban–rural variation in leukemia mortality during the years 1931–1955 at ages under 60. At older ages, however, a gradient according to degree of urbanization was evident throughout the period under study (Figs. 4 and 5).

Estimates have been made of the mortality from leukemia in Scotland during the years 1939 to 1956. Excessive deaths were observed in two urban areas, Aberdeen and Edinburgh, and a deficient death rate in another urban area, Glasgow (Court-Brown et al., 1960b). These findings again suggest that it is not urbanization, per se, but one or more associated variables, which may account for the observed geographic patterns of leukemia mortality. This is demonstrated once again, in the results of a survey of leukemia prevalence in the province of Milan (Eridani et al., 1964). The failure of the leukemia cases to distribute themselves according to degree of regional industrialization is plainly evident (Fig. 6).

Finally, brief mention should be made of a study of leukemia mortality in three midwestern states (Kansas, Missouri, and Oklahoma) from 1950 to 1959. Death rates, specific for five gradations of community size, indicated no clear relationship to degree of urbanization (Martin et al., 1966).

Although the smallest communities (rural communities) had the lowest death rates in all three states, the highest age-adjusted mortality was found in communities of 2500 to 4900 persons in Missouri and Oklahoma and in communities of 10,000 to 49,000 in Kansas. The large metropolitan areas in these states did not have the highest rates. The investigators suggested that these mortality patterns might be a function of the sizable nonwhite populations of these states which were not taken into account. However, MacMahon and Koller (1957) have shown that the commonly observed discrepancy between white and nonwhite leukemia death rates tends to disappear when allowance is made for social and economic (rather than racial) differences between white and nonwhite. Previously, the Registrar General's report for 1930 to 1932 demonstrated a positive association of leukemia mortality in England and Wales with high social and occupational class (Registrar General, 1938). In addition, the data of Sacks and Seeman (1947) substantiate the correlation of this disease with economic level.

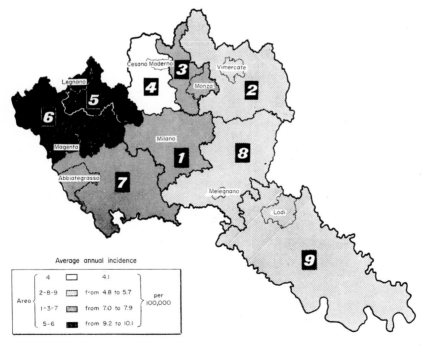

FIG. 6. Average annual incidence of hospitalized cases of leukemia by districts in Province of Milan, 1959–1961. 1, Industrial; 2–5, partly industrial; 6–7, partly agricultural; 8–9, agricultural. (From Eridani et al., 1964.)

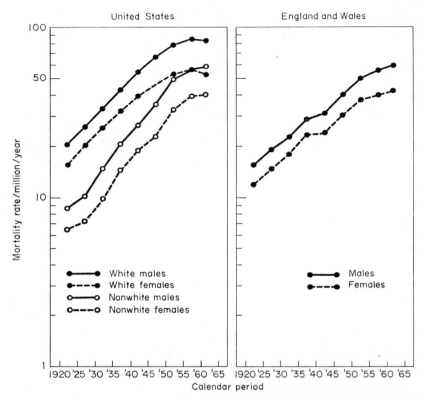

Fig. 7. Leukemia mortality rates by sex and calendar period in the U.S. white and nonwhite populations, and in England and Wales, 1921–1964, for all ages (age-adjusted to U.S. population of 1950). (From Fraumeni and Miller, 1967a.)

C. Secular Trend

Since the inception of the publication of vital records, most published data on leukemia mortality experience in many countries suggest a marked increase. In the United States the crude leukemia death rate (per 100,000) rose from 1.0 in 1900 to 4.3 in 1944 (Sacks and Seeman, 1947) to 7.0 in 1965 (U.S. Public Health Service, 1967). During this time period similar increases occurred in England and Wales (Registrar General, 1900–1965) and in Australia (Lancaster, 1955). The trend in Japan has also been upward, but at a lower level (Takeda, 1960). Comparable figures are available for only one other country, New Zealand; these show a 35-year period of apparently stable rates (1908–1943) followed by a period of rising mortality (Gunz, 1966). In Denmark (Clemmesen and Sorensen, 1958), Sweden (Nordenson and Asplund, 1956), and Ontario (Sloman and Sellers, 1959) leukemia death rates have risen steadily since the 1930's. In all countries where mortality has been tabulated by the World Health Organization the leukemia trend has been upward from 1940 to 1960 (Grais, 1962), although actual rates have varied considerably between countries. Despite this temporal increase in leukemia mortality, the rate of increase began to level off about 1940 among United States whites and about 1955 among U.S. nonwhites (Gilliam and Walter, 1958) and in England and Wales (Fraumeni and Miller, 1967a) (Fig. 7). In more recent years, declines in death rates have appeared in the Netherlands, Denmark, Germany, Australia (Segi and Kurihara, 1966) and in the region of Omsk, U.S.S.R. (Demchenko, 1965).

Leukemia runs an almost invariably fatal course and one is tempted to infer from the mortality trend that the incidence has increased as well.

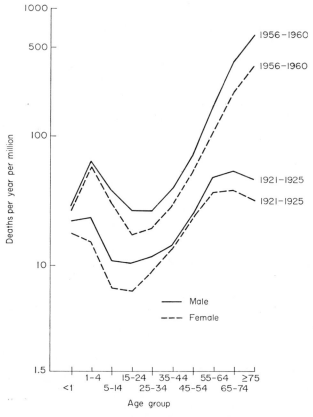

FIG. 8. Age- and sex-specific average annual United States leukemia death rates for the period 1921–1925 and 1956–1960. (From Rucknagel, 1966.)

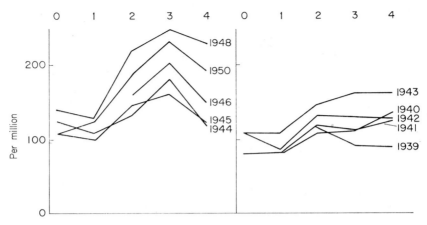

FIG. 9. Childhood incidence of leukemia in the United States by cohorts of children born in the years shown. (From Burnet, 1958.) Abscissa—age in years.

Such an inference would have considerable theoretical importance, implying the introduction (or intensification) in the environment of a carcinogen potent enough to have caused an increase in mortality relatively greater than for any other disease in western nations except lung cancer and coronary thrombosis (Witts, 1957). A complete resolution of this question is not now possible, but there is no reason to doubt that the observed time trend, or at least the magnitude of it, has been exaggerated by concomitant improvements in diagnostic accuracy, cause-of-death certification, and survivorship from competing (infectious) causes of death.

D. AGE

Most studies agree that the leukemia death rate rises to a minor peak during the first 5 years of life, falls to a minimum during young adulthood, and then rises to a maximum in old age. The leukemia pattern in Japan appears to be unique in the absence of a clear-cut peaking in old age (Segi and Kurihara, 1966). Within age categories, however, the death rates have exhibited variable rates of increase over time. In general, rates have increased most rapidly among the very young and the very old (Fig. 8), i.e., precisely those age groups that would be expected to have benefited most from improvements over time in leukemia diagnosis, cause-of-death certification, and quality of medical care.

A childhood peak in leukemia mortality (ages 2–4) was first recorded in England and Wales during the 1920's (Court-Brown and Doll, 1961) and became more pronounced during the 1940's (Hewitt, 1955). In the United States, a comparable peak did not emerge among white males until the early 1940's and not among white females until the late 1940's (Gilliam and Walter, 1958). An analysis by birth cohort (Fig. 9) indicates that this peak initially appeared among children born between 1943 and 1944 (Burnet, 1958). On the other hand, hospital data have long shown a prevalence peak in leukemia during the third and fourth years of life (Cooke, 1942). In the period since 1960, a peak has begun to develop among Japanese children (Miller, 1967a) and, less definitively, among U.S. non-whites as well (Fraumeni and Miller, 1967a) (Fig. 10). These trends, if valid, suggest that an environmental leukemogen was introduced or became more prevalent among English children around 1920 and among white American children around 1940. United States nonwhite and Japanese children may have had a more recent exposure. The nature of the agent, if in fact any exists, remains conjectural—a viral factor, a cytogenetic defect acting prezygotically, a change during gestation, or an early postnatal exposure are all possibilities. It is interesting to note that a childhood peak is found in Burkitt's lymphoma which, except for a maximum at age 5 years, is strikingly similar to that noted in childhood leukemia (Fig. 11).

The body of evidence opposed to the view that the childhood peak reflects an increased incidence of leukemia is not inconsiderable. Ederer *et al.* (1965a) point out that the childhood mortality peak is not unique to leukemia; similar, though somewhat less pronounced peaks are seen in

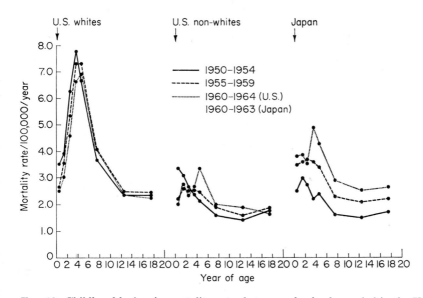

Fig. 10. Childhood leukemia mortality rates by age and calendar period in the U.S. (1950–1964) and Japan (1950–1963). (From Fraumeni and Miller, 1967a.)

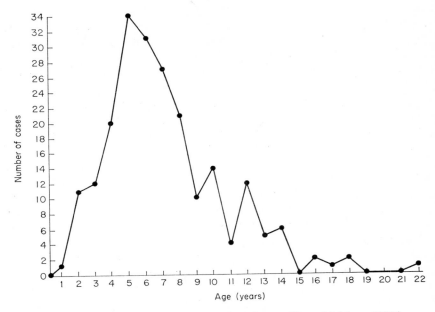

Fɪɢ. 11. Age distribution of Burkitt's lymphoma. (From Meighan, 1965.)

neuroblastoma and in Wilms' tumor. Slocumb and MacMahon (1963) attribute the peaking more to an increase in the average duration of survivorship of leukemia among infants rather than to a rise in childhood rates. It is their view, that the changing mortality pattern can best be explained by a postponement of death from infancy to early childhood, although they concede that it "antedated any specific therapy known to increase survival of leukemic patients." They cite the data of Gilliam and Walter (1958) which show that a leveling off in the rate of increase in white infant leukemia death rates took place shortly after 1940 and that by 1946–1950 there occurred an actual decline; this became evident among nonwhite infants a decade later. Thus, the peaking of mortality at ages 2 to 4 coincided approximately with declines in death rates in infancy.

Hewitt (1964) offers another explanation for the peaking, namely, a gradual reduction over time in the proportion of childhood anemias misdiagnosed as leukemia. He points out that "if the number of deaths certified as anemia can be taken as roughly proportional to the number of occasions on which a fatal blood condition had to be diagnosed (that is, the number of opportunities for a misdiagnosis of leukemia), it is easy to account both for the apparent excess of leukemia in white American infants as compared with those of England and Wales and also for the recent reduction of that excess." Although Hewitt's hypothesis cannot be tested directly, he was able to demonstrate that the infant leukemia mortality rate declined the most (from 1950–1954 to 1955–1959) in the five states with the highest proportion of infant deaths attributed to anemia, and declined the least in the six states with the lowest anemia death rate among infants. Deaths from infectious diseases have an age distribution in childhood very similar to that for anemia and have undergone roughly comparable declines over time (Hewitt, 1964). The decrease in this competing risk of death among infants may explain the childhood leukemia peak, which may or may not be independent of the anemia hypothesis.

Leukemia and certain infectious diseases appear to have parallel prevalence patterns in adolescence as well as in early childhood (Fig. 12). This similarity has been offered as an explanation for another interesting age pattern in leukemia, the adolescent peak. Lee (1961) analyzed leukemia mortality by single years of age for England and Wales, Scotland, Canada, and the United States. In each of these countries the male death rate declines from its childhood peak to a minimum at about age 13 and then rises to a new peak at about age 17; in females there is evidence of a similar

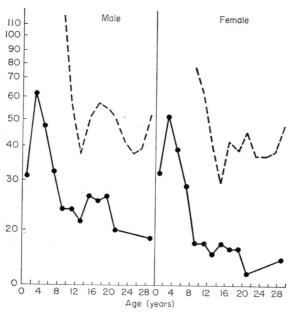

Fig. 12. Leukemia and acute lower respiratory infections. Hospital admissions for bronchitis and pneumonia, National Hospital In-Patient Inquiry, England and Wales, 1953-1956 (dashed lines). Leukemia death rates, England and Wales, 1945–1957 (solid lines). (From Lee, 1961.)

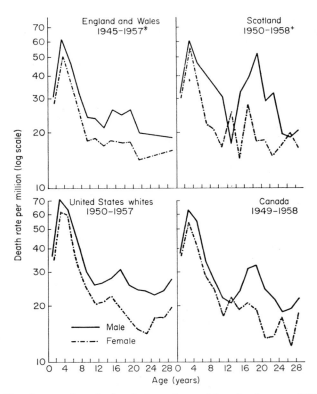

FIG. 13. Death rates from leukemia in males and females by age. * Five-year age groups, 20–24 and 25–29, due to lack of official population estimates. + based on small numbers. (From Lee, 1961.)

though less pronounced trend (Fig. 13). In England and Wales the adolescent peak has been present in nine out of the ten quinquenniums between 1911 and 1959 in males, but in only four quinquenniums in females (Court-Brown and Doll, 1961). These peaks of excess mortality appear to be comprised primarily of acute myeloid leukemia cases with unusually short clinical courses before hospital admission. Lee has noted that adolescent mortality peaks are not limited to leukemia (Lee, 1962b). A number of other diseases, including bone tumors, various infections, and congenital defects also show excessive mortality during this age period. Whether the adolescent peak is related in any way to the hormonal or other physiological changes associated with sexual maturation remains conjectural.

Leukemia mortality (and, in all likelihood, incidence) falls to a minimum during the third decade of life. Thereafter it rises continuously into old age (Fig. 8), except, as previously noted, in Japan. Graphs of leukemia mortality by age sometimes show an apparent decline after the age of 80 or so. This disappears when the analysis is by birth cohort (Hewitt, 1955) and is, therefore, most likely a transient feature attributable to some aspect of the cross-sectional nature of the population studied.

All adult age groups have participated in the upward trend of leukemia mortality during the past four decades, though not equally. By far the greatest increase has occurred among the elderly (Fig. 14). The trends in the average annual age-specific rates among U.S. whites are given in Fig. 15, which is drawn in semilogarithmic scale to reflect the rates of change. In addition to the slope reversal in infant leukemia mortality which has already been noted, a leveling off in the trend is evident among all other age groups except those 75 and over. When the percent change in age-specific leukemia death rates during this time-span is calculated, it is seen that the 75 and over age group also shows a decline in the rate of increase

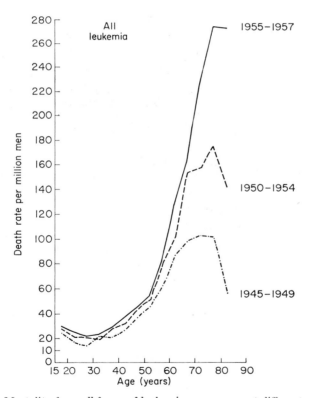

FIG. 14. Mortality from all forms of leukemia among men at different ages (from 15 years upward) in England and Wales in 1945–1949, 1950–1954, and 1955–1957. (From Court-Brown and Doll, 1959.)

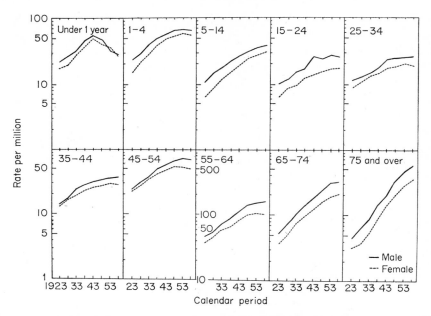

FIG. 15. Trends in average annual age-specific leukemia death rates among white males and females, United States, 1921–1960. (From Fraumeni and Wagoner, 1964.)

(Table IV). Allowing for the variability expected from data based upon the relatively small numbers of cases in young adults, it appears that the decline in the leukemia trend began among white U.S. infants around 1940 and gradually came to affect all older groups. The reason for this pattern is not known. It may somehow be related to the gradual disappearance or abatement of a once prevalent leukemogenic agent. This would be consistent with the suggestion that "the mortality experience of young children is the most sensitive indicator of environmental leukemogens" (Fraumeni and Miller, 1967b). The trends for U.S. nonwhites are more irregular because of the smaller numbers. However, they also show a leveling off during the past decade.

E. SEX

The male preponderance of leukemia mortality in infancy* and childhood has fallen while in adulthood and old age it has increased (Fig. 16). This may also be seen as a convergence of sex-specific death rates in the

*In England and Wales, leukemia mortality among infants under 1 year has been similar in both sexes since 1911 (Court-Brown and Doll, 1961); in the United States, male infants showed a slight excess in mortality until the 1940's (Gilliam and Walter, 1958).

TABLE IV

PERCENT CHANGE[a] IN AGE-SPECIFIC LEUKEMIA DEATH RATES;
U.S. DEATH REGISTRATION STATES, 1931–1963[b]

Age group (years)	1931 to 1940	1940–1944 to 1945–1949	1945–1949 to 1950–1954	1950–1954 to 1955–1959	1955–1959 to 1960–1963
Under 1	+75	−10	−20	−25	−7
1–4	+55	+11	+10	−5	−4
5–14	+46	+14	+21	+7	+3
15–24	+50	+6	+5	+5	0
25–34	+33	+11	+5	0	0
35–44	+37	+7	+14	+3	−6
45–54	+53	+8	+11	−2	−2
55–64	+64	+23	+13	+4	−2
65–74	+59	+27	+33	+18	−2
75 and over	+126	+48	+55	+25	+14
All ages	+61	+20	+17	+9	0

[a] Figures age-adjusted to U.S. Census 1940, except for 1931 to 1940.

[b] Sacks and Seeman (1947) data for 1931–1940; *Statist. Bull.*, Metropolitan Life Ins. Co. (1966), data for 1940–1963.

young and a divergence of rates in the old (Fig. 15). These trends in the sex ratio have coincided with early increases and gradual stabilization of leukemia death rates among the young and with a much longer period of rising mortality among the elderly. From this, Fraumeni and Wagoner (1964) concluded that an equal number of males and females have contributed to the overall increase in childhood leukemia, whereas males have been selectively affected by adult leukemia. This conclusion, if valid, could have interesting etiological implications, perhaps the possible selective exposure of males to environmental factors, occupational or otherwise. However, among nonwhites the sex ratios have not shown consistent trends.

F. TYPES OF LEUKEMIA

It is important to distinguish between the various cytological and clinical types of leukemia because of their divergent distributions by age, sex, and race. Unfortunately, the various methods used to classify leukemia deaths have not been and still are not completely satisfactory. Prior to 1949, leukemia deaths were classified only as "leukemia" or "aleukemia." The subsequently adopted *6th Revision of the International List of Diseases and Causes of Death* (World Health Organization, 1948) assigned them to five rubrics: lymphatic, myeloid, monocytic, acute (unspecified), and other and unspecified. This classification does not permit an analysis by clinical types of leukemia (acute or chronic) according to cytological types. The *7th*

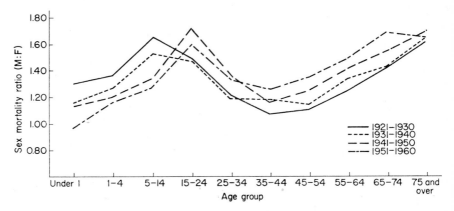

FIG. 16. Trends in sex ratios (M/F) of average annual age-specific leukemia death rates among white population, United States, 1921–1960. (From Fraumeni and Wagoner, 1964.)

Revision of the International List of Diseases and Causes of Death places all acute leukemias, irrespective of cell type, into one rubric. It is not until the eighth revision, adopted for use in 1968, that leukemia deaths were coded according to each of the possible clinical and cytological types. Some years will have to pass, however, before the number of deaths is sufficient for a detailed mortality analysis.

Leukemia mortality statistics depend upon the accuracy and care with which the physician records the underlying cause of death. Certification practices among physicians vary and improvements should be encouraged. The proportion of English and Welsh leukemia deaths in which cytological or clinical type was incompletely specified decreased from 54.3% in 1945–1949 to 17.4% in 1958–1961 following the Registrar General's inquiries concerning omissions (Court-Brown *et al.*, 1964).

Recent data show that the acute leukemias account for somewhat more than half of all deaths (Court-Brown *et al.*, 1964; Wells and Lau, 1960). Of the remainder, the chronic lymphatic form appears to be more prevalent than the myeloid in western nations; in the Orient, however, the reverse is true, chronic lymphatic leukemia is quite rare (Table V). These observations must be interpreted with great caution in view of the inadequacies of census and mortality data from most countries of the Far East. These inadequacies make it necessary, in calculating these ratios, to utilize relative frequencies of identified leukemia cases rather than morbidity or mortality rates relating to the populations at risk. In view of the known relationship of chronic lymphatic leukemia with age (Fig. 17), it is likely that, to some extent, the observed differences in leukemia frequency stem

TABLE V

RATIO OF CHRONIC LYMPHATIC TO CHRONIC MYELOID LEUKEMIA AND PERCENT
POPULATION 65 YEARS AND OVER FOR VARIOUS SELECTED COUNTRIES

Investigator	Country and time period	Percent of population 65 and over	Frequency measure used	CL/CM ratio[c]
Kessler (1968)	United States (whites) 1959–1961	9.7[a]	Standardized rates	1.42
Kessler (1968)	United States (nonwhites) 1959–1961	6.1[a]	Standardized rates	1.36
Court-Brown et al. (1964)	England and Wales 1958–1961	11.9[b]	Standardized rates	1.07
Court-Brown et al. (1964)	Norway 1957–1959	10.9[b]	Standardized rates	1.21
Court-Brown et al. (1964)	Finland 1957–1961	7.2[b]	Standardized rates	1.45
Nelson and Merrett (1966)	Northern Ireland 1957–1963	9.7[b]	Average annual rates	1.49
Jhala and Tilak (1967)	India 1960–1964	—	Relative frequencies	0.24
Sonnet et al. (1966)	Congolese Bantu 1958–1963	—	Relative frequencies	1.29
Magnússon (1964)	Iceland 1957–1961	—	Relative frequencies	1.86
Seno (1964)	Japan 1957–1961	5.8[b]	Relative frequencies	0.21
Wells and Lau (1960)	Singapore 1949–1958	—	Relative frequencies	0.08

[a] Calculated from U.S. Bureau of the Census (1964).
[b] Calculated from World Health Organization (1963).
[c] CL = chronic lymphatic; CM = chronic myeloid.

from differences in the age distributions of the respective populations. Japan, with a low ratio of chronic lymphatic to chronic myeloid (CL/CM) leukemia, also has the lowest proportion of persons aged 65 and over among the listed countries with published census data. No reliable census data are available for India or Singapore for the computation of death rates. However, some indication of the mortality experience can be obtained from an analysis of proportionate mortality by age. In Singapore, 25.2% of all deaths in 1960 occurred among persons aged 65 and over; the analogous figures for Norway, Finland, and Iceland were 70.5, 57.5, and 62.9%, respectively. Apparently the oriental nations have relatively fewer persons at risk of chronic lymphatic leukemia than those in the West. Differences in

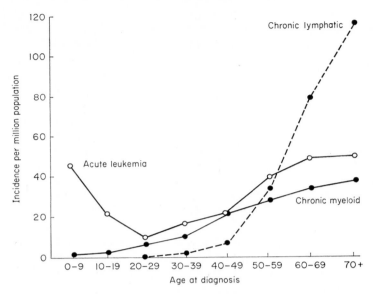

Fig. 17. Age incidence of leukemia by type in Brooklyn, 1943–1952. (From Witts, 1957.)

age distribution alone, however, are insufficient to explain the differences in the CL/CM ratios; for example, Japan's aged population is only slightly smaller (as a proportion of the total) than U.S. nonwhites. Yet the difference in the CL/CM ratio is sevenfold. On the other hand, England and Wales have the highest proportion of elderly among the listed countries, but also have the lowest CL/CM ratio of the western nations. Differences in access to medical care and practices in cause-of-death certification are no doubt other factors that play a role. It is believed, for example, that Asians prefer to leave the hospital in the terminal stages of a fatal illness in order to die at home (Wells and Lau, 1960). Whether this can explain the relative rarity of chronic lymphatic leukemia which has been recently noted among Orientals in the United States as well (Shimkin and Loveland, 1961; Buell and Dunn, 1965) is not known. The observation that Japanese normally have higher peripheral lymphocyte counts than Caucasians (Tomonaga, 1966) suggests another possibility, namely, a biological or racial difference of some kind. The relatively high CL/CM ratio among the Congolese Bantu and the low ratios among the Caucasians of India cast doubt on the importance of a racial difference. The possibility of a biological basis for the differences is suggested by the considerable sex differences in CL/CM ratios: 1.61 and 1.19 among U.S. white males and females, respectively, and 1.60 and 1.09 among U.S. nonwhites.

The frequency distributions by age of the various clinical types of leu-kemia vary with the definitions employed. When definitions corresponding to those of the last two *International List of Diseases and Causes of Death* are applied, the findings are that (*1*) chronic lymphatic leukemia increases rapidly with age after 50; (*2*) chronic myeloid leukemia increases less rapidly with age almost continuously throughout the life-span; and (*3*) acute leukemia shows a bimodal distribution with peaks in early childhood and in old age (Fig. 17).

When the leukemia definition stresses cytological type rather than clinical form, a somewhat different distribution appears (Fig. 18): (*1*) lymphatic leukemia shows a bimodal distribution with peaks at the extremes of age; (*2*) myeloid leukemia is the predominant disease in adulthood; and (*3*) acute, unspecified leukemia is relatively more common in childhood and declines throughout the remainder of life.

The two frequency distributions just examined are not incompatible; in fact, when considered together they suggest a consistent pattern of leu-kemia incidence, one which is supported by the well-designed surveys of leukemia mortality in England and Wales (Doll, 1961) and of leukemia incidence in Brooklyn, New York (MacMahon and Clark, 1956). The bimodal lymphatic leukemia curve in Fig. 18 consists of a childhood peak of acute lymphatic leukemia and an old age peak of chronic lymphatic leukemia. The high, sustained myeloid leukemia curve in Fig. 18 reflects

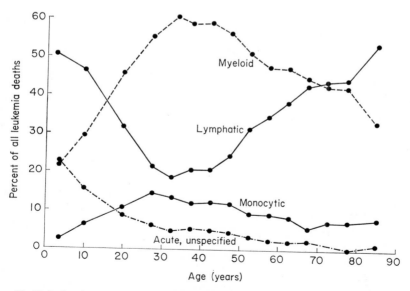

FIG. 18. Relative frequency of leukemia deaths by type and age. (From Hewitt, 1955.)

the prevailing forms of the disease in adults: acute and chronic myeloid leukemia. The downward sloping acute, unspecified leukemia curve probably reflects the dominant cytological type at each age: acute, lymphatic leukemia in childhood and old age and acute myeloid leukemia in adulthood.

Until recently it has not been possible to examine time trends in leukemia mortality by specific cell type. An opportunity to do this was provided by the Registrar General of England and Wales when he extracted pertinent information from the records of all persons certified as dying of leukemia between 1945 and 1957. It was found that an increase had occurred among children in the mortality attributable to both acute lymphatic and acute myeloid leukemia, but that this was largely the result of a reduction in the attribution of deaths to other and unspecified leukemias (Lee, 1961). Among adolescents and young adults (ages 15–29) there was evidence of a real, though modest, increase in both acute and chronic myeloid leukemia. During this time period, small, perhaps insignificant, decreases took place in the relatively high sex ratios common in children and young adults.

The time trends in later adulthood and old age have been more remarkable. Between 1945–1947 and 1955–1957, male mortality from acute leukemia increased at all ages beyond young adulthood but especially in the older ages (Fig. 19). Chronic lymphatic leukemia increased in the older ages (Fig. 20). The same was true for chronic myeloid leukemia, which, in

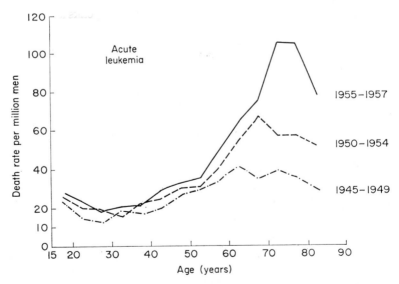

Fig. 19. Estimated mortality from acute leukemia among men at different ages (from 15 years upward) in England and Wales, in 1945–1949, 1950–1954, and 1955–1957. (From Court-Brown and Doll, 1959.)

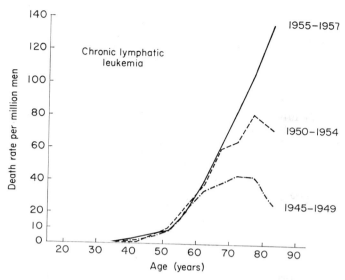

Fig. 20. Estimated mortality from chronic lymphatic leukemia among men at different ages (from 15 years upward) in England and Wales in 1945–1949, 1950–1954, and 1955–1957. (From Court-Brown and Doll, 1959.)

addition, showed a rise among male adults under age 60 (Fig. 21). Among women the corresponding death rates also rose, excepting that for chronic myeloid leukemia in adults under 60 years (Court-Brown and Doll, 1959). The direction and magnitude of these time trends is summarized in Table VI.

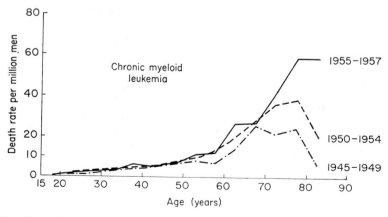

Fig. 21. Estimated mortality from chronic myeloid leukemia among men at different ages (from 15 years upward) in England and Wales in 1945–1949, 1950–1954, and 1955–1957. (From Court-Brown and Doll, 1959.)

TABLE VI

MEAN OF RATIOS[a] OF 1955 TO 1957 AGE-SPECIFIC DEATH RATES FOR
LEUKEMIA TO SIMILAR DEATH RATES FOR 1945 TO 1949,
BY SEX, AGE GROUPS, AND TYPE[b]

| | Age groups | | | |
| | 30–59 | | 60 and over | |
Type of leukemia	Males	Females	Males	Females
Chronic lymphatic	1.02	0.68	2.56	1.82
Chronic myeloid	1.34	0.93	3.38	1.74
Acute	1.29	1.32	2.51	3.04

[a] $\text{Ratio} = \dfrac{1955\text{--}1957 \text{ death rate}}{1945\text{--}1949 \text{ death rate}}$.

[b] Calculated from data of Court-Brown and Doll (1959).

Because leukemias of all types in both sexes have increased so rapidly among the elderly during this time period, it is likely that the observed trend among the elderly stems more from enhanced case ascertainment rather than from increased disease incidence. This view is compatible with the recent leveling off in the rate of leukemia increase among the aged (Table IV). It is also consistent with the marked declines which have been recorded in the mortality attributed to senility among the older age groups during this period (Table VII). The reduction in the frequency of certification of causes of death to senility is generally thought to reflect improvements in the accuracy of death certificates (Doll, 1961). It is noteworthy that such reductions become greater with increasing age and are much greater among nonwhites than whites.

Acute leukemia, as distinct from the chronic forms, has increased in all adult and elderly age groups, though more so among the latter, suggesting that it may, in part, reflect a real increase in incidence. Whether this is attributable in some measure to increased exposure to environmental carcinogens is, of course, not known. However, it is of some interest that of the chronic forms of leukemia only the myeloid type has increased among adults under 60 years, though only in males. It is the myeloid form of (chronic) leukemia which has been associated with the effects of radiation (Stewart et al., 1962).

A time trend analysis of leukemia mortality by cytological type was recently undertaken in the United States (Fraumeni and Miller, 1967a). From 1958–1960 to 1961–1964 a slight decrease in age-specific mortality occurred among white males and females under age 75. Death rates fell for all types of leukemia except the acute form which showed a slight increase

TABLE VII

CHANGE IN AGE-SPECIFIC MORTALITY PER 1,000,000 MALES ATTRIBUTED TO
SENILITY AND LEUKEMIA, ENGLAND AND WALES AND
UNITED STATES, 1947–1956

| Age groups | England and Wales[a] | | United States[b] | | | |
| | | | Whites | | Nonwhites | |
	Senility	Leukemia	Senility	Leukemia	Senility	Leukemia
65–69	−89	+66	−45	+96	−207	+165
70–74	−620	+98	−168	+124	−731	+138
75–79	−2465	+195	−586[c]	+183[c]	−1100[c]	+132[c]
80 and over	−10103	+243	−3636[c]	+326[c]	−5663[c]	+195[c]

[a] Doll (1961).

[b] Calculated from Vital Statistics of the U.S., 1947–1956 (U.S. Public Health Service, 1949, 1958) and from U.S. Census of Population, 1950 (U.S. Bureau of Census, 1953).

[c] The age distribution of males over 74 in the 1960 U.S. Census used to partition the 1947 population into age groups 75–79 and 80 and over.

over 44 years of age. In general, mortality from the lymphatic and myeloid forms of leukemia declined to the same degree. It, therefore, appears unlikely that the recent decline in leukemia mortality in the United States is attributable to decreased radiation exposure, although the narrowness of the time period studied precludes any firm conclusions.

As already indicated, high sex ratios for leukemia mortality have been reported in many countries. The time trends of these ratios have also been described. No comparably standardized data broken down by specific type of leukemia have become available to date except for England and Wales, Northern Ireland, and the United States. For several other countries it was possible to calculate sex ratios based upon observed numbers of cases rather than on morbidity or mortality rates. Although such calculations are affected by differences in the reference population, the resulting sex ratios are, for the most part, similar to those derived from standardized death rates (Table VIII). Thus, males have a 10–70% increment in acute leukemia, 10–60% in chronic myeloid leukemia, and 40–200% in chronic lymphatic leukemia if the more deviant values for Iceland and the Congo Republic are ignored. Ratios for the latter two countries are based upon 57 and 35 cases, respectively.

The data from England and Wales and the United States indicate that sex differentials are greatest for chronic lymphatic leukemia and least for chronic myeloid leukemia. From the known relationships of the chronic leukemias to age, these differences in sex ratios might be attributed to a factor acting differentially upon the sexes in the older ages. Such a factor

TABLE VIII

Sex Ratios[a] for Leukemia by Type from Various Selected Studies

Investigator	Country and time period	Basis for sex ratio	Sex ratio			
			Acute leukemia	Chronic myeloid	Chronic lymphatic	
Court-Brown et al. (1964)	England and Wales 1958–1961	Age-adjusted death rates	1.5	1.1	2.0	
Lilienfeld et al. (1968)	United States 1959–1961	Age-adjusted death rates	1.4	1.4	2.1	
Nelson and Merrett (1966)	Northern Ireland 1957–1963	Age-adjusted death rates	1.4	0.9	1.4	
Magnússon (1964)	Iceland 1957–1961	No. of cases	3.1	1.3	2.3	
Jhala and Tilak (1967)	India 1960–1964	No. of cases	—	1.3	2.0	
Seno (1964)	Japan 1957–1961	No. of cases	1.7	1.6	1.2	
Gunz (1964)	New Zealand 1958–1961	No. of cases	1.1	1.3	2.0	
Sonnet et al. (1966)	Congo Republic 1958–1963	No. of cases	3.3	6.0	2.0	

[a] Calculated from data of above studies.

might be an environmental agent to which males are selectively exposed or to which they are unusually susceptible. Alternatively, the factor might be related to greater case ascertainment among males, although no obvious reason for this is apparent.

III. Distribution in Time and Space

A. Leukemia Clusters

The secular trends in leukemia and the differences in its prevalence between the various countries and states within the United States indicate that this disease varies over time and over space. In recent years some interest has been focused on the possible clustering of leukemia cases within both time and space together. This was stimulated by the accumulating evidence that, at least in certain animals, leukemia is caused by viruses. If human leukemia were caused by an infectious agent, then one might expect it to be transmitted in the fashion of other communicable diseases, some of which (e.g., poliomyelitis and infectious hepatitis) occur in space–time clusters.

In the past few years a number of clinical reports of apparent "micro-epidemics" of leukemia have appeared (Table IX). These are almost invariably the result of the occurrence, within a given locality, of more than the usual number of leukemia cases over a given time period. The number of such cases is always very small and a statistical analysis of the significance of the "clustering" is usually impossible. First of all, this is because an analysis is done after the observations have been made. Glass et al. (1968) graphically illustrate the effect of analyzing "gerrymandered" areas. Secondly, case ascertainment is usually more complete in the area of the suspected cluster than elsewhere. From such studies it is not possible to distinguish between true disease clusters and the occasional concurrence of cases which one might expect to observe in a few of the thousands of localities at risk of more than a single case over a given time-span.

More refined analytic statistical methods have been developed to determine whether leukemia cases tend to cluster in time and space. Most of these proceed from an analysis of all possible pairs of spatially and temporally separated cases and are distinguished by "their applicability even in the absence of knowledge about the underlying population or underlying disease rates" (Mantel, 1967). Unfortunately, variations of findings and inferences derived therefrom probably reflect the differences in the statistical methods used in analyzing the data. The methods and results of the major investigations of leukemia clustering in the United States are summarized in Table X; those of England and elsewhere are presented in Table XI.

TABLE IX

CLINICAL REPORTS OF LEUKEMIA CLUSTERS

Investigator	Geographic area	Time	No. of patients	Type of leukemia	Additional details
U.S. Department of Health, Education, and Welfare (1967), Leukemia Surveillance Program Report	Warwick, New York (Population: 12,551)	1967	2	Acute granulocytic adult	Both cases noted within same month; in persons working at same automobile factory
U.S. Department of Health, Education, and Welfare (1967), Leukemia Surveillance Program Report	Beulah, North Dakota (Population: 1318)	1966	2	Acute adult	Expected number of cases = 1 in 10 years; both cases noted within same month in next-door neighbors
U.S. Department of Health, Education, and Welfare (1967), Leukemia Surveillance Program Report	Metuchen, New Jersey (Population: 13,581)	1963–1965	3	Acute and chronic	Expected number of cases = 0.1 or less; three cases in residents of same block
Colon (1966)	Friend, Nebraska	1962–1964	3	Acute childhood	Onsets within 15 months of each other; no known contacts between cases; only 1 parent of the 6 under age 40
Medical News Item (1968)	Prairie Village, Kansas	1961–1967	2	Acute and chronic	Both cases resided in same house
Medical News Item (1968)	North Kansas City, Missouri	1961–1967	2	Acute	Both cases residing in same apartment house
Heath and Manning (1964)	Louisville, Illinois (Population under age 15: 300)	1961	2	Acute childhood	Expected number of cases = 0.1; children lived on adjoining farms and attended the same school
Heath et al. (1964)	Orange, Texas (Population: 25,605)	1960	3	Acute childhood	Onsets within 8 months of each other; no known contacts between cases; 5 newborn infants died with congenital

heart disease between July and October, 1961

Reference	Location	Number	Type	Years	Comments
U.S. Department of Health, Education, and Welfare (1967), Leukemia Surveillance Program Report	Douglas, Georgia (Population: 8736)	3	Acute and chronic	1958–1966	Three cases in successive occupants of one house
Heath and Hasterlik (1963)	Niles, Illinois (Population: 20,393)	8	Acute childhood	1957–1960	Observed incidence 5× expected rate; onset of 3 cases within 8 months of each other, 5 cases within 10 months; 7 of the 8 children had contacts in one school and a "rheumatic-like" illness occurred there at the same time; 7 infant deaths with congenital heart lesions occurred from 1955 to 1960
U.S. Department of Health, Education, and Welfare (1967), Leukemia Surveillance Program Report	Parowan and Paragonah, Utah (Population: 1786)	4	Acute (3 teenagers, 1 adult)	1956–1967	Expected number of cases = 1.4; onset of 2 cases within 10 months of each other and of 2 other cases within 4 months; 3 patients students at same school
U.S. Department of Health, Education, and Welfare (1967), Leukemia Surveillance Program Report	Monticello, Utah (Population: 1845)	4	Acute childhood	1956–1965	Expected number of cases = 0.34; onset of 2 cases within 8 months of each other; patients all students at same school; town site of uranium mill, 1949–1960
Heath and Manning (1964)	Cheyenne, Wyoming (Population under age 15: 15,000)	4	Acute childhood	1956–1957	Expected number of cases = 0.6; onsets within 10 months of each other; no known contacts between cases
Heath and Manning (1964)	Waldwick, New Jersey (Population under age 15: 8000)	4	Acute childhood	1956	Expected number of cases = 0.3; no known contacts between cases

TABLE X
ANALYTIC STUDIES OF LEUKEMIA CLUSTERS IN THE UNITED STATES

Investigator	Geographic area	Time	No. and type of cases	Sources of case data	Definition of cluster	Investigator's findings	Remarks
Glass et al. (1968)	Los Angeles, Calif.	1960–1964	298 children	Death records	By method of Ederer et al. (1964)	No clusters found at first. But, after "gerrymandering" the spatial partition, significant, though spurious, clustering was found	
Lundin et al. (1966)	Pittsburgh, Penn.	1953–1962	165 children and adults	Death records	Observed number of paired leukemia deaths during a given time interval which exceeds the number expected on basis of constant probability of death over the interval	No clustering was observed over the entire observation period. However, an excessive number of leukemia deaths occurred between 6 and 8 years apart	Authors' assumption of constant probability of death over time was substantiated by their analysis of mortality pattern of paired decedents from diseases not known to aggregate in space and/or time
Meighan and Knox (1965)	Portland, Oregon	1950–1961	69 children	Death records and University Hospital records	By method of Knox (1964)	Excessive clustering of paired cases closer than 250 days and 4 km. apart; also for cases closer than 365 days and 1 km. apart	
Mustacchi (1965)	San Francisco, Calif.	1946–1955	639 children and adults	Hospital records and death records	Observed number of leukemia cases in 1949 to 1955 which exceeds number expected on basis of reported incidence in 1946 to 1948 for city tracts in which at least 1 case occurred	Leukemia cases in 1949 to 1955 tended to cluster in those tracts where cases had previously occurred in 1946 to 1948. These findings were independent of variations	Populous tracts with low leukemia rates can qualify as "with leukemia" areas and small tracts with high leukemia incidence might fail to do so

Author	Location	Years	Number	Source	Criteria	Results	Comments
					in 1946 to 1948		between city tracts in race, religion, and economic status, but might be a function of crowded living conditions
Ederer et al. (1964, 1965c)	Connecticut	1945–1949	2610 children and adults	State cancer registry	Observed number of cases occurring in 1 year or in 2 successive years in total of each 5-year town unit, which exceeds expected number calculated by combinatorial methods	No significant differences between observed and expected numbers of cases in either 1- or 2-year clusters for either children or total cases	This method showed significant clustering when applied to poliomyelitis and to infectious hepatitis data
Pinkel and Nefzger (1959)	Buffalo, New York	1943–1956	137 children (95 in central city)	Local and state cancer registries	2 or more reported cases within 2 years and $\frac{1}{3}$ mile of each other	16 clusters found ($p = 0.15$). This is "suggestive" of clustering effect in central city	1. Author's probability model has been questioned because of the apparent lack of independence between pairs 2. Author's assumption of uniform population density in Buffalo is questionable 3. Method may not distinguish between spatial, temporal, and spatial–temporal clustering
Pinkel et al. (1963)	Buffalo, New York	1943–1956	95 children	Local and state cancer registries	Average ridit <0.50 for time–space distribution of paired cases less than 1 mile apart. (Average ridit for paired cases 1 or more miles apart $= 0.50$)	Average ridits for paired cases were significantly less than 0.50, when the pairs were less than $\frac{1}{2}$ mile apart. This is indicative of clustering	Time was calculated to the nearest year; thus, clustering over shorter periods could not be examined

TABLE XI

ANALYTIC STUDIES OF LEUKEMIA CLUSTERS IN ENGLAND AND ELSEWHERE

Investigator	Geographic area	Time	No. and type of cases	Sources of case data	Definition of cluster	Investigator's findings	Remarks
Moszczyński (1968)	Brzesko, Poland	1962–1966	87 patients "with cancer and leukemia"	Not stated	By method of Knox (1964)	Clustering within 30 days and 1 km. of each other	Details are lacking
Barton et al. (1965)	Liverpool, England	1957–1962	84 acute	Cancer registry	Value of Q (a B-function measure of space variation within time clusters) significantly less than 1.00, for time clusters, defined as adjacent cases with an intervening time interval of less than the ratio total time period/No. of cases + 1	$Q = 0.8883$ (no significant clustering)	1. This method showed evidence of significant clustering for measles and poliomyelitis
	Bristol, England	1956–1962	57 acute	Cancer registry		$Q = 1.0493$ (no clustering)	2. Method has been criticized by Mantel (1967)
	Birmingham, England	1954–1961	118 acute	Cancer registry		$Q = 1.0959$ (no clustering)	
	Sheffield, England	1954–1961	73 acute	Cancer registry		$Q = 0.8381$ (no significant clustering)	
	Northumberland and Durham, England	1951–1960	96 children under 6 years	Data of Knox (1964)		$Q = 1.0430$ (no clustering)	
	Cornwall, England	1947–1962	85 acute	Cancer registry		$Q = 0.8036$ (no significant clustering)	
Goldenberg and Zarowski (1967)	Manitoba, Canada	1956–1964	674 children and adults	Cancer registry and death records	By method of Mustacchi (1965)	In urban Manitoba leukemia (1959–1964) tended to cluster in tracts where cases had previously occurred (1956–1958). This was especially true for Winnipeg North where	Author suggests possibility of leukemia vacuities, i.e., areas of reduced incidence

Reference	Place	Years	Number	Source	Method	Results	Comments
Mainwaring (1966)	Liverpool, England	1955–1964	74 children	2 children's hospitals and death records	By method of Knox (1964)	Excessive clustering of paired cases with short distances and short times apart, especially for pairs closer than 300 days and 4 km. apart. there was also a marked deficiency of leukemia cases in 1959–1964 in those tracts showing a previous absence of cases (1956–1958)	Authors found evidence of clustering for only 3 out of 12 combinations of critical times and critical distances apart
Till et al. (1967)	Greater London, England	1952–1961	483 children	Death records	By method of Knox (1964)	Weak evidence of clustering for lymphoblastic leukemia (under 75 days and $\frac{1}{4}$ km.).	
Knox (1964)	Northumberland and Durham, England	1951–1960	185 children	Local hospitals, cancer registry, and death records	By method of Barton and David (1966) Observed number of paired cases occurring in less than an empirically determined critical space–time distance, which exceeds expected number calculated as a Poisson variable	No evidence of clustering found. Cases of children under 6 years clustered in distances under 1 km. and under 2 months time. No clustering was observed for myeloblastic leukemia cases of any age, nor for lymphoblastic cases over age	1. The age, time, and space limits chosen tend to maximize the observed clustering 2. Confirmation of the validity of the Knox method has been offered by Barton and David (1966)

It may be seen that with the method of Ederer *et al.* (1964) no significant clustering was found in Connecticut or in Los Angeles. Negative findings are also reported from studies of New York City and San Francisco data (Fraumeni and Miller, 1967a). The method of Barton and David (1966) also led to negative findings in a number of English towns and cities. Yet both of these methods found significant clustering for poliomyelitis and other viral diseases. On the other hand, the method of Pinkel *et al.* (1963) and of Knox (1964) tended to show significant clustering. From these often contradictory results it is not possible to infer whether clustering in leukemia does or does not occur. It is also important to remember that the occurrence of clustering would not, per se, substantiate the viral etiology of leukemia because other factors (e.g., radiation exposure and environmental leukemogens) might also be associated with clustering. By the same reasoning, the absence of clustering need not rule out the viral etiology of this disease if it has a long or variable latent period or if the units of time and space examined are larger than those in which the clustering has occurred. In light of this, the observation by Lundin *et al.* (1966) of an excessive number of leukemia deaths 6–8 years apart is suggestive. Note should also be taken of the results based upon the method of Mustacchi (1965) which tend to implicate certain characteristics of space, rather than time, in the clustering of leukemia cases.

B. SEASONAL INCIDENCE

Diseases that vary in frequency with the season of the year are of interest because of the etiological implications of such incidence patterns. The periodicity of the arthropod-borne virus infections, for example, is related to the life cycles of insect vectors. The seasonal variation of human leukemia has been investigated in numerous studies, no doubt a reflection of the tenacious interest in its possible viral etiology.

Leukemia is not an acute, self-limited infectious disease, however, and there are inherent difficulties in studying its seasonality in the classic epidemiological manner. In contrast to the acute infectious diseases, leukemia lacks a clearly defined time of onset and even the acute forms come to medical attention at varying clinical stages of the disease. For this reason, in the various studies and reports the onset date for leukemia has varied from the first symptom noted by the patient or his family to the first clinical sign noted by a physician, the date of the histological diagnosis, or the date of first hospitalization. In acute leukemia, a month or more may elapse between first symptom and hospitalization, and as a result cyclical fluctuations between periods of this length may elude detection.

Methods for case ascertainment have also varied widely in studies of seasonality in leukemia. Studies based upon prevalent cases for any given geographic area are few. Instead, cases treated at one or more hospitals are usually analyzed or, alternatively, a group of patients has been identified from death records. Various combinations of hospitalized and decedent patients have also been utilized.

Because leukemia is a rare disease, the number of patients upon which the studies are based is naturally quite small, rarely does it exceed 100 per year. This undoubtedly contributes to the variability of the observed findings reported in the different studies.

The most recent studies on the seasonal fluctuation of leukemia in the United States are summarized in Table XII. No consistent pattern is evident. In a study of childhood leukemics treated at twelve different medical centers, there was a tendency for the onset of symptoms to occur with greater frequency in the winter and spring (Fraumeni, 1963). Similar findings had been reported earlier from one other hospital studied (Hayes, 1961). On the other hand, no seasonal pattern was found in a rather complete survey of childhood leukemia mortality in Oregon (Meighan and Knox, 1965) and in two other hospital surveys (Steinberg, 1960; Lauriault and Jim, 1966).

Several studies in the United Kingdom have found seasonal peaks for leukemia in the summer (Table XIII). Especially noteworthy are the studies of Lee (1962a, 1963) which were based upon the nearly 4600 cases reported to the National Cancer Registration Scheme from 1946 to 1960. Although no explanation is forthcoming for the summer peaking, it is possible to speculate on the reason for Lee's observation of a winter peak for leukemia, a peak which increased with age and was more prominent in the lymphoid form of the disease. This could be attributed to the greater prevalence of respiratory infections during the winter which are often prodromes of the leukemic process. Of course, one would still have to account for the absence of winter peaks in the other studies.

Other countries have also contributed several reports on the seasonality of leukemia; these are summarized in Table XIV. The absence of a clear-cut seasonal fluctuation in leukemia incidence is, perhaps, the only inference which can be derived from them.

C. Season of Birth

Newborn and very young animals are commonly believed to be unusually susceptible to carcinogenic agents, including viruses (Bailar and Gurian, 1964). Toth (1968), however, has critically reviewed many of the studies of chemical carcinogenesis in newborn animals and has concluded that "the issue is more complex than was anticipated, and is still open to controversy." The idea of the susceptibility of the young together with the previously mentioned childhood peak in leukemia mortality, suggests the

TABLE XII

SUMMARY OF STUDIES ON THE SEASONAL INCIDENCE OF LEUKEMIA IN THE UNITED STATES

Investigator and year	Geographic area and time	Leukemia cases or deaths		Type of leukemia	Leukemia onset dated from	Seasonal pattern noted by investigator	Monthly incidence graphed
		No.	Age				
Fraumeni (1963)	12 U.S. hospitals (National Cooperative Leukemia Survey) 1958-1961	541	Under 16	All	Clinical signs	Winter and spring peaking for both lymphatic and myeloid leukemias	
Lauriault and Jim (1966)	1 hospital in Honolulu, 1954-1964	42	Under 16	Acute	Not stated	None	

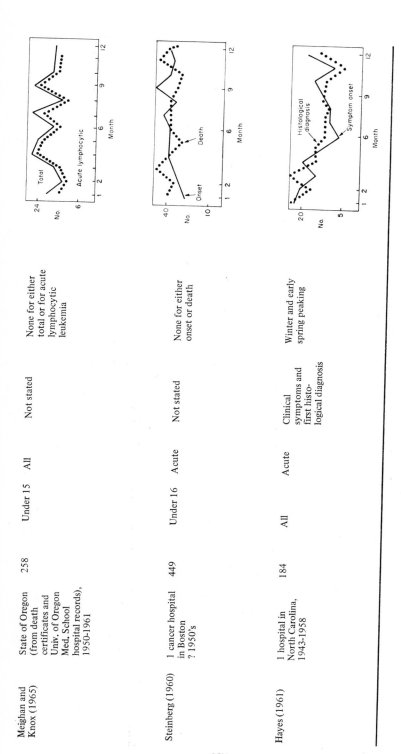

Meighan and Knox (1965)	State of Oregon (from death certificates and Univ. of Oregon Med. School hospital records), 1950-1961	258	Under 15	All	Not stated	None for either total or for acute lymphocytic leukemia
Steinberg (1960)	1 cancer hospital in Boston ? 1950's	449	Under 16	Acute	Not stated	None for either onset or death
Hayes (1961)	1 hospital in North Carolina, 1943-1958	184	All	Acute	Clinical symptoms and first histological diagnosis	Winter and early spring peaking

267

TABLE XIII

SUMMARY OF STUDIES ON THE SEASONAL INCIDENCE OF LEUKEMIA IN THE UNITED KINGDOM

Investigator and year	Geographic area. and time	Leukemia cases or deaths		Type of leukemia	Leukemia onset dated from	Seasonal pattern noted by investigator	Monthly incidence graphed
		No.	Age				
Mainwaring (1966)	Liverpool (its 2 children's hospitals and death certificates), 1955–1964	74	Under 15	Acute	Clinical signs and diagnosis date	May–October slightly greater than Nov.–April especially for lymphatic leukemia and in children under 5	
Swan (1963)	1 London hospital, 1953–1962 ?	56	Adults	Acute	Clinical signs	Winter and spring peaks noted, whether clinical onset, diagnosis or death date employed	

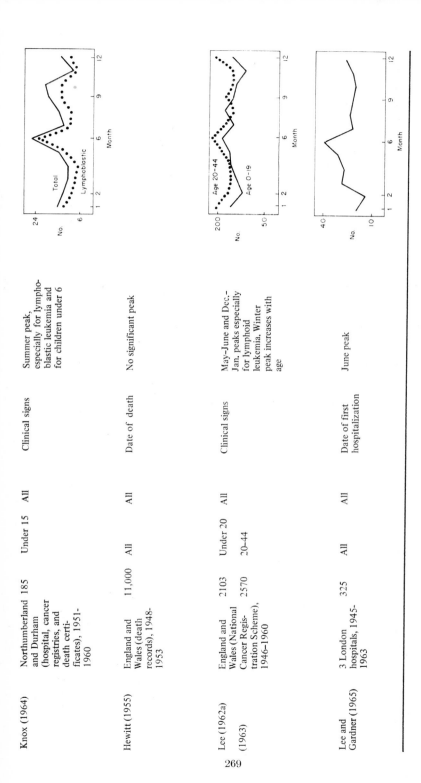

Knox (1964)	Northumberland and Durham (hospital, cancer registries, and death certificates), 1951-1960	185	Under 15	All	Clinical signs	Summer peak, especially for lymphoblastic leukemia and for children under 6
Hewitt (1955)	England and Wales (death records), 1948-1953	11,000	All	All	Date of death	No significant peak
Lee (1962a) (1963)	England and Wales (National Cancer Registration Scheme), 1946-1960	2103 2570	Under 20 20-44	All	Clinical signs	May-June and Dec.-Jan. peaks especially for lymphoid leukemia. Winter peak increases with age
Lee and Gardner (1965)	3 London hospitals, 1945-1963	325	All	All	Date of first hospitalization	June peak

269

TABLE XIV

OTHER STUDIES ON THE SEASONAL INCIDENCE OF LEUKEMIA

Investigator and year	Geographic area and time	Leukemia cases or deaths No.	Age	Type of leukemia	Leukemia onset dated from	Seasonal pattern noted by investigator	Monthly incidence graphed
Gunz (1966)	New Zealand (Survey), 1959-1963	400	Adults	Acute	Clinical signs	No peak for children; summer peak for adults only (in December)	
	1954-1963	286	Under 15	All			
Lee (1964)	New Zealand Victoria, Australia, 1958-1961, 1946-1959	543 987	All	All	Clinical signs	Summer peak (Nov.–Dec.)	
Goldenberg and Zarowski (1967)	Manitoba (cases reported to cancer registry), 1956-1964	700+	All	All	Date reported to registry	Oct.-Dec. peak (coincides with pattern for all neoplasms)	
Radujkov et al. (1965)	Novi Sad Clinic, 1953-1964 ?	118	All	Acute	First clinic visit ?	Spring and fall peaks	

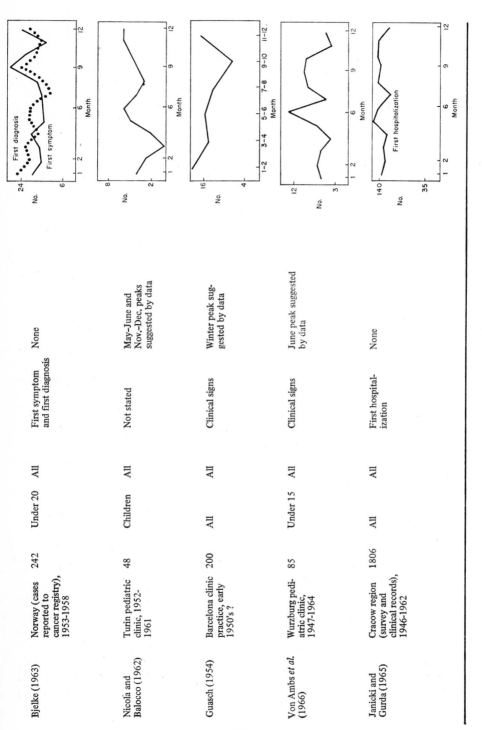

Bjelke (1963)	Norway (cases reported to cancer registry), 1953-1958	242	Under 20	All	First symptom and first diagnosis	None
Nicola and Balocco (1962)	Turin pediatric clinic, 1952-1961	48	Children	All	Not stated	May-June and Nov.-Dec. peaks suggested by data
Guasch (1954)	Barcelona clinic practice, early 1950's ?	200	All	All	Clinical signs	Winter peak suggested by data
Von Ambs et al. (1966)	Wurzburg pediatric clinic, 1947-1964	85	Under 15	All	Clinical signs	June peak suggested by data
Janicki and Gurda (1965)	Cracow region (survey and clinical records), 1946-1962	1806	All	All	First hospitalization	None

271

possibility of an intrauterine or early postnatal viral infection in the pathogenesis of childhood leukemia. If such is the case, and if the viral leukemogen is periodically virulent, then the birth dates of leukemic children would, indeed, be expected to show seasonal or secular fluctuations.

Bailar and Gurian (1964) examined the birth months of all 20,451 persons dying with cancer in Connecticut from 1957 to 1961. The observed distribution by month did not differ substantially from the expected age–sex distribution of cancer mortality rates among persons born in different months. When the Connecticut data for childhood leukemia were augmented with data from four other studies, the distribution by birth month did not differ from that of a sample of United States births. Additional stratification by geographic region and by smaller age categories did not alter the results.

Ederer *et al.* (1965b) analyzed the month of birth among 961 white infants who died of leukemia and among 1552 white infants who died from other neoplasms in 1950 to 1959 in the United States. By restricting the analysis to infants, they hoped to maximize the likelihood of detecting a seasonal agent acting *in utero* or soon after birth to influence leukemia. When compared to total United States births, the leukemic infants showed an excess of May–June births and a deficiency of October–November births. When compared to the infants dying of other neoplasms, the leukemic infants showed similar seasonal differences of statistically significant magnitude. The authors admit that the observed seasonality might have been the result of other factors unrelated to leukemia, including differential survivorship, competing causes of death, and death certification practices. It is also not improbable that the diversity of climatic and other conditions throughout the United States could very well act to obscure the seasonal behavior of a viral leukemogen in any particular geographic subregion.

Stewart and Hewitt (1965b) examined the birth dates of 135 children dying of leukemia before their first birthday and found a significant excess of births in the first half of the calendar year. The authors then collected data on an additional 270 infants and reported no significant seasonality. They offer as a suggestion for the occurrence of seasonal patterns in the birth dates of infants with leukemia and with other neoplasms the following: These infants might come from "a population in which the risk of intrauterine death is exceptionally high, and since foetal death rates in general vary between different seasons, one might well expect some seasonal pattern in the birth dates of live-born members of this particular population."

Some human viruses have periodicities of longer duration than a single season. Fraumeni *et al.* (1966) examined the records of 616 leukemic children under age 5 who were born in New York from 1943 to 1957 and looked for evidence of clustering by birth year within a specific town. No year–town clustering was found, indicating that childhood leukemia does not follow a secular pattern with periods of one calendar year. It should be noted that leukemia under age 15 was found to cluster according to the year of report to the state cancer registry, but that artifacts related to the registration process were probably responsible for this.

An analysis somewhat similar to that of Fraumeni *et al.* (1966) in New York was conducted by Stark and Mantel (1967) in Michigan among 375 leukemic children born during 1950 to 1959 who died in the first 5 years of life. No unusual annual, seasonal or monthly variations in birth date were found, whether the state as a whole or individual counties were considered. Restriction of the analysis to infants dying in the first year of life did not affect the results.

These studies on birth dates of leukemic children have nearly all been based upon the complete or nearly complete ascertainment of cases within given geographic areas. The sizes of the populations studied and the methods employed were adequate to detect evidence of seasonality or secular epidemicity if present. The failure of most of these studies to find periodicity suggests that if a virus initiates the leukemic process in children, it does so independently of the season or the year of birth.

IV. Exposure to Physical and Chemical Agents

A. Ionizing Radiation

Following the sporadic case reports of leukemia developing among individuals working with radiation and the experimental production of leukemia among mice exposed to X-rays, epidemiological studies have also shown that leukemia in humans can be caused by exposure to ionizing radiation. Many of these studies have recently been reviewed by Lilienfeld (1966), and Table XV summarizes the three types of epidemiological studies on radiation leukemogenesis. There is no need to review all of the studies

TABLE XV
Types of Epidemiological Studies on Radiation Leukemogenesis[a]

A. Leukemia in Japanese A-bomb survivors
B. Leukemia in radiologists
C. Leukemia in groups with medical radiation exposures
    1. Ankylosing spondylitis patients
    2. Children radiated for "enlarged thymus"?
    3. Medical internal radiation exposures—^{32}P
    4. Therapeutic and diagnostic radiation in adults
    5. Prenatal diagnostic radiation

[a] Lilienfeld (1966).

in detail; it is generally accepted that ionizing radiation administered in sufficient dose postnatally is leukemogenic. However, there are still several issues of this problem that are not as yet resolved.

One concerns the possible leukemogenic effect of prenatal radiation. Many retrospective studies on this relationship have been carried out and reported on. In these studies, either childhood leukemia cases or deaths were selected and compared to various types of control groups with respect to the frequency of prenatal radiation exposure (Table XVI). It is clear from Table XVI that the most extensive study, judged on the basis of size (Stewart, 1961), shows a relative risk of 1.8. Four additional studies of intermediate size (Ford et al., 1959; Kaplan, 1958; Polhemus and Koch, 1959) show relative risks ranging from 1.3 to 1.7, which are clearly consistent with Stewart's results. Of the four remaining studies, only one had a relative risk greater than 1 (1.9). However, it is also evident that even in the three remaining small studies, the 95% confidence limits indicate that their relative risks are consistent with those of the larger studies. In addi-

TABLE XVI

RELATIVE LEUKEMIA RISK IN RETROSPECTIVE STUDIES OF CHILDREN DYING OF LEUKEMIA AFTER DIAGNOSTIC IRRADIATION in Utero[a]

Reference	Age (years) of leukemics at death	Time of death for leukemics	Mothers receiving abdominal irradiation during pregnancy		Relative risk, 95% limits in parentheses
			Leukemics	Controls	
Stewart (1961)	<10	1953–1955	96/780 (12.3%)	117/1638 (7.1%)	1.8 (2.4–1.4)
Ford et al. (1959)	<10	1951–1955	20/70 (28.6%)	48/247 (19.4%)	1.7 (2.9–0.8)
Kaplan (1958)	?	1955–1956	37/150 (24.7%)	24/150 (16.0%)	1.7 (3.7–1.0)
Kaplan (1958)	?	1955–1956	34/125 (27.2%)	27/125 (21.6%)	1.4 (2.5–0.7)
Polhemus and Koch (1959)	?	1950–1957	72/251 (28.7%)	58/251 (23.1%)	1.3 (2.0–0.9)
Kjeldsberg (1957)	?	1946–1956	5/55 (9.1%)	8/55 (14.5%)	0.6 (2.0–0.2)
Murray et al. (1959)	<20	1940–1957	3/65 (4.6%)	3/65 (4.6%)	1.0 (12.0–0.6)
Murray et al. (1959)	<20	1940–1957	3/65 (4.6%)	7/93 (7.5%)	0.6 (2.4–0.1)
Murray et al. (1959)	<20	1940–1957	3/65 (4.6%)	2/82 (2.4%)	1.9 (40.0–1.1)

[a] United Nations Scientific Committee on the Effects of Atomic Radiation (1964).

tion, when one considers the diversity of the selected control groups and the sampling variability, the results are remarkably consistent in showing an excess frequency of leukemia among children of radiation-exposed mothers. These results were once again obtained by Graham *et al.* (1966) in a large-scale retrospective study of leukemia in three states of the United States.

There has been considerable interest in the relationship of intrauterine radiation to leukemia because it provides information on the possible effect of low-dose radiation. Several prospective and cohort studies have been carried out because of inherent difficulties in the reported retrospective studies (Lilienfeld *et al.*, 1967). An uncontrolled study by Court-Brown *et al.* (1960a) did not confirm the relationship. A retrospective cohort study by MacMahon (1962), which had some but not all of the advantages of a prospective study, indicated that offspring of mothers exposed to prenatal radiation had a frequency of leukemia that was about 40% higher than the non-X-rayed control group. A preliminary report of a prospective study by Diamond (1968) of 19,348 X-ray-exposed white and Negro women with single births and 34,754 nonexposed white and Negro women offers some interesting findings. Among white exposed women the death rate of their offspring was 1.84× higher than of the controls, whereas among Negro women no differences were noted (Table XVII). Of special interest was the excess death rate in the exposed group which prevailed for practically all causes of death. The relative risk for leukemia deaths in the white group was 2.86 and for neoplasms in general, 1.29. The absence of a relationship in Negroes and the presence of an excess mortality for all causes of death as well as for leukemia among the white exposed group is difficult to interpret. This does suggest, however, that the observed relationship of leukemia to intrauterine radiation may not be causal but indirect.

These relationships noted in Diamond's (1968) study continued to persist after adjustments for operative procedure at delivery and complications of pregnancy. Nevertheless, it is felt that the following selective factors may be involved in this indirect association:

1. Among whites, X-ray exposure may more likely be associated with definite indications for such a procedure while among Negroes, X-ray exposure may more likely be a random event.

2. Women of lower socioeconomic levels may more likely have conditions of pregnancy or past histories leading to X-ray exposure, and the lower socioeconomic level is probably associated with a higher perinatal and childhood mortality. Thus, exposed whites and all Negroes may more likely experience a higher mortality.

3. Women of lower socioeconomic levels probably receive poorer prenatal medical care, and their children poorer postnatal care. This may

TABLE XVII

NUMBER OF DEATHS AND DEATH RATES PER 100,000 PERSON YEARS AT RISK BY CAUSE[a,b]

Cause (ISC[c] code No.)	White				Negro			
	Exposed		Controls		Exposed		Controls	
	No.	Rate	No.	Rate	No.	Rate	No.	Rate
Infective and parasitic diseases (001–138)	7	8.0	11	6.3	11	14.2	21	15.4
Neoplasms (140–205)	11	12.5	17	9.7	3	3.9	11	8.1
(Leukemia)	(7)	(8.0)	(5)	(2.8)	(0)	(0.0)	(4)	(2.9)
Diseases of the nervous system and sense organs (330–398)	13	14.8	14	8.0	16	20.7	24	17.6
Diseases of the respiratory system (470–527)	42	47.9	31	17.7	56	72.4	89	65.4
Diseases of the digestive system (530–587)	11	12.5	11	6.3	14	18.1	24	17.6
Congenital malformations (750–759)	25	28.5	37	21.1	13	16.8	30	22.0
Accidents, poisonings, and violence (800–999)	28	31.9	27	15.4	31	40.1	67	49.2
Other	11	12.5	13	7.4	13	16.8	34	25.0
Total	148	168.7	161	91.7	157	203.1	300	220.4
No. of person years	87,740		175,608		77,295		136,146	

[a] For those found alive or dead after 28 days only.
[b] Diamond (1968).
[c] International Statistical Classification.

also contribute to higher mortality in the white exposed and in all Negroes.

These questions will continue to be explored through analyses of existing study data as well as special analyses of additional data which will be collected for subsamples of the study population. In addition, other variables which may have a relation to mortality will be investigated, including maternal age, parity, previous prenatal and childhood mortality in the sibs of the study children, length of gestation, birth weight, and birth order.

Clearly, the issue of the relationship of prenatal radiation to leukemia is far from settled. Continued study is certainly indicated, although it is not completely clear which approach would be most fruitful. It is possible that an interaction of X-ray exposure with another etiological factor is necessary to produce leukemia; this possibility will be discussed later.

Of interest is the finding of Graham et al. (1966) who observed in the Tri-State Leukemia Study that mothers of children with leukemia gave a more frequent history of exposure to diagnostic radiation prior to the conception of the child than did the control group (Table XVIII). The data were adjusted for different combinations of factors shown to have a possible association with either leukemia or preconception radiation. This association was absent with regard to the history of preconception radiation of the father. A similar observation for maternal exposure was made earlier by Stewart et al. (1958) and co-workers but attracted very little attention. Fraumeni and Miller (1967b) suggest that the causal relationship between

TABLE XVIII

ADJUSTED PERCENTAGE OF MOTHERS EXPOSED TO DIAGNOSTIC RADIATION
PRIOR TO CONCEPTION, OF CASES AND CONTROLS, WITH
ESTIMATED RELATIVE RISK OF LEUKEMIA[a]

| | Percent irradiated | | | |
| | Cases (313) | Controls (853) | Relative risk | Probability |
Adjusted for				
Year of birth, age of mother, and birth order	46.0	36.4	1.55	0.003
Year of birth, age of mother, and pregnancy order	46.2	36.5	1.56	0.003
Year of birth, age of mother, miscarriages and stillbirths	46.7	36.2	1.60	<0.001
Age of mother, miscarriages and stillbirths, and birth order	47.1	34.0	1.73	<0.001
Age of mother, miscarriages and stillbirths, and pregnancy order	46.9	34.1	1.73	<0.001

[a] Graham et al. (1966).

preconception radiation and leukemia is doubtful. They point out that a prospective investigation of 17,700 children by the Atomic Bomb Casualty Commission (ABCC) failed to show any increase in leukemia after preconception radiation, despite the very heavy exposure (Hoshino *et al.*, 1967). However, the sample size in the ABCC study was such that only a fourfold excess risk would have been detected, whereas in the study by Graham *et al.* (1966) the relative risk was of the order of 1.55 to 1.73. Clearly, the ABCC study did not include a sufficiently large sample in order to detect a 1.73 risk.

If there is a relationship between chromosomal abnormality and leukemia, it is not biologically unreasonable to suspect a possible relationship between preconception radiation and leukemia. It is conceivable that radiation of the ovary may produce chromosomal damage in the ova. Additional epidemiological studies of sufficient size would be in order to evaluate this relationship. It would also be advantageous to study this issue directly by histological examination, as well as tissue culture examination, of ovarian tissue. These observations should be studied to determine their possible relationship to a history of prior radiation exposure.

B. OTHER AGENTS

The evidence that certain chemicals have an effect on the bone marrow suggests the possibility that chemicals may be leukemogenic. However, supporting evidence for such an effect is meager. Clinical observations do suggest that benzene exposure is leukemogenic (Vigliani and Saita, 1964; Cronkite, 1961). Case reports, reviewed by McCarthy and Chalmers (1964), have also suggested that phenylbutazone therapy may result in leukemia, and Fraumeni and Miller (1967a) have also reported that chloramphenicol therapy may have such an effect. The totality of all of the results of these reports can only be regarded as suggestive. Detailed and systematic investigation by well designed, large-scale epidemiological studies are needed.

V. Association with Mongolism and Other Chromosomal Abnormalities

A firmly established epidemiological relationship is that of leukemia with mongolism. This has been determined by the study of (*1*) the frequency of mongoloids among cases with leukemia and (*2*) the frequency of mortality from leukemia among mongoloids. These studies have been recently reviewed by Lilienfeld (1969) and summarized in Tables XIX and XX describing the methods of selection, the comparison groups, and the results.

Table XIX summarizes seven studies that report on the frequency of mongoloids among cases of leukemia, which ranges from 1.3 to 7.2% as compared to 0.03 to 0.3% among the comparison groups. The degree of excess of mongoloids among leukemic children ranged from 6 to 100×.

Variations in the estimates of the excess frequency of mongoloids are probably the result of differences in diagnostic criteria as well as in the methods of selection of leukemia cases and comparison groups. Table XX summarizes four studies on the frequency of leukemia among mongoloids compared to the observed frequency in a comparison group or frequency expected on the basis of mortality experience. In general, the frequency of leukemia among mongoloids is about 8 to 18× greater than expected. Once again, the variations no doubt reflect differences in the diagnostic criteria of leukemia and in the frequency of leukemia in the different geographic areas selected for study. However, it should be noted that only two studies used a comparative group and in no study was a control group actually selected in a systematic random fashion (Holland et al., 1962; DeWolff, 1964).

Turner (1962) reported on the results of a study in Pennsylvania in which he found the leukemia mortality rate among mongoloids to be 2.2 per 1000 males and 1.7 for females as compared with 0.08 per 1000 male and 0.04 for other female mental defectives. Of interest are his observations that the increased risk of leukemia in the mongoloid population is present throughout life and not limited to any specific type of leukemia but does involve the type appropriate to the age of the affected individual.

Another aspect of the relationship of mongolism with leukemia is the familial aggregation of these two conditions. There are reports on the occurrence of leukemia among family members of mongoloids and of mongolism among family members of children with leukemia (Miller et al., 1961; Buckton et al., 1961). The mortality experience of the parents of 1620 mongoloid children was analyzed and compared with that expected from the national death rates in England and Wales by Holland et al. (1962). The mortality experience of parents from all causes was somewhat lower than expected; 3 deaths occurred from leukemia where 1.2 were expected and 57 deaths from other forms of cancer where 64 were expected. In a national cooperative study of leukemia in the United States, Miller (1963) reported 5 cases of mongolism among 1000 sibs of leukemic children as compared to an expectancy of 1.4—a difference which was considered to be statistically significant. Stark (1963) had consistent findings in a smaller series. In contrast, Barber and Spiers (1964) did not observe such an excess frequency in their study of the sibs of 1795 leukemia cases in England: 5.9 mongoloids were to be expected and 7 were actually observed.

The relationship of mongolism to leukemia is of considerable interest in view of the following observations in mongoloids: (1) the nuclei of the polymorphonuclear cells have fewer lobes than normal (Turpin and Bernyer, 1947; Shapiro, 1949; Lüers and Lüers, 1954; Mittwoch, 1957), (2) there is a shift to the left of the polymorphonuclear leukocytes and a decrease in

TABLE XIX

SUMMARY OF STUDIES SHOWING FREQUENCY OF MONGOLOIDS AMONG CASES OF LEUKEMIA AND A COMPARISON GROUP[a]

Investigator	Years of study	Methods of selection	Leukemia cases			Comparison group				Degree of excess
			Total No.	Mongoloids No.	%	Type	Total No.	Mongoloids No.	%	
Iverson (1960)	1946–1957	Case records throughout Denmark of patients of 0 to 14 years admitted to hospitals for first time with diagnosis of leukemia	273	5	1.8	Expected on basis of mongolism incidence of 1/600	—	0.5	—	10
Knox (1964)	1951–1960	Leukemia in children with onset before 15th birthday in the north of England	185	9	4.9	—	—	—	—	—

Reference	Period	Study population	No.	Obs.	Rate	Comparison group	No.	Obs.	Rate	Ratio
Stewart et al. (1958)	1953–1955	Deaths from leukemia or cancer in children under 10 years of age in England and Wales	667	17	2.5	Deaths from other cancers of childhood	739	1	0.1	25
						Live children matched for sex, age, locality	1416	0	0	—
Ager et al. (1965)	1953–1957	Deaths 0–4 years of age from leukemia in Minnesota	124	9	7.2	Highest recorded incidence of mongolism	—	—	0.3	21
Barber and Spiers (1964)	1953–1960	Deaths from leukemia and other childhood cancers in England and Wales before age of 10 years	1795	49	2.7	Deaths from other cancers of childhood	1985	3	0.2	10–100
						Live children matched for sex, age, locality	3778	1	0.03	—
Wald et al. (1961)	1955–1959	Leukemia deaths in Pennsylvania	—	21	—	Expected on basis of mongolism incidence of 1.5 per 1000	—	2	—	10
Miller (1963)	1958–1961	Children with leukemia under 16 years of age in 12 medical groups in U.S. (white children)	459	6	1.3	Neighborhood controls matched by age, birth order, family size, and race	459	0 (1 expected based on incidence data)	0	6

a Lilienfeld (1969).

TABLE XX

SUMMARY OF STUDIES SHOWING FREQUENCY OF LEUKEMIA AMONG MONGOLOIDS AND A COMPARISON GROUP OR EXPECTED FREQUENCY BASED ON MORTALITY EXPERIENCE[a]

Investigator	Years of study	Mongoloids			Comparison group					Degree of excess
		Methods of selection	Total No.	Leukemia		Type	Total No.	Leukemia		
				No.	%			No.	%	
Merrit and Harris (1956)	1930–1955	Cases diagnosed at Duke University Hospital	255	4	1.6	None	—	—	—	—
Carter (1958)	1944–1955	Survey of children who attended The Hospital for Sick Children in London to determine survivorship of mongoloids	725	3	0.4	None	—	—	—	—

Investigators	Period	Description	No.	Observed		Expected number of deaths from leukemia from national mortality rates			
Holland et al. (1962)	1944–1955	Children at The Hospital for Sick Children in London	738	5	0.7	—	—	0.19	—
	1946–1957	Children notified to Medical Officer of Health or to Mental Health Dept. of Middlesex County Council	365	0	0	—	—	0.06	—
	1948–1959	Patients diagnosed or admitted to 1 of 5 mental deficiency hospitals (survivorship)	930	2	0.2	(Same as above)	—	0.14	—
Total			—	7					
DeWolff (1964)	1945–1961	Children examined at Hospital for Sick Children in Aarau (Switzerland)	134	5	3.7	Frequency of leukemia hospital patients over 7-year period 10,171	45	0.39 / 0.4	18 / 8-9

[a] Lilienfeld (1969).

the number of large lymphocytes, and (3) a decrease in the frequency of drumsticks (nuclear appendages) in their polymorphonuclear leukocytes. Related to this is a finding in a great majority of cases of chronic granulocytic leukemia of what has been described as the Ph^1 (Philadelphia) chromosome. It is a specific abnormality in which chromosome No. 21 has lost approximately one-half of one of its arms; the cause or causes are unknown.

Explanations of the relationship of mongolism to leukemia are at present speculative. It has been suggested that a gene located on the trisomic chromosome No. 21 may control granulopoiesis. It has also been postulated that the relationship is indirect, that is, each disease may be a result of the same etiological agent. For example, radiation could produce nondisjunction and result in trisomy 21 and independently produce leukemia. Since the nondisjunction would have to occur prior to or immediately after conception, one would expect that mongoloids with leukemia would be most prevalent and perhaps even limited to the younger age groups. The only available data for evaluating this is that of Turner (1962) indicating that the excess leukemia risk is present throughout life.

TABLE XXI

CONGENITAL CYTOGENETIC DISORDERS AND LEUKEMIA-LYMPHOMA[a]

Congenital disorder	Cytogenetic defect	Associated leukemia-lymphoma
Down's syndrome (mongolism)	Trisomy-21	Risk of leukemia known to be 20-fold or greater
Klinefelter's syndrome (seminiferous tubule dysgenesis)	XXY or mosaic	Case reports: 1 acute myelogenous leukemia 1 chronic myelogenous leukemia 1 acute lymphocytic leukemia 2 reticulum cell sarcomas 1 acute undifferentiated leukemia
D-trisomy (Pātau's syndrome of multiple anomalies)	Trisomy in group 13–15	Case reports: 1 congenital myeloblastic leukemia 1 acute myelogenous leukemia
Bloom's syndrome (low birth weight, stunted growth, sun-sensitive telangiectatic erythema of face)	Chromosome breakage and rearrangement of cultured blood cells	23 cases reviewed by Sawitsky et al.[b]; 2 acute myelogenous leukemias; 1 acute leukemia
Fanconi's syndrome (congenital pancytopenia with multiple anomalies)	Chromosome breakage and rearrangement of cultured blood cells	2 case reports with acute monocytic leukemia

[a] Fraumeni and Miller (1967a).
[b] Sawitsky et al. (1966).

TABLE XXII

CASE REPORTS OF AGGREGATION OF CONGENITAL CHROMOSOMAL
ABNORMALITIES AND LEUKEMIA IN FAMILIES[a]

Type of leukemia	Chromosomal abnormality	Reference
Sibships[b]		
Acute lymphocytic and acute myelogenous	XX/XXY mosaicism	Baikie *et al.* (1961)
Acute lymphocytic	Down's syndrome (15/21 translocation)[c] in 3 sibs	Buckton *et al.* (1961)
Acute lymphocytic	Down's syndrome in 2 sibs	Karhausen and Hutchison (1966)
Acute stem cell	Down's syndrome in 2 sibs	Conen *et al.* (1966)
Families		
Chronic lymphocytic (in father)	Son with XXXXY sex-chromosome complement; sister and niece with Down's syndrome (trisomy-21)	
Leukemia (5 cases)[d]	Down's syndrome in 1 child[d]	Miller *et al.* (1961); Heath and Moloney (1965)

[a] Miller (1966).

[b] 1 diagnosis per child.

[c] Mother 15/21-translocation carrier.

[d] Over three generations.

Pertinent to this hypothesis is the recently published report of an experiment in which 7,12-dimethylbenz[a]anthracene (DMBA) in repeated doses produced trisomy of one group of chromosomes and leukemia in rats; this occurred in 10 or 43% of leukemic rats in three series of experiments (Sugiyama *et al.*, 1967). This confirmed a previous report of a similar experiment where in a different rat strain one case was produced by 7,12-DMBA.

Another possible explanation is that individuals with chromosomal abnormalities in general are more susceptible to specific environmental agents that produce leukemia, as well as malignancies in general (DeGrouchy, 1966). Recently, Fraumeni and Miller (1967a), in discussing various epidemiological aspects of leukemia, indicated that there is suggestive evidence of an increased risk of leukemia in other clinical syndromes with chromosomal abnormalities, for example, the syndromes of Bloom and Fanconi, although the other chromosomal disorders do not demonstrate as great an increase in risk (Table XXI).

Another approach to a better understanding of this issue was presented by Miller (1966), who summarized case reports suggesting the presence of familial aggregation of several chromosomal abnormalities and leukemia (Table XXII).

Conceptually, Fraumeni and Miller's (1967a) hypothesis is an attractive one. Unfortunately, the statistical significance of individual case reports on the association of diseases in an individual or within a family is difficult to evaluate since these cases are no doubt selectively reported. In view of the importance of this hypothesis, systematic epidemiological studies of these relationships are clearly indicated.

Recently, Turner's observations in Pennsylvania were supplemented by Jackson et al. (1968) to include California; the mortality experience of mongoloids in California state hospitals for 1952 to 1962 were compared with mongoloids in Pennsylvania state and private hospitals for 1945 to 1959. In California, they observed 5 deaths from leukemia as compared to an expected 0.426 on the basis of age-specific mortality rates, a twelve-fold excess, whereas in Pennsylvania, the observed number was 17 with an expectancy of 0.279, a sixty-one-fold excess. In addition, the California leukemia deaths were limited to the 5–9 year age group in contrast to Pennsylvania where they included all ages.

Jackson et al. (1968) explained that the different mortality experience in these two states may be the result of differences in the occurrence of leukemogenic agents in the environments of the two populations which act on the same genetic substrate, namely mongolism. Of course, it is possible to postulate another explanation not mentioned by Jackson et al. Perhaps the causes of nondisjunction which result in mongolism differ in these two populations and such causes differentially result in leukemia. Although this explanation appears unlikely, it deserves consideration in the evaluation of these data.

Despite this reservation, these observations are of considerable interest and indicate that similar studies should be carried out in other geographic areas. It might then be possible to delineate high and low rate areas and compare such areas on as many epidemiological and environmental characteristics as possible. The necessity for a sufficient number of cases would probably require a national study, but the results might well warrant the effort.

VI. Maternal Age and Birth Order

The prevailing interest in a possible relationship between childhood leukemia and maternal age at time of birth and birth order reflects a general interest in the relationship of these factors to childhood diseases. This interest has been intensified by the confirmed relationship of leukemia to mongolism and of mongolism to maternal age.

Manning and Carroll (1957), in their study of 188 children with leukemia, 42 with lymphoma, 93 with other malignancies, and 50 controls selected from an orthopedic clinic, noted that the mean age of the mothers was higher at birth than that of the other groups and the children with leukemia were more frequently of the birth order of 3 and over. In the Oxford survey, Stewart et al. (1958) reported that 6.9% of their leukemic children were born to mothers over 40 years of age as compared to 3.5% of children with other malignancies. They also found a 10% excess of first born children in their leukemia group as compared to the national birth data. In contrast to these findings, however, Steinberg (1960), in his study of 249 children with leukemia using an internal method of analysis without a control group, reported no relationship with either maternal age or birth order.

The studies just discussed were not specifically designed as an analysis of birth characteristics, but they did stimulate an intensive investigation of this issue by MacMahon and Newill (1962). They were able to study 4198 children who had died from malignant diseases in New England or the Middle Atlantic States. These investigators estimated from their data that first births had a childhood mortality from leukemia that was 50% higher than fifth and later births and that children with mothers 40 years of age and over had almost a 40% higher mortality than mothers under 20 years of age. No other childhood malignancy studied showed any similar relationships with maternal age or birth order.

Ager et al. (1965), in a study of 112 children 0–4 years of age with leukemia, confirmed these findings on the relationship to maternal age; the age at birth of child for mothers of leukemic children was higher on the average by 2 years than were the controls. In the case–control comparison, they did not note any differences in birth order, but when a comparison was made between the birth order distribution of their cases and of all of the births in Minnesota during the same time period, they observed a slight excess of low-order births among the leukemics.

These findings for both maternal age and birth order were not confirmed by Graham et al. (1966) in their Tri-State Leukemia Study, with the exception of their leukemic children born prior to 1950 who were more frequently first born than were the controls (52.1 vs. 33.8%).

The most recent study of this problem was made by Stark and Mantel (1966), who analyzed the leukemia mortality experience for Michigan for the period 1950–1964 by maternal age and birth order. Their detailed statistical analysis of these data indicated that the risk of death from childhood leukemia increased with advancing maternal age and decreased with advancing birth order. They also noted that the risk of death from all causes in childhood increased with advancing birth order and decreased with advancing maternal age until 34 years of age—after this age the death rate increased slightly. In view of these different patterns, they suggested that the variables of maternal age and birth order may be closely associated with the etiological agents of childhood leukemia.

It is clear that the results of the different studies have been inconsistent. However, for the most part and particularly in the better controlled studies, there does appear to be an effect of maternal age and birth order. Further investigation is necessary, preferably with a large series of leukemia deaths similar to that used by Stark and Mantel (1966). A study covering several states would undoubtedly be necessary in order to arrive at a more definitive answer to this problem. The issue is pertinent today because of the suggestive relationship of leukemia to chromosomal abnormalities. For example, the finding that leukemia mortality increases with maternal age at birth is an epidemiological characteristic that is consistent with the chromosomal hypothesis since the frequency of such chromosomal abnormalities as mongolism does increase with maternal age. On the other hand, an inverse relationship of leukemia with birth order is difficult to explain on this basis and another explanation must be sought. A more definitive study would help expedite a clearer understanding of the relationship between leukemia, maternal age, and birth order.

VII. Familial Aggregation

The conventional approach to the search for possible genetic implications of a disease is to investigate the familial aggregation of the disease. The studies of familial aggregation of leukemia have been recently reviewed by Kolmeier and Bayrd (1963) and Rucknagel (1966) and, therefore, a detailed review at this time does not seem justified.

There have been many case reports of familial leukemia in the literature—about 100. The interpretation of such reports is difficult because of possible selective biases, and a more systematic approach utilizing samples of cases and controls is necessary. Videbaek (1947), in the first large-scale familial study, compared 209 leukemia patients to 200 healthy controls and found 17 cases of leukemia among 4041 relatives of patients as compared to 1 case among 3641 relatives of the control patients. Busk (1954), however, in a critical evaluation of Videbaek's study, pointed out some of the biases that were probably present in Videbaek's study design. In addition, he carried out some additional computations using data from the Danish Cancer Registry and concluded that Videbaek's data do not actually show familial aggregation.

Videbaek's report was followed by reports of similar studies by Amiotti (1953), Morganti and Cresseri (1954), Guasch (1954), Kaliampetos (1954), and Steinberg (1957), all of whom reported no familial aggregation of leukemia. These studies are all vulnerable to criticism on the basis of inadequate selection of control or comparison groups. Two of these studies

(Amiotti, 1953; Steinberg, 1957) were limited to leukemia in children. In attempting to explain the reports in the literature of familial cases of leukemia, Steinberg did some interesting computations. He determined that the probability of developing leukemia by age 35—from U.S. life tables and age-specific death rates—was about 0.001. If a patient had 10 relatives who have on the average survived age 35, the estimated probability of at least 1 having leukemia is about 0.01. In 1956, there were 11,396 deaths from leukemia in the United States, and one would expect about 100 of these patients to have had a relative with leukemia. Therefore, the reports in the literature of a fair number of families with 2 or more cases of leukemia are not unexpected.

However, Steinberg goes on to point out that there are repeated instances of families in which there is a high concentration of leukemia occurrence. For example, Steinberg reports on three families in one of which 5 of 8 children died of acute leukemia, in another 3 of 7, and another 4 of 12. Calculations indicate that such occurrences are highly improbable—the probability being less than 1×10^{-6}. Steinberg emphasizes that "very rarely . . . heredity may be of importance in determining susceptibility to acute leukemia. In general, however, it does not seem to play a significant role."

More recently two epidemiological studies on childhood leukemia were able to provide some information on familial aggregation. In the Oxford Survey of Childhood Cancers, which included 780 cases of leukemia, Stewart (1961) reported an increased frequency of leukemia "fraternities" in the case group as compared with the controls. However, it was not possible from the published data to determine the actual frequencies among case and control relatives.

In a national study in the United States of almost 450 leukemic children and matched controls, out of 1000 sibs of leukemic cases, 5 had leukemia as compared to none among 956 sibs of the control children (Miller, 1963). In addition, Miller noted an excess frequency of Down's syndrome among sibs of the cases (5 as compared to about 1.4 expected).

Once again, from the published data, it is difficult to definitely state that leukemia aggregates in families. There is suggestive evidence from the more recent studies (Stewart, 1961; Miller, 1963) on childhood leukemia that there is a degree of familial aggregation, although it must be granted that it is not large. A major difficulty in evaluating the published results of many of these studies stems from the inadequacy of selection of control groups and the problems of diagnosis. In addition, it would be extremely desirable to include in an analysis of such data specific cytological types of leukemia.

In the Tri-State Leukemia Study (Graham *et al.*, 1966), information was collected on the mortality experience of relatives of cases and controls. These data are being analyzed at present and the results should soon be forthcoming.

As previously indicated, studies of familial aggregation have been oriented primarily toward a search for a genetic basis for leukemia. However, these data also have value from the viewpoint of a viral hypothesis since familial aggregation, if limited to immediate family members, represents one aspect of the study of "clustering."

One can extend the concept of family to include nonbiologically related family members such as husbands and wives in order to evaluate nongenetic "clustering" in families. Milham (1965) analyzed the death certificates of 876 spouses of widows and widowers who died of leukemia in upstate New York during 1951 to 1961 and compared them with a control group of deaths matched for age, sex, race, marital status, township of residence, and date of death (within 4 weeks). Seven deaths from leukemia were ascertained among the spouses of the 876 leukemia deaths as compared to 5 among the matched controls. Milham concluded that the results were consistent with the hypothesis that "adult leukemia is not contagious in the usual sense." This approach is interesting and the results should be confirmed in a larger study because a moderate degree of association would not be detected with a sample of this size.

VIII. Twin Studies

Over the years case reports have appeared of concordant pairs of twins with leukemia. It is impossible to evaluate adequately the degree of selective bias in such reports, and, unfortunately, it is impossible to use these data on twins for information on any existing genetic influences in leukemia; however, an initial attempt at a systematic study was made by MacMahon and Levy (1964) who assembled a series of 72 twin sets, in which one member had leukemia. The investigators matched birth and death certificates of children born between 1947 and 1960 in the northeastern United States; and included 3 additional series of twin children with leukemia who had been interviewed in other studies. In 5 of these sets, both members were affected; a concordance frequency of 11% for like-sex pairs and a frequency of 25% for probable monozygotic pairs was estimated. The authors also noted a similarity between pair members who were concordant for leukemia in the ages of onset and of death.

In an effort to confirm these observations, Hewitt et al. (1966) analyzed the data collected in the Oxford Survey of Childhood Cancers with negative results. Miller (1968) analyzed the death certificates for all children (21,659) under 15 years of age who had died of cancer in the United States between 1960 and 1964 and observed five pairs of like-sexed twins with leukemia, all under 6 years of age. He was unable, however, to obtain concordance rates since he did not know the number of twin pairs at risk according to sex or zygosity. He did, nevertheless, estimate that a 20% concordance rate for monozygotic twin pairs (suggested by MacMahon and Levy) would result in nine like-sexed concordant pairs, and, therefore, his data confirm those of MacMahon and Levy.

MacMahon and Levy reported in their study that about 25 pairs of twins with both members affected with leukemia had been reported in the world's literature by 1964, the year of their report. Twenty-two of these 25 pairs were reported as monozygotic. It is of interest that during 1966 to 1967, several investigators (Goh *et al.*, 1967; Goh and Swisher, 1965; Woodliff *et al.*, 1966; Jacobs *et al.*, 1966) who were studying the relationship of chromosomal abnormalities to leukemia, reported four monozygotic twin pairs, one member of which had leukemia and the other who did not.

One can thus readily appreciate the difficulty in evaluating the results of the twin studies reported thus far. Individual case reports are far from satisfactory. Estimating concordance frequencies indirectly leaves a great deal to be desired. In order to utilize observations of the disease in twins, it is clearly essential to obtain the necessary data from a registry of twins, or from a national study of twin pairs. In a study satisfying these requirements one could select all members of twin pairs with leukemia and first determine the zygosity, using objective and standard methods and then the presence of leukemia. A large-scale collaborative effort is required. Perhaps data will become available from the several existing twin registries. At present it is necessary to use caution and refrain from making any judgment on possible inferences from the reported studies to date.

IX. Overview

A. CONCEPTUAL MODELS

Several investigators exploring the epidemiological aspects of leukemia have developed models or conceptual frameworks in an attempt to explain the various epidemiological features of this disease. Miller (1967a) presented one such model which attempted to delineate those groups with an exceptionally high risk of leukemia (Table XXIII). He pointed out that despite the cytogenetic diversity of these groups, there is a common denominator present in each high risk group, either a genetic or chromosomal characteristic, which may play a role in leukemogenesis (Table XXIV). It is noteworthy that the high risk groups not characterized by exposure to environmental agents, such as radiation, were children, whereas the radiation–exposed groups were adults. Perhaps, there is a need to distinguish between childhood and adult leukemia; childhood leukemia

TABLE XXIII
GROUPS AT EXCEPTIONALLY HIGH RISK OF LEUKEMIA[a]

Group	Approximate risk	Time interval	References
Identical twins of children with leukemia	1 in 5[b]	Weeks or months	MacMahon and Levy (1964)
Radiation-treated polycythemia vera	1 in 6	10–15 years	Modan and Lilienfeld (1965)
Bloom's syndrome	1 in 8[c]	<30 years of age	Sawitsky et al. (1966)
Hiroshima survivors who were within 1000 meters of the hypocenter	1 in 60	12 years	Brill et al. (1962)
Down's syndrome	1 in 95	<10 years of age	Barber and Spiers (1964)
Radiation-treated patients with ankylosing spondylitis	1 in 270	15 years	Court-Brown and Doll (1965)
Sibs of leukemic children	1 in 720	10 years	Miller (1963), Stewart (1961)
U.S. Caucasian children <15 years of age	1 in 2880	10 years	National Center for Health Statistics (1964)

[a] Miller (1967b).

[b] Of 22 identical twins with leukemia, the co-twin was affected in 5 instances.

[c] Three leukemics among 23 persons with Bloom's syndrome.

may be genetically or chromosomally determined, whereas adult leukemia may be, to a large degree, environmentally determined. This inference would suggest that the direction of epidemiological studies should differ in adults and children.

A more detailed type of model was presented by Stewart and Hewitt (1965a) from their analysis of data on childhood leukemia. They categorized

TABLE XXIV
DISTINCTIVE GENETIC FEATURES OF GROUPS AT HIGH RISK OF LEUKEMIA[a]

High-risk category	Genetic feature
Identical twin of child with leukemia	Genetically identical
Bloom's and Fanconi's syndromes	Genetically induced chromosomal fragility
Radiation-treated polycythemia	Aneuploidy prior to radiation; chromosomal breaks subsequently
Exposure to ionizing radiation or benzene	Long-persisting chromosomal breaks
Down's syndrome	Congenital aneuploidy

[a] Miller (1967b).

TABLE XXV

Provisional List of Some Components of Childhood Leukemia Mortality[a]

Component	Typical age at death (years)	Possible time of origin
Familial cases	0, 1	Prezygotic
"Excess" cases in first born children	2, 3	?
Nongranular cases	2, 3, 4, 5	?
"Normal" childhood leukemia (including mongoloid cases?)	3, 4	?
Radiogenic cases		
A. Obstetric radiology	4, 5	Third trimester of pregnancy
"Clustered" cases	8	?
	0–5	?
Radiogenic cases		
B. Postnatal treatment of thymus, etc.	5–9	Infancy

[a] Stewart and Hewitt (1965a).

the various components of childhood leukemia mortality by typical age at death and possible time of origin (Table XXV). The etiological implications are apparent although it must be granted that many of these inferences are speculative.

Burch (1962, 1964, 1965), in a series of papers, has developed a mathematical model for leukemogenesis based on the assumption that a given number of mutations of genes and chromosomes are required for the development of leukemia. By applying this model to existing epidemiological data, he has inferred that various combinations of inherited, somatic mutations and possible nongenetic factors will produce the different types of leukemias. For example, leukemias in childhood and adolescence generally develop from one inherited and two somatic mutations together with a nongenetic factor; the nongenetic factor could be an infection with a virus. In contrast, chronic lymphatic leukemia in adults would develop from a combination of one inherited and three somatic mutations. Although such a model is conceptually fascinating, its value for suggesting particular directions for research is not clear; also, it is not clear what the biological mechanism may be by which the number of different mutations can result in different cell types of leukemia.

The most recent attempt to integrate, at least for childhood leukemia, all the findings on the different possible etiological factors using actual epidemiological data was made by Gibson et al. (1968). They used data collected as part of the Tri-State Leukemia Study (see above) for leukemic children, 1–4 years of age, who represented 51% of 319 leukemia cases under 15 years of age (Graham *et al.*, 1966). They tried to evaluate the contributions to the risk of developing leukemia of the following four risk factors: preconception radiation, reproductive wastage (history of miscarriages and stillbirths) prior to conception of subject, *in utero* radiation, and history of childhood virus diseases contracted more than 12 months prior to the diagnosis of leukemia. Estimated relative risks of developing leukemia for combinations of these risk factors are presented in Table XXVI (Gibson *et al.*, 1968).

There is an overall pattern of increasing relative risk with increasing combinations of "pathological" and "radiological" exposures. This is more clearly shown in Table XXVII, where the data are arranged according to whether the risk factor was a pathological or radiological event and by the number of such events. Three types of relationships appear from this table. Whenever there is only one factor, i.e., radiological or pathological, the risks are low. In this instance, they are either 1.01 or 1.13. For two factors of the same type, the risks are only slightly higher (1.21 or 1.56). The combination of one pathological and one radiological factor results in a relative risk of 1.62, which is higher than the preceding risks, but not yet statistically significant. Combinations of multiple pathological and/or radiological factors produce risks that are all significantly higher than the nonexposed group; the lowest risk is 2.69 and the highest risk, consisting of two pathological and two radiological factors, is 4.64× that of the nonexposed group.

These data suggest that an increase in the number of radiological factors or pathological factors alone does not significantly increase the risk for leukemia. However, when exposure, either radiological or pathological, is followed by some exposure to the other type of factor, there is a significant increased risk for leukemia. These findings, although of considerable interest, can only be considered as suggestive. Confirmation is necessary for the leukemic children in this same age group, but other age groups should also be investigated. It should be noted that these findings conform in a general conceptual way to the multistage model of leukemogenesis presented by Burch (1962, 1965).

B. RESEARCH NEEDS

The existing body of knowledge on leukemia which has been reviewed raises more questions than it answers about the nature of this disease. If such questions are properly formulated they can become hypotheses for testing by well-designed epidemiological studies. We should like to suggest a number of areas for such research.

The viral hypothesis of leukemogenesis is in need of further testing. It

TABLE XXVI

RELATIVE RISKS FOR LEUKEMIA IN CHILDREN 1–4 YEARS OF AGE
(WEIGHTED FOR SEX) FOR ALL COMBINATIONS OF
FOUR RISK FACTORS[a]

No. and type of risk factors[b]	No. with exposure[c]		Weighted X^2	Probability	Relative risk
	Case	Control			
No exposure	21	42	—	—	1.00
Pathological					
CV only	13	25	<1.00	0.91	1.07
RW only	8	12	<1.00	0.62	1.33
RW + CV	3	6	<1.00	0.89	1.21
Radiological					
PC only	22	44	<1.00	0.92	1.04
IU only	10	20	<1.00	0.95	1.06
PC + IU	17	22	1.19	0.28	1.56
Single pathological and radiological					
CV + PC	11	19	<1.00	0.71	1.20
CV + IU	3	4	<1.00	0.49	1.75
RW + PC	8	9	1.44	0.23	1.90
RW + IU	3	0	5.11	0.02	7.71
Multiple pathological and radiological					
RW + IU + CV	1	1	<1.00	0.62	1.97
RW + IU + PC	5	5	1.07	0.30	1.97
PC + IU + CV	13	8	5.90	0.015	3.20
RW + CV + PC	7	4	5.11	0.02	4.13
RW + CV + IU + PC	6	2	5.36	0.02	4.64

[a] Gibson et al. (1968).

[b] CV—child virus diseases of subject; RW—mother's reproductive wastage prior to conception of subject; PC—mother's irradiation prior to conception of subject; IU—in utero irradiation of subject.

[c] The total number in these columns does not include those persons who had insufficient data on one or more of the variables being tested.

has not as yet been substantiated by the studies on space–time clustering or by the efforts to isolate viruses in cases of human leukemia. One possibility is the study of leukemia incidence in large groups of contacts and suitably chosen controls. For example, school children developing leukemia might be identified and their classroom contacts followed for several years to determine their risk of developing leukemia. Classmates of other school-children without leukemia could serve as controls. In view of the low incidence of leukemia, such a study would have to include large numbers of children, probably from several metropolitan school systems. The ad-

TABLE XXVII

PATTERN OF ESTIMATED RELATIVE RISKS FOR LEUKEMIA IN CHILDREN
AGED 1–4 YEARS WHEN CONSIDERING BOTH THE TYPE AND NUMBER
OF RISK FACTORS (WEIGHTED FOR DIFFERENCE IN SEX)[a]

No. of pathological factors	No. of radiological factors		
	0	1	2
0	1.00	1.01	1.56
1	1.13	1.62	2.69[b]
2	1.21	3.36[b]	4.64[b]

[a] Gibson et al. (1968).
[b] Significant at the 0.05 level.

vantage of this approach lies in the investigation of an explicitly defined population at risk of developing leukemia.

Systematic studies of familial or household aggregation in leukemia can provide another test of the viral hypothesis. The relevance of both of these approaches, however, depends upon the assumption that the hypothesized viral leukemogen acts in the conventional fashion of infective microorganisms. If this is not so—for example, if the virus is irreversibly altered during its transmission—then these studies would not serve as an adequate test of the viral hypothesis. Of course, clustering may also reflect common environmental exposure to disease factors other than living agents. The studies of school contacts and household aggregation are also valid for the investigation of these factors.

Epidemiological tests of the possible role of the genetic material in leukemia are clearly called for. Heritable factors as well as environmental agents acting pre- or postzygotically on the genome must be sought. The following studies illustrate the many possibilities for testing the genetic hypothesis:

1. Measurement of the prevalence of chromosomal abnormalities in a large group of leukemic patients compared with neighborhood controls of the same age.

2. Prospective investigation of leukemia incidence or mortality in large groups of persons with and without karyotypic abnormalties. (This study would depend upon the availability of an effective method for the mass screening of karyotype.)

3. Measurement of leukemia risk in monozygous and dizygous twins identified from large twin registries.

4. Investigation of the aggregation of leukemia cases among close relatives of a previously identified leukemic group compared with that in relatives of neighborhood controls.

5. Determination of the maternal and paternal ages at birth of leukemic children compared with the parental ages at birth of similarly aged neighborhood control children.

6. Comparison of the incidence of congenitally malformed offspring among adult leukemics of both sexes with the incidence among normal adults.

7. Studies of associated space–time clustering of newly diagnosed cases of childhood leukemia and of congenitally malformed infants.

Unless (or until) the genetic or the viral hypothesis is substantiated it will be necessary to continue the search for other environmental factors in leukemia. As is true for other diseases, clues to the etiology of this disease can probably be derived from observations on geographic and ethnic differences in its distribution. By comparing the mortality experience of resident and migrant groups of the same nativity, the effects of geography and ethnos can then be differentiated.

The frequent use of mortality figures in epidemiological studies of leukemia requires special comment. Before differences in mortality rates are accepted as indicating differences in degree of leukemogenic exposure, one must demonstrate that the incidence of leukemia is reflected by its mortality. To accomplish this, one might select several geographic areas which have high, average, and low reported death rates from leukemia. Death certificates, hospital charts, and physicians' records could then be examined in order to determine whether the observed geographic differences were real (i.e., reflecting differences in incidence or prevalence) or whether they were artifactual (i.e., due to differences in cause-of-death certification practices and diagnostic variation). If it were concluded that the geographic differences in mortality were real, then studies might be designed to seek possible explanations.

Among the other epidemiological observations on leukemia which are in need of further elucidation are the following:

1. The high sex ratio in adult leukemia.

2. The apparently different ratios of lymphoid and myeloid leukemia in Occidentals and Orientals.

3. The apparent childhood and adolescent peaks in leukemia mortality.

REFERENCES

Ager, E. A., Schuman, L. M., Wallace, H. M., Rosenfield, A. B., and Gullen, W. H. 1965. *J. Chronic Diseases* **18**, 113–132.

Amiotti, P. L. 1953. *Minerva Pediat.* **5**, 449–450.

Baikie, A. G., Court-Brown, W. M., Buckton, K. E., and Harnden, D. G. 1961. *Lancet* **ii**, 1003–1004.

Bailar, J. C., III, and Gurian, J. M. 1964. *J. Natl. Cancer Inst.* **33**, 237–242.

Barber, R., and Spiers, P. 1964. *Progr. Rept. II, Monthly Bull., Min. Health,* **23,** 46–52.
Barton, D. E., and David, F. N. 1966. *In* "Research Papers in Statistics" (F. N. David, ed.), pp. 445–459. Wiley, New York.
Barton, D. E., David, F. N., and Merrington, M. 1965. *Ann. Human Genet.* **29,** 97–102.
Bjelke, E. 1963. *Cancer* **17,** 248–255.
Brill, A. B., Tomonaga, M., and Heyssel, R. M. 1962. *Ann. Internal Med.* **56,** 590–609.
Buckton, K. E., Harnden, D. G., Baikie, A. G., and Woods, G. E. 1961. *Lancet* **i,** 171–172.
Buell, P., and Dunn, J. E., Jr. 1965. *Cancer* **18,** 656–664.
Burch, P. R. J. 1962. *Nature* **195,** 241–243.
Burch, P. R. J. 1964. *Ann. N.Y. Acaa. Sci.* **114,** 213–222.
Burch, P. R. J. 1965. *Proc. Roy. Soc. (London)* **B162,** 223–287.
Burnet, M. 1958. *New Engl. J. Med.* **259,** 423–431.
Busk, T. 1954. *Proc. 2nd Natl. Cancer Conf., 1952* pp. 1087–1101.
Carter, C. O. 1958. *J. Mental Deficiency* **2,** 64–74.
Clemmesen, J. 1965. "Statistical Studies in the Aetiology of Malignant Neoplasms. Part I: Review and Results," 543 pp. Munksgaard, Copenhagen.
Clemmesen, J., and Sorensen, J. 1958. *Danish Med. Bull.* **5,** 73–128.
Colon, V. F. 1966. *Nebraska State Med. J.* **51,** 137–140.
Conen, P. E., Erkman, B., and Laski, B. 1966. *Arch. Internal Med.* **117,** 125–132.
Cooke, J. V. 1942. *J. Am. Med. Assoc.* **119,** 547–550.
Court-Brown, W. M., and Doll, R. 1959. *Brit. Med. J.* **i,** 1063–1069.
Court-Brown, W. M., and Doll, R. 1961. *Brit. Med. J.* **i,** 981–988.
Court-Brown, W. M., and Doll, R. 1965. *Brit. Med. J.* **ii,** 1327–1332.
Court-Brown, W. M., Doll, R., and Bradford Hill, A. 1960a. *Brit. Med. J.* **ii,** 1539–1545.
Court-Brown, W. M., Spiers, F. W., Doll, R., Duffy, B. J., and McHugh, M. J. 1960b. *Brit. Med. J.* **i,** 1753–1759.
Court-Brown, W. M., Doll, R., and Bradford Hill, A. 1964. *Pathol. Microbiol.* **27,** 644–654.
Cronkite, E. P. 1961. *Arch. Environ. Health* **3,** 297–303.
DeGrouchy, J. 1966. *Ann. Internal Med.* **65,** 603–607.
Demchenko, A. P. 1965. *Probl. Gematol. i Pereliv. Krovi* **10,** 53–55.
DeWolff, E. 1964. *Ann. Paediat. Suppl.* **202,** 1–47.
Diamond, E. L. 1968. Presented at Society for Epidemiologic Research, Washington, D.C., unpublished observations.
Doll, R. 1961. *In* "Scientific Basis of Medicine, Annual Research" (J. Paterson Ross, ed.), 96 pp. Oxford Univ. Press (Athlone), London and New York.
Ederer, F., Myers, M. H., and Mantel, N. 1964. *Biometrics* **20,** 626–638.
Ederer, F., Miller, R. W., and Scotto, J. 1965a. *J. Am. Med. Assoc.* **192,** 97–100.
Ederer, F., Miller, R. W., Scotto, J., and Bailar, J. C., III. 1965b. *Lancer* **ii,** 185–186.
Ederer, F., Myers, M. H., Eisenberg, H., and Campbell, P. C. 1965c. *J. Natl. Cancer Inst.* **35,** 625–629.
Eridani, S., Tiso, R., and Kluzer, G. 1964. *Haematol. Latina (Milan)* **7,** 9–41.
Ford, D. D., Paterson, J. C. S., and Treuting, W. L. 1959. *J. Natl. Cancer Inst.* **22,** 1093–1104.
Fraumeni, J. F., Jr. 1963. *Brit. Med. J.* **ii,** 1408–1409.
Fraumeni, J. F., Jr., and Miller, R. W. 1967a. *J. Natl. Cancer Inst.* **38,** 593–605.
Fraumeni, J. F., Jr., and Miller, R. W. 1967b. *Science* **155,** 1126–1127.
Fraumeni, J. F., Jr., and Wagoner, J. K. 1964. *Public Health Rept. (U.S.)* **79,** 1093–1100.

Fraumeni, J. F., Jr., Ederer, F., and Handy, V. H. 1966. *Cancer* **19**, 996–1000.
Gibson, R. W., Bross, I. D. J., Graham, S. L., Lilienfeld, A. M., Schuman, L. M., Levin, M. L., and Dowd, J. E. 1968. *New Engl. J. Med.* **279**, 906–909.
Gilliam, A. G., and Walter, W. A. 1958. *Public Health Rept. (U.S.)* **73**, 773–784.
Glass, A. G., Hill, J. A., and Miller, R. W. 1968. *J. Pediat.* **73**, 101–107.
Goh, K. O., and Swisher, S. N. 1965. *Arch. Internal Med.* **115**, 475–478.
Goh, K. O., Swisher, S. N., and Herman, E. C. 1967. *Arch. Internal Med.* **120**, 214–219.
Goldenberg, G. J., and Zarowski, V. S. 1967. *Cancer* **20**, 2200–2212.
Graham, S., Levin, M. L., Lilienfeld, A. M., Schuman, L. M., Gibson, R., Dowd, J. E., and Hempelmann, L. 1966. *Natl. Cancer Inst. Monograph* **19**, 347–371.
Grais, M. 1962. *Bull. World Health Organ.* **26**, 683–688.
Guasch, J. 1954. *Sang* **25**, 384–421.
Gunz, F. W. 1964. *Pathol. Microbiol.* **27**, 697–704.
Gunz, F. W. 1966. *New Zealand Med. J. Suppl.* **65**, 857–862.
Haenszel, W., and Chiazze, L., Jr. 1965. *J. Natl. Cancer Inst.* **34**, 85–101.
Hayes, D. M. 1961. *Cancer* **14**, 1301–1305.
Heath, C. W., Jr., and Hasterlik, R. J. 1963. *Am. J. Med.* **34**, 796–812.
Heath, C. W., Jr., and Manning, M. D. 1964. *Lancet* **i**, 1394.
Heath, C. W., Jr., and Moloney, W. C. 1965. *New Engl. J. Med.* **272**, 882–887.
Heath, C. W., Jr., Manning, M. D., and Zelkowitz, L. 1964. *Lancet* **ii**, 136–137.
Hewitt, D. 1955. *Brit. J. Prevent. Social Med.* **9**, 81–88.
Hewitt, D. 1960. *Acta, Unio Intern. Contra Cancrum* **16**, 1643–1647.
Hewitt, D. 1964. *New Engl. J. Med.* **270**, 932–935.
Hewitt, D., Lashof, J. C., and Stewart, A. M. 1966. *Cancer* **19**, 157–161.
Holland, W. W., Doll, R., and Carter, C. O. 1962. *Brit. J. Cancer* **16**, 177–184.
Hoshino, T., Kato, H., Finch, S. C., and Hrubec, Z. 1967. *Blood* **30**, 719–730.
Iverson, T. 1960. *Acta Paediat.* **49**, 167–170.
Jackson, E. W., Turner, J. H., Klauber, M. R., and Norris, F. D. 1968. *J. Chronic Diseases* **21**, 247–253.
Jacobs, E. M., Luce, J. K., and Cailleau, R. 1966. *Cancer* **19**, 869–876.
Janicki, K., and Gurda, M. 1965. *Polski Tygod. Lekar.* **20**, 304–305.
Jhala, C. I., and Tilak, S. S. 1967. *Indian J. Med. Sci.* **21**, 163–168.
Kaliampetos, G. 1954. *Deut. Med. Wochschr.* **79**, 1783–1785.
Kaplan, H. S. 1958. *Am. J. Roentgenol. Radium Therapy Nucl. Med.* **80**, 696–706.
Karhausen, L. W., and Hutchison, G. B. 1966. Unpublished data cited in Miller (1966).
Kessler, I. I. 1968. Unpublished observations.
Kjeldsberg, H. 1957. *Tidsskr. Norske Laegeforen.* **77**, 1052–1053.
Knox, G. 1964. *Brit. J. Prevent. Social Med.* **18**, 17–24.
Kolmeier, K. H., and Bayrd, E. D. 1963. *Proc. Staff Meetings Mayo Clinic* **38**, 523–531.
Lancaster, H. O. 1955. *Med. J. Australia* **2**, 1064.
Lauriault, C. D., and Jim, R. T. S. 1966. *Hawaii Med. J.* **26**, 125–126.
Lee, J. A. H. 1961. *Brit. Med. J.* **i**, 988–992.
Lee, J. A. H. 1962a. *Brit. Med. J.* **i**, 1737–1738.
Lee, J. A. H. 1962b. *In* "Epidemiology Reports on Research and Teaching" (J. Pemberton, ed.), pp. 32. Oxford Univ. Press, London and New York.
Lee, J. A. H. 1963. *Brit. Med. J.* **ii**, 623.
Lee, J. A. H. 1964. *Pathol. Microbiol.* **27**, 772–776.
Lee, J. A. H., and Gardner, M. J. 1965. *In* "Current Research in Leukemia" (F. G. J. Hayhoe, ed.), pp. 266–299. Cambridge Univ. Press, London and New York.
Lilienfeld, A. M. 1966. *Yale J. Biol. Med.* **39**, 143–164.

Lilienfeld, A. M. 1969. "Epidemiology of Mongolism." Johns Hopkins Press, Baltimore, Maryland.
Lilienfeld, A. M., Pederson, E., and Dowd, J. E. 1967. "Cancer Epidemiology: Methods of Study." Johns Hopkins Press, Baltimore, Maryland.
Lilienfeld, A. M., Levin, M. L., and Seltser, R. 1968. Unpublished observations.
Lüers, T., and Lüers, H. 1954. *Arztl. Forsch.* **8**, 263–267.
Lundin, F. E., Jr., Fraumeni, J. F., Jr., Lloyd, J. W., and Smith, E. M. 1966. *J. Natl. Cancer Inst.* **37**, 123–133.
McCarthy, D. D., and Chalmers, T. M. 1964. *Can. Med. Assoc. J.* **90**, 1061–1067.
MacMahon, B. 1957. *Public Health Rept. (U.S.)* **72**, 39–46.
MacMahon, B. 1962. *J. Natl. Cancer Inst.* **28**, 1173–1191.
MacMahon, B., and Clark, D. 1956. *Blood* **11**, 871–881.
MacMahon, B., and Koller, E. K. 1957. *Blood* **12**, 1–10.
MacMahon, B., and Levy, M. 1964. *New Engl. J. Med.* **270**, 1082–1085.
MacMahon, B., and Newill, V. A. 1962. *J. Natl. Cancer Inst.* **28**, 231–244.
Magnússon, S. 1964. *Pathol. Microbiol.* **27**, 705–707.
Mainwaring, D. 1966. *Brit. J. Prevent. Social Med.* **20**, 189–194.
Manning, M. D., and Carroll, B. E. 1957. *J. Natl. Cancer Inst.* **19**, 1087–1094.
Mantel, N. 1967. *Cancer Res.* **27**, 209–220.
Martin, D. C., Chin, T. D. Y., Larsen, W. E., Roth, A. E., and Werder, A. A. 1966. *J. Kansas Med. Soc.* **67**, 361–365.
Meadors, G. F. 1956. *Public Health Rept. (U.S.)* **71**, 103–108.
Medical News Item. 1968. *J. Am. Med. Assoc.* **203**, 25.
Meighan, S. S. 1965. *Med. Times* **93**, 1068–1079.
Meighan, S. S., and Knox, G. 1965. *Cancer* **18**, 811–814.
Merrit, D. H., and Harris, J. S. 1956. *A.M.A. J. Diseases Children* **92**, 41–44.
Milham, S., Jr. 1965. *Science* **148**, 98–100.
Miller, O. J., Breg, W. R., Schmickel, R. D., and Tretter, W. 1961. *Lancet* **ii**, 78–79.
Miller, R. W. 1963. *New Engl. J. Med.* **268**, 393–401.
Miller, R. W. 1966. *New Engl. J. Med.* **275**, 87–93.
Miller, R. W. 1967a. *Tohoku J. Exptl. Med.* **91**, 103–107.
Miller, R. W. 1967b. *Cancer Res.* **27**, 2420–2423.
Miller, R. W. 1968. *New Engl. J. Med.* **279**, 122–126.
Mittwoch, U. 1957. *J. Mental Deficiency Res.* **1**, 26–31.
Modan, B., and Lilienfeld, A. M. 1965. *Medicine* **44**, 305–344.
Morganti, G., and Cresseri, A. 1954. *Sang* **25**, 421–453.
Moszcyński, P. 1968. *Lancet* **i**, 1378.
Murray, R., Heckel, P., and Hempelmann, L. H. 1959. *New Engl. J. Med.* **261**, 585–589.
Mustacchi, P. 1965. *Cancer* **18**, 362–368.
National Center for Health Statistics. 1964. "Vital Statistics of the United States, Annual Report, 1964." U.S. Govt. Printing Office, Washington, D.C.
Nelson, M. G., and Merrett, J. D. *Irish J. Med. Sci.* **489**, 361–366.
Newill, V. A. 1961. *J. Natl. Cancer Inst.* **26**, 405–417.
Nicola, P., and Balocco, A. 1962. *Minerva Pediat.* **14**, 1531–1546.
Nordenson, N. G., and Asplund, A. G. 1956. *Acta Med. Scand.* **154**, 31–40.
Pinkel, D., and Nefzger, D. 1959. *Cancer* **12**, 351–358.
Pinkel, D., Dowd, J. E., and Bross, I. D. J. 1963. *Cancer* **16**, 28–33.
Polhemus, D. W., and Koch, R. 1959. *Pediatrics* **23**, 453–461.
Radujkov, Z., Borota, R., and Lucic, A. 1965. *Med. Pregled. (Novi Sad)* **18**, 19–21.

Registrar General's Decennial Supplement, England and Wales. 1938. 1931 Occupational Mortality, Part II. H. M. Stationery Office, London.

Registrar General's Statistical Review of England and Wales, 1902–1967 (for the Years 1900 to 1965). H. M. Stationery Office, London.

Rucknagel, D. L. 1966. *New Zealand Med. J.* **65,** 869–874.

Sacks, M. S., and Seeman, I. 1947. *Blood* **2,** 1–14.

Sawitsky, A., Bloom, D., and German, J. 1966. *Ann. Internal Med.* **65,** 487–495.

Segi, M., and Kurihara, M. 1966. "Cancer Mortality for Selected Sites in 24 Countries (1962–1963)," No. 4, 358 pp. Dept. of Public Health, Tohoku Univ. School of Med., Sendai, Japan.

Seno, S. 1964. *Pathol. Microbiol.* **27,** 684–696.

Shapiro, A. 1949. *J. Mental Sci.* **95,** 689.

Shimkin, M. B., and Loveland, D. B. 1961. *Blood* **17,** 763–766.

Slocumb, J. C., and MacMahon, B. 1963. *New Engl. J. Med.* **268,** 922–925.

Sloman, J. G., and Sellers, A. H. 1959. *Can. J. Public Health* **50,** 518.

Sonnet, J., Michaux, J. L., and Hekster, C. 1966. *Trop. Geograph. Med.* **18,** 272–286.

Stark, C. R. 1963. Ph.D. Thesis in Public Health, Univ. of Michigan, Ann Arbor, Michigan.

Stark, C. R., and Mantel, N. 1966. *J. Natl. Cancer Inst.* **37,** 687–698.

Stark, C. R., and Mantel, N. 1967. *Cancer Res.* **27,** 1729–1775.

Stark, C. R., and Oleinick, A. 1966. *J. Natl. Cancer Inst.* **37,** 369–379.

Statistical Bulletin, Metropolitan Life Insurance Co. 1966. Vol. 47, data for 1940–1963.

Steinberg, A. G. 1957. *Proc. 3rd Natl. Cancer Conf., 1956* pp. 353–356.

Steinberg, A. G. 1960. *Cancer* **13,** 985–999.

Stewart, A. 1961. *Brit. Med. J.* **i,** 452–460.

Stewart, A., and Hewitt, D. 1965a. *Current Topics Radiation Res.* **1,** 223–253.

Stewart, A. M., and Hewitt, D. 1965b. *Lancet* **ii,** 789–790.

Stewart, A., Webb, J., and Hewitt, D. 1958. *Brit. Med. J.* **i,** 1495–1508.

Stewart, A., Pennybacker, W., and Barber, R. 1962. *Brit. Med. J.* **ii,** 882–890.

Sugiyama, T., Kurita, Y., and Nishizuka, Y. 1967. *Science* **158,** 1058–1059.

Swan, A. 1963. *Brit. Med. J.* **ii,** 1063–1064.

Takeda, K. 1960. *Acta, Unio Intern. Contra Cancrum* **16,** 1629–1642.

Till, M. W., Hardisty, R. M., Pike, M. C., and Doll, R. 1967. *Brit. Med. J.* **3,** 755–758.

Tomonaga, M. 1966. *New Zealand Med. J.* Haematol. Suppl., **65,** 863–869.

Toth, B. 1968. *Cancer Res.* **28,** 727–738.

Turner, J. H. 1962. Thesis, Sci.D. Hyg., Univ. of Pittsburgh, Pittsburgh, Pennsylvania.

Turpin, R., and Bernyer, G. 1947. *Rev. Hematol.* **2,** 190–206.

United Nations Scientific Committee on the Effects of Atomic Radiation. 1964. Suppl. 14, a/5814.

U.S. Bureau of Census. 1943. Census of the United States: 1940. Vol. II, Characteristics of the Population. U.S. Govt. Printing Office, Washington, D.C.

U.S. Bureau of Census. 1953. U.S. Census of Population: 1950. Vol. II, Characteristics of the Population. Part 1. Summary. Govt. Printing Office, Washington, D.C.

U.S. Bureau of Census. 1964. U.S. Census of Population: 1960. Vol. I, Characteristics of the Population. Part 1. Summary. U.S. Govt. Printing Office, Washington, D.C.

U.S. Department of Health, Education, and Welfare. Bureau of Disease Prevention and Environmental Control, National Communicable Disease Center. 1967. Leukemia Surveillance Program Report No. 2. U.S. Govt. Printing Office, Washington, D.C.

U.S. Public Health Service, National Office of Vital Statistics. 1949. Vital Statistics of the United States, 1947. Part 1. Natality and Mortality Data for the U.S. U.S. Govt. Printing Office, Washington, D.C.

U.S. Public Health Service, National Office of Vital Statistics. 1958. Vital Statistics of the United States, 1956. Vol. II. Mortality Data. U.S. Govt. Printing Office, Washington, D.C.

U.S. Public Health Service, National Center for Health Statistics. 1967. Vital Statistics of the United States, 1965. Vol. II. Mortality. Part A. U.S. Govt. Printing Office, Washington, D.C.

Videbaek, A. 1947. "Heredity in Human Leukemia and its Relation to Cancer," 279 pp. Lewis, London.

Vigliani, E. C., and Saita, G. 1964. *New Engl. J. Med.* **271,** 872–876.

Von Ambs, E., Ströder, J., and Ferneding, M. 1966. *Arch. Kinderheilk.* **173,** 149–159.

Wald, N., Borges, W. H., Li, C. C., Turner, J. H., and Harnois, M. C. 1961. *Lancet* **i,** 1228.

Walter, W. A., and Gilliam, A. G. 1956. *J. Natl. Cancer Inst.* **17,** 475–480.

Wells, R., and Lau, K. S. 1960. *Brit. Med. J.* **i,** 759–763.

Witts, L. J. 1957. *Brit. Med. J.* **i,** 1197–1202.

Woodliff, H. J., Dougan, L., and Onesti, P. 1966. *Nature* **211,** 533.

World Health Organization. 1948. Manual of the International Statistical Classification of Diseases, Injuries and Causes of Death, 6th Revision. World Health Organ., Geneva.

World Health Organization. 1963. Annual Epidemiological and Vital Statistics, 1960. World Health Organ., Geneva.

AUTHOR INDEX

Numbers in italic refer to the pages on which the complete references are listed.

Jeejeebhoy, H. F., 107, *134*
Jenkins, V. K., 4, *96*
Jensen, F., 114, 115, 116, 117, 122, *133, 134*
Jensen, F. C., *163*
Jerkofsky, M., 120, *135*, 156, *164*
Jerne, K., 193, *220*
Jevleva, E. S., 109, *135*
Jhala, C. I., 249, 256, *299*
Jim, R. T. S., 265, 266, *299*
Johanovsky, J., 109, *134*
Johns, L. W., 4, *98*
Jonsson, N., 6, *99*, 126, 128, *134, 136*, 147, *161*
Jordan, W. P., 4, 13, 18, *95*

K

Kaliampetos, G., 288, *299*
Kaliss, N., 22, *96*, 196, *220*
Kaloczky, M., 4, *98*
Kaplan, H. S., 4, *97*, 274, *299*
Kara, J., 114, 117, 119, *136*
Karhausen, L. W., 285, *299*
Karon, M., 59, *96*
Karush, F., 208, *220*
Kassanis, B., 158, *163*
Kato, H., 278, *299*
Katz, M., 110, *136*, 171, *223*
Kelloff, G., 141, *163*
Kessler, I. I., 230, 231, 249, *299*
Ketcham, A. S., 173, 188, *221*
Kim, J. H., 195, *221*
King, A. S., 149, *161*
Kirschstein, R. L., 152, 156, *162, 164*
Kit, S., 116, 117, 121, *132*
Kitahara, T., 113, 116, *135*, 154, *164*
Kite, J. H., 176, *222*
Kjeldsberg, H., 274, *299*
Klauber, M. R., 286, *299*
Klein, E., 3, 6, 8, 9, 12, 13, 14, 17, 18, 19, 22, 24, 25, 26, 29, 30, 31, 33, 35, 47, 48, 49, 83, 88, 89, *96, 97, 99*, 102, 107, 108, 109, 110, 129, *134, 136*, 169, 171, 173, 175, 177, 182, 185, 188, 194, 195, 196, 203, 205, 206, 210, 213, *217, 218, 219, 220, 222*
Klein, G., 3, 6, 8, 9, 12, 13, 14, 17, 18, 19, 24, 25, 26, 29, 30, 31, 35, 47, 48, 49, 83, 88, 89, *96, 97, 99*, 102, 104, 105, 107, 108, 109, 110, 123, 127, 129, *132, 134, 136*, 152, *164*, 168, 169, 170, 171, 173,

177, 182, 183, 185, 188, 192, 194, 195, 196, 204, 205, 206, 209, 213, 214, *217, 218, 220, 222, 223*
Klement, V., 147, 148, *163, 164*
Kluchareva, T. E., 106, 110, 111, 115, 124, 125, 127, 128, 130, 131, *133, 134,* 199, *218*
Kluzer, G., 236, 237, *298*
Knox, G., 260, 262, 263, 264, 265, 267, 269, 280, *299, 300*
Kobayashi, H., 13, 60, *97*
Koch, M. A., 6, *97,* 104, 116, *134, 135,* 152, *164*
Koch, R., 274, *300*
Kodama, T., 60, *97*
Kolb, W. P., 209, 210, *218, 220*
Koldovsky, P., 6, 9, 16, 22, 23, 33, 79, 80, *95, 97,* 104, *134,* 175, 197, *217, 220*
Koller, E. K., 237, *300*
Kolmeier, K. H., 288, *299*
Kolodny, R. L., 179, *219*
Koprowska, J., 117, *134*
Koprowski, H., 107, 108, 113, 114, 115, 116, 117, *133, 134, 135,* 153, *163,* 176, *220*
Koskinies, D., 177, *223*
Kourilsky, F. M., 109, 110, *134,* 173, 188, *220*
Krischke, W., 46, 84, *96*
Kronman, B. S., 180, *217*
Krüger, G., *220*
Kryukova, I. N., 128, *134,* 147, *165*
Kurihara, M., 226, 227, 229, 230, 231, 239, 240, *301*
Kurita, Y., 285, *301*

L

Lacy, S., 153, *163*
Lancaster, H. O., 238, *299*
Lane, W. T., 75, *96,* 150, 151, 157, *163, 164,* 172, *219*
Larsen, W. E., 236, *300*
Larson, V. M., 130, *133,* 199, *218*
Lasfargues, J. C., 60, *99*
Lashof, J. C., 290, *299*
Laski, B., 285, *298*
Latarjet, R., 121, 122, *134,* 147, 153, *162, 163*
Lau, K. S., 249, 250, *302*
Lauriault, C. D., 265, 266, *299*
Lavrin, D. H., 126, *132*

Winn, H. J., 108, *136,* 172, 175, 182, 196, 205, *222, 223*
Winocour, E., 117, 121, *133,* 152, 153, *161*
Witts, L. J., 240, 250, *302*
Wood, D. A., 171, 193, 194, *221*
Woodliff, H. J., 291, *302*
Woodruff, M. F. A., 201, 205, *223*
Woods, G. E., 279, 285, *298*
Wright, B. S., 60, *99*

Y

Yang, J. P. S., 187, 191, 198, 204, 216, *219*
Yoshida, K., 8, 58, 59, *98*

Yoshida, T. O., 108, *136,* 183, *223*
Youn, J. K., 60, *95*
Young, R. D., 123, 125, 130, *133,* 199, *218*
Yumoto, T., 2, *99*

Z

Zarowski, V. S., 262, 270, *299*
Zeigel, R. F., 46, 55, *95, 99*
Zeithlin, E. M., 121, *132*
Zelkowitz, L., 258, *299*
Zilber, L. A., 102, 109, 112, *135, 136,* 147, *165*
Zueva, Y. N., 13, 21, 29, 30, 36, 37, 38, *99*

SUBJECT INDEX

315